Principles of
Molecular Virology

3rd Edition

For
Joe and Jules

Principles of
Molecular Virology
3rd Edition

Alan J. Cann
University of Leicester, UK

ACADEMIC PRESS

A Harcourt Science and Technology Company

San Diego   London   Boston
New York   Sydney   Tokyo   Toronto

Copyright © 2001 by ACADEMIC PRESS

Academic Press
A Harcourt Science and Technology Company
Harcourt Place, 32 Jamestown Road, London NW1 7BY, UK
http://www.academicpress.com

Academic Press
A Harcourt Science and Technology Company
525 B Street, Suite 1900, San Diego, California 92101-4495, USA
http://www.academicpress.com

ISBN (Standard Edition) 0-12-158533-6
ISBN (Instructors' Edition) 0-12-158535-2
ISBN (Standard CD-ROM) 0-12-158534-4
ISBN (Instructors' CD-ROM) 0-12-158536-0

A catalogue record for this book is available from the British Library

Typeset by J&L Composition Ltd, Filey, North Yorkshire.
Printed in Great Britain by the Bath Press, Somerset, UK
01 02 03 04 05 06 BP 9 8 7 6 5 4 3 2 1

CONTENTS

PREFACE TO THE THIRD EDITION

This edition of *Principles of Molecular Virology* seeks to build on the success of the first and second editions. In addition to complete updating, numerous additions (and hopefully, enhancements) have been made to the text. These include new sections on 'Viruses and Apoptosis' (Chapter 6) and 'Bacteriophages and Human Disease' (Chapter 7), the addition of learning objectives for each chapter and a new appendix describing key events in the history of virology (Appendix 3). However, probably the first change most readers will notice is a new format with the addition of colour illustrations to enhance understanding of key points.

An exciting new development has been the inclusion of an electronic companion to the book in the form of the enclosed CD. In addition to interactive learning resources on the CD which complement each chapter, the 'Virology Online' section has been written to encourage readers with access to the internet to go beyond reading the text of the book to find more information online.

I would like to extend my thanks to all of my academic colleagues who have helped with the preparation of this edition, but in particular I value the contribution of the many people who have contacted me with suggestions and comments regarding the previous editions. I hope that readers of this edition will continue to do so. I would also like to thank the editorial staff of Academic Press for their support and assistance during the preparation of the book. Finally, I would like to thank my family for respecting the sign which has spent many hours on the door of my study, 'I am working. Please don't come in'. It's OK now kids, I've taken the sign down.

Alan J. Cann
Department of Microbiology & Immunology
University of Leicester
June 2000

PREFACE TO THE SECOND EDITION

Much has changed since the first edition of *Principles of Molecular Virology* was published in 1993, but the need for this book is now stronger than ever. This edition is completely revised and updated and contains many new figures and tables. As a result, it is somewhat longer, but not, I hope, so long that it loses sight of the original objective – to present the concerns of contemporary virology to students in a concise and digestible manner.

Many people should be thanked for helping inspire this edition, but I will single out a few for particular mention. I am very grateful to all those who provided feedback on the first edition and I have tried to include as many of their comments/requests as possible; in particular, coverage of the rapidly developing area of plant virology has been greatly expanded. I am also grateful to my teaching colleagues in Leicester and elsewhere for their suggestions. Finally, the person who should perhaps receive most thanks is my long-suffering editor at Academic Press, Tessa Picknett

Alan J. Cann
Department of Microbiology & Immunology
University of Leicester
July 1996

PREFACE TO THE FIRST EDITION

This book came about through my own need for a text to augment my under-graduate lectures on virology. Not that there is a particular shortage of books on virology, but even during my own relatively short career, the subject has expanded so rapidly that most professionals feel pressurized by the the task of keeping up with current trends, let alone the responsibility of initiating a new generation in such a rapidly changing discipline. Many excellent and recent texts exist that deal with the subject in a detailed and somewhat traditional manner; the second edition of *Fields' Virology* (Raven Press, 1990), the third edition of Matthews' *Plant Virology* (Academic Press, 1991) and, in a more general sense, the second edition of *Molecular Biology of the Cell* (Garland Press, 1989) immediately spring to mind. Unfortunately, these books have two major disadvantages for their use in teaching. First, the volume of material they contain is overwhelming for a student discovering the sub-ject for the first time and who may be unable to sort out the information they require from the mountain of detail they encounter. Second, in these times, few students can afford to purchase one of these tomes. Even persuading university libraries, whose budgets are under constant pressure, to purchase more than one or two copies is difficult and an inadequate solution in a time of expanding student numbers. Better then to reserve these texts for the reference purpose for which they are best suited and to introduce students to the subject in a gentler way.

In discussion with many of my colleagues at this and other universities, it was clear that most felt there was a place for a text which would cover the current emphasis and concerns of virology. In these conversations, there was no doubt as to what was required. My contemporaries have no difficulty with the label 'molecular virology,' but most when pressed would have difficulty in expressing a comprehen-sive definition. Perhaps the best way to describe how I have approached the subject here is consider it as 'virology at a molecular level' or even better, 'molecules and viruses.' Having already damned the 2000-page reference source as unsuitable for my purpose and yet such an all-embracing definition of 'molecular virology,' the problem was therefore how to resolve these two apparently conflicting issues. My chosen solution is to outline the *principles* of the subject with reference to specific *examples* chosen to illustrate the matter under discussion. The onus is therefore firmly on the reader to pursue particular matters on which he or she requires more information in more detailed 'reference texts' or in the immense volume of research publications appearing annually.

I would like to have spent much more time discussing the history of virology in Chapter 1, a subject I find to be a fascinating as well as a valuable insight as to how we got to where we are today. In the event, it was only possible to provide a brief overview and to refer the reader to one of the many other texts which have been published on this subject — perhaps the one area of virology where an author's work does not become outdated in a short period. It is only my intention to arm readers with the framework that makes it possible for them to achieve this task succesfully. Anyone who complains that this book does not spend sufficient time dealing with (or even mention) their pet area of interest has therefore missed the point.

To disarm the jargon (which I have avoided wherever possible) and unavoidable technical terms, I have included a glossary as an appendix to the book. Terms shown in the text in **bold** print are defined in this glossary.

Cliché it may be, but there are genuinely too many people to acknowledge for the creation of this book to make it possible to do this individually. It will have to suffice for me to thank all my colleagues in Leicester and elsewhere for helpful discussions; all the people who have helped and influenced my career over the years, and the undergraduates on whom I have field-tested the material, and for whom this book is intended.

Alan J. Cann
Microbiology Department
University of Leicester
October 1992

THE PRINCIPLES OF MOLECULAR VIROLOGY CD

Wherever the ✇ icon appears in the text, an accompanying learning resource can be found on the compact disk (CD) included with this book. To use the CD, put it in a computer and use your favourite web browser (Netscape or Internet Explorer) to open the file 'START.htm'. If you need further help, click on the file 'README.txt'.

The CD contains interactive learning resources which complement each chapter of the book. However, to gain the maximum benefit from the disk, you will need internet access. The resources in the 'Virology Online' section have been selected to encourage you to move beyond the text of the book and find information about any topic you may wish to investigate. Not sure what any word or name in the text means? Type it into the search forms listed in 'Virology Online' and you will be surprised how much information is available.

However, readers should be aware that the quality and accuracy of information they may find on the internet varies greatly. All of the resources suggested on the CD are of the highest quality, although neither the author nor Academic Press can guarantee that they will remain freely available indefinitely. Information accessed through search engines is another matter – it is up to users to judge the quality of resources found in this way:

- Who wrote the information? A knowledgeable academic in a respected university or a teenager in their bedroom?
- When did they write it? This year or six years ago – is there even a date on the page?
- What is their motivation for making the information available? Commercial or non-commercial?

By considering these quality issues, readers can expand the capacity of this book indefinitely.

CHAPTER 1

INTRODUCTION

'Those who cannot remember the past are condemned to repeat it.'
(George Santayana)

Learning Objectives

On completing this chapter, you should be able to:
- Understand what a virus is and explain how viruses differ from all other organisms
- Summarize the history of virology and explain how the present state of our knowledge of viruses was achieved
- Describe the techniques most frequently used to study viruses.

There is more biological diversity within viruses than in all the rest of the bacterial, plant and animal kingdoms put together. This is the result of the success of viruses in parasitizing all known groups of living organisms, and understanding this diversity is the key to comprehending the interactions of viruses with their hosts. This book deals with 'molecular virology' in a rather broad sense – that is, 'virology at a molecular level', or perhaps even, 'molecules and viruses'. Protein–protein, protein–nucleic acid and protein–lipid interactions determine the structure of virus particles, the synthesis and expression of virus **genomes** and the effects of viruses on the host cell. This is virology at a molecular level.

However, before exploring the subject further, it is necessary to understand the nature of viruses. It would also be useful to know something of the history of virology, or more accurately, how virology as a discipline in its own right arose, in order to understand its current concerns and future directions. These are the purposes of this introductory chapter. The principles behind certain techniques mentioned in this chapter may not be familiar to some readers. It may be helpful to use the Further Reading at the end of this chapter to become conversant with these methods. In this and the subsequent chapters, terms in **bold blue** within the text are defined in the glossary (Appendix 1) ⊘ (the CD icon in the text indicates that you can find an interactive learning resource on the accompanying CD).

VIRUSES ARE DISTINCT FROM LIVING ORGANISMS

Viruses are submicroscopic, obligate intracellular parasites. This simple but useful definition goes a long way towards describing and differentiating viruses from all other groups of living organisms. However, this short definition is in itself inadequate. Clearly, there is no problem in delimiting viruses from higher macroscopic organisms. Even within a broad definition of microbiology encompassing **prokaryotic** organisms and microscopic **eukaryotes** such as algae, protozoa and fungi, in most cases it will suffice. There are, however, a few groups of prokaryotic organisms that have specialized intracellular parasitic life cycles and which confound the above definition. These include the *Rickettsiae* and *Chlamydiae* – obligate intracellular parasitic bacteria which have evolved to be so cell-associated that they can exist outside the cells of their hosts only for a short period of time before losing viability. Therefore it is necessary to add further clauses to the definition of what constitutes a virus:

- Virus particles are produced from the assembly of pre-formed components, whereas other agents grow from an increase in the integrated sum of their components and reproduce by division
- Virus particles (**virions**) themselves do not grow or undergo division
- Viruses lack the genetic information which encodes apparatus necessary for the generation of metabolic energy or for protein synthesis (ribosomes).

No known virus has the biochemical or genetic potential to generate the energy necessary to drive all biological processes (e.g. macromolecular synthesis). They are therefore absolutely dependent on the host cell for this function. It is often asked whether viruses are alive or not. One view is that inside the host cell, viruses are alive, whereas outside it they are merely complex assemblages of metabolically inert chemicals. That is not to say that chemical changes do not occur in extracellular virus particles, as will be explained elsewhere, but these are in no sense the 'growth' of a living organism.

A common mistake is to assume that viruses are smaller than bacteria. While this is true in most cases, size alone does not serve to distinguish between them. The largest virus particles (e.g. granuloviruses) are 120–300 nm in diameter and 300–500 nm long while the smallest bacteria (e.g. *Mycoplasma*, *Ralstonia pickettii*) are only 200–300 nm long. Although there will always be some exceptions and uncertainties in the case of organisms which are too small to see and in many cases difficult to study, for the most part, the above guidelines will suffice to determine the definition of a virus.

A number of novel, pathogenic entities possess properties which confound the above definition, yet are clearly more similar to viruses than other organisms. These are the entities known as **viroids**, **virusoids** and **prions**. Viroids are very small (200–400 nucleotides) circular RNA molecules with a rod-like secondary structure. They have no **capsid** or **envelope** and are associated with certain plant diseases. Their replication strategy is like that of viruses – they are obligate intra-cellular parasites. Virusoids are satellite, viroid-like molecules, somewhat larger than viroids (e.g. approximately 1000 nucleotides), which are dependent on the pres-ence of virus replication for multiplication (hence '**satellite**'); they are packaged into virus capsids as passengers. **Prions** are infectious agents generally believed to consist of a single type of protein molecule with no nucleic acid component. Confusion arises from the fact that the prion protein and the gene which encodes it are also found in normal 'uninfected' cells. These agents are associated with 'slow virus diseases' such as Creutzfeldt-Jakob disease in humans, scrapie in sheep and bovine spongiform encephalopathy (BSE) in cattle. Chapter 8 deals with these subviral infectious agents in more detail. Moreover, molecular genetics has shown that perhaps 5–10% of the **eukaryotic** cell **genome** is composed of mobile retrovirus-like elements (**retrotransposons**), which may have had a considerable role in shaping these complex genomes (Chapter 3). Furthermore, certain **bac-teriophage** genomes closely resemble bacterial **plasmids** in their structure and in the way they are replicated. Therefore, research has revealed that the relation-ship between viruses and other living organisms is perhaps more complex than was previously thought.

THE HISTORY OF VIROLOGY

It is easy to regard events that occurred prior to our own personal experience as pre-historic. Much has been written about virology as a 'new' discipline in biology, and as far as the formal recognition of viruses as distinct from other living organisms is concerned this is true. However, we now realize that ancient peoples were not only aware of the effects of virus infection, but in some instances also carried out active research into the causes and prevention of virus diseases. Perhaps the first written record of a virus infection appears in a hieroglyph from Memphis, the capital of Ancient Egypt, drawn in approximately 3700 BC, which depicts a temple priest showing typical clinical signs of paralytic poliomyelitis. The Pharoh Ramses V, who died in 1196 BC and whose extraordinarily well-preserved mummified body is now in a Cairo Museum, is believed to have succumbed to smallpox – the similarity between the pustular lesions on the face of the mummy and those of more recent patients is startling.

Smallpox was **endemic** in China by 1000 BC. In response, the practice of **variolation** was developed. Recognizing that survivors of smallpox outbreaks were protected from subsequent infection, the Chinese inhaled the dried crusts from smallpox lesions like snuff, or in later modifications, inoculated the pus from a lesion into a scratch on the forearm. Variolation was practised for centuries and was shown to be an effective method of disease prevention, although risky because the outcome of the inoculation was never certain. Edward Jenner was nearly killed by variolation at the age of seven! Not surprisingly, this experience spurred him on to find a safer alternative treatment. On 14 May 1796, Jenner used cowpox-infected material obtained from the hand of Sarah Nemes, a milkmaid from his home village of Berkeley in Gloucestershire, England, to successfully vaccinate 8-year-old James Phipps. Although initially controversial, **vaccination** against smallpox was almost universally adopted worldwide during the nineteenth century.

The early success of vaccination, although a triumph of scientific observation and reasoning, was not based on any real understanding of the nature of infectious agents; this arose separately from another line of reasoning. When Antony van Leeuwenhoek (1632–1723), a Dutch merchant, constructed the first simple microscopes he was able to identify bacteria as the 'animalcules' he saw in his specimens. However, it was not until Robert Koch and Louis Pasteur in the 1880s jointly proposed the 'germ theory' of disease that the significance of these organisms became apparent. Koch defined the four famous criteria now known as Koch's postulates which are still generally regarded as the proof that an infectious agent is responsible for a specific disease:

- The agent must be present in every case of the disease.
- The agent must be isolated from the host and grown *in vitro*.
- The disease must be reproduced when a pure culture of the agent is inoculated into a healthy susceptible host.
- The same agent must be recovered once again from the experimentally infected host.

Subsequently, Pasteur worked extensively on rabies, which he identified as being caused by a 'virus' (from the Latin for 'poison') but despite this, he did not discriminate between bacteria and other agents of disease. In 1892, Dimitri Iwanowski, a Russian botanist, showed that extracts from diseased tobacco plants could transmit disease to other plants after passage through ceramic filters fine enough to retain the smallest known bacteria. Unfortunately, he did not realize the full significance of these results. A few years later, in 1898, Martinus Beijerinick confirmed and extended Iwanowski's results on *Tobacco mosaic virus* and was the first to develop the modern idea of the virus, which he referred to as contagium vivum fluidum ('soluble living germ'). In the same year, Freidrich Loeffler and Paul Frosch showed that a similar agent was responsible for foot-and-mouth disease in cattle, but despite the realization that these new-found agents caused disease in animals as well as plants, there was resistance to the idea that they might have anything to do with human diseases. This was finally dispelled by Karl Landsteiner and Erwin

Popper in 1909, who showed that poliomyelitis was caused by a 'filterable agent' – the first human disease to be recognized as being caused by a virus.

Frederick Twort (1915) and Felix d'Herelle (1917) were the first to recognize viruses which infect bacteria, which d'Herelle called **bacteriophages** (eaters of bacteria). In the 1930s and subsequent decades, pioneering virologists such as Salvador Luria, Max Delbruck and many others used these viruses as model systems to investigate many aspects of virology, including virus structure (Chapter 2), genetics (Chapter 3), replication (Chapter 4), etc. These relatively simple agents have since been very important to our understanding of all types of viruses, including those of humans which are much more difficult to propagate and study. The further history of virology is the story of the development of experimental tools and systems with which viruses could be examined and by which whole new areas of biology were opened up, including not only the biology of the viruses themselves, but inevitably also the biology of the host cells on which these agents are entirely dependent.

LIVING HOST SYSTEMS

In 1881, Louis Pasteur began to study rabies in animals. Over several years, he developed methods of producing attenuated virus preparations by progressively drying the spinal cords of rabbits experimentally infected with the agent. When inoculated into animals, these preparations would protect them from challenge with virulent virus. In 1885, he inoculated a child, Joseph Meister, with this, the first artificially produced virus **vaccine** (since the ancient practice of **variolation** and Jenner's use of cowpox virus for **vaccination** relied on naturally occurring viruses). Whole plants have been used to study the effects of plant viruses ever since *Tobacco mosaic virus* was first discovered by Iwanowski. Usually such studies involve rubbing preparations containing virus particles into the leaves or stem of the plant.

During the Spanish–American War of the late nineteenth century and the subsequent building of the Panama Canal, American deaths due to yellow fever were colossal. The disease also appeared to be spreading slowly northward into the continental United States. Through experimental transmission to mice Walter Reed, in 1900, demonstrated that yellow fever was caused by a virus spread by mosquitoes. This discovery eventually enabled Max Theiler in 1937 to propagate the virus in chick embryos and to produce an attenuated vaccine – the 17D strain – which is still in use today. The success of this approach led many other investigators from the 1930s to the 1950s to develop animal systems to identify and propagate pathogenic viruses.

Eukaryotic cells can be grown *in vitro* (tissue culture) and viruses can be propagated in these cultures, but these techniques are expensive and technically quite demanding. Some viruses, such as influenza virus, will replicate in the living tissues of developing embryonated hens' eggs. Egg-adapted strains of influenza virus replicate well in eggs and very high virus **titres** can be obtained. Embryonated hens' eggs were first used to propagate viruses in the early decades of the twentieth century. This method has proved to be highly effective for the isolation and culture of many viruses, particularly strains of influenza virus and various poxviruses (e.g. *Vaccinia virus*). Counting the 'pocks' on the chorioallantoic membrane of eggs produced by the replication of *Vaccinia virus* was the first quantitative assay for any virus.

Today, animal host systems still have their uses in virology:

- To produce viruses which cannot be propagated *in vitro*, e.g. *Hepatitis B virus*
- To study the pathogenesis of virus infections, e.g. coxsackieviruses
- To test vaccine safety, e.g. oral poliovirus vaccine.

Nevertheless, they are increasingly being discarded for the following reasons:

- Breeding and maintenance of animals infected with pathogenic viruses is expensive
- Whole animals are complex systems, in which it is sometimes difficult to discern events
- Results obtained are not always reproducible, due to host variation
- Unnecessary or wasteful use of experimental animals is morally repugnant
- They are rapidly being overtaken by 'modern science' – cell culture and molecular biology.

The use of whole plants as host organisms does not give rise to the same moral objections as the use of living animals and continues to play an important part in the study of plant viruses. However, such systems are sometimes slow to deliver results and can be expensive to maintain.

In recent years, an entirely new technology has been employed to study the effects of viruses on host organisms. This involves the creation of **transgenic** animals and plants by inserting all or part of the virus **genome** into the DNA of the experimental organism, resulting in expression of virus **mRNA** and proteins in somatic cells (and sometimes in the cells of the germ line). Thus the pathogenic effects of virus proteins, individually and in various combinations, can be studied in living hosts. An important example of this technology is the use of 'SCID-hu' mice constructed from immunodeficient lines of animals transplanted with human tissue. These mice provide an intriguing model for the study of the pathogenesis of *Human immunodeficiency virus* (HIV) since there is no real alternative to studying the properties of this important virus *in vivo*. While these transgenic techniques often raise the same moral objections as the 'old-fashioned' experimental infection of animals by viruses, they are immensely powerful new tools for the study of virus pathogenicity. A growing number of plant and animal virus genes have been analysed in this way, although the results have not always been as expected, and in many cases it has proved difficult to equate the observations obtained with those gathered from experimental infections. Nevertheless, this method will undoubtedly become much more widely used as more of the technical difficulties associated with the construction of **transgenic** organisms are solved.

CELL CULTURE METHODS

Cell culture began early in the twentieth century with whole-organ cultures, then progressed to methods involving individual cells, either **primary cell** cultures (somatic cells from an experimental animal or taken from a human patient which can be maintained for a short period in culture) or **immortalized** cell lines, which, given appropriate conditions, continue to grow in culture indefinitely.

In 1949, John Enders and his colleagues were able to propagate *Poliovirus* in primary human cell cultures. This opened what many regard as the 'Golden Age of Virology' – the identification and isolation during the 1950s and 1960s of many viruses and their association with human diseases, for example, many enteroviruses and respiratory viruses, such as adenoviruses. Widespread virus isolation led to the realization that subclinical virus infections were very common; for example, even in **epidemics** of the most virulent strains of *Poliovirus*, there are approximately 100 subclinical infections for each paralytic case of poliomyelitis.

Renato Dulbecco in 1952 was the first to quantify accurately animal viruses using a **plaque** assay. In this technique, dilutions of the virus are used to infect a cultured cell **monolayer**, which is then covered with soft agar to restrict diffusion of the virus, resulting in localized cell killing and the appearance of plaques after the monolayer is stained (Figure 1.1). Counting the number of plaques directly determines the number of infectious virus particles applied to the plate. The same technique can also be used biologically to clone a virus, i.e. isolate a pure form from a mixture of types. This technique had been in use for some time to quantify the number of infectious virus particles in **bacteriophage** suspensions applied to confluent 'lawns' of bacterial cells on agar plates, but its application to viruses of **eukaryotes** enabled rapid advances in the study of virus replication to be made. Plaque assays largely replaced earlier endpoint dilution techniques, such as the $TCID_{50}$ (tissue culture infectious dose) assay, which are statistical means of measuring virus populations in culture. However, endpoint techniques may still be used in certain circumstances, for example, for viruses which do not replicate in culture, or which are not cytopathic and do not produce plaques, e.g. *Human immunodeficiency virus* (HIV).

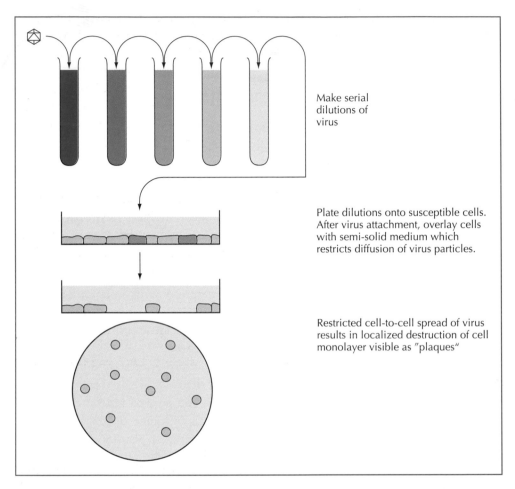

Make serial
dilutions of
virus

Plate dilutions onto susceptible cells.
After virus attachment, overlay cells
with semi-solid medium which
restricts diffusion of virus particles.

Restricted cell-to-cell spread of virus
results in localized destruction of cell
monolayer visible as "plaques"

Figure 1.1 Plaque assays are performed by applying a suitable dilution of a virus preparation to a confluent or semi–confluent adherent monolayer of susceptible cells. After allowing time for virus attachment to and infection of the cells, liquid medium is replaced by a semi-solid culture medium containing a polymer such as agarose or carboxymethyl cellulose, which restricts diffusion of virus particles from infected cells. Only direct cell to-cell spread can occur, resulting in localized destruction of the monolayer. After a suitable period, the medium is usually removed and the cells stained to make the holes in the monolayer (plaques) more easily visible. Each plaque therefore results from infection by a single plaque–forming unit (p.f.u.).

SEROLOGICAL/IMMUNOLOGICAL METHODS

As the discipline of virology was emerging, the techniques of immunology were also developing and, as with molecular biology more recently, the two disciplines have always been very closely linked. Developing an understanding of the mechanisms of immunity to virus infections has, of course, been very important. In recent years the role that the immune system itself plays in pathogenesis has become known (see Chapter 7). Immunology as a discipline in its own right has contributed many classical techniques to virology (Figure 1.2).

George Hirst, in 1941, observed **haemagglutination** of red blood cells by influenza virus (see Chapter 4). This proved to be an important tool not only in the study of influenza, but also with several other groups of viruses, for example, *Rubella virus*. In addition to measuring the **titre** (i.e. relative amount) of virus present in any preparation, this technique can also be used to determine the antigenic type of the virus. Haemagglutination will not occur in the presence of antibodies which bind to and block the virus haemagglutinin. If an antiserum is titrated against a given number of haemagglutinating units, the haemagglutination inhibition titre and specificity of the antiserum can be determined. Also, if antisera of known specificity are used to inhibit haemagglutination, the antigenic type of an unknown virus can be determined. In the 1960s and subsequent years, many improved detection methods for viruses were developed, for example:

- Complement fixation tests
- Radioimmunoassays
- Immunofluorescence (direct detection of virus antigens in infected cells or tissue)
- Enzyme-linked immunosorbent assays (ELISAs)
- Radioimmune precipitation
- Western blot assays.

These techniques are sensitive, quick and quantitative.

In 1975, George Kohler and Cesar Milstein isolated the first monoclonal antibodies from clones of cells selected *in vitro* to produce an antibody of a single specificity directed against a particular antigenic target. This enabled virologists to look not only at the whole virus, but at specific regions – epitopes – of individual virus antigens (Figure 1.3). This ability has greatly increased our understanding of the function of individual virus proteins. Monoclonal antibodies are also finding increasingly widespread application in other types of serological assay (e.g. ELISAs), to increase their reproducibility, sensitivity and specificity.

It would be inappropriate here to spend too long on the technical details of what is also a very rapidly expanding field of knowledge. However, I recommend strongly that readers who are not familiar with the serological and immunological techniques mentioned above should familiarize themselves thoroughly with this subject by reading one or more of the texts given in the Further Reading for this chapter. Time spent in this way will repay the reader throughout the rest of this book.

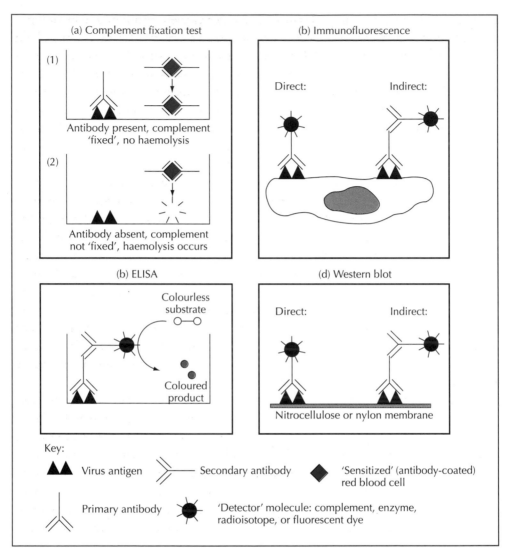

Figure 1.2 It is hard to overestimate the importance of serological techniques in virology. Four assays illustrated by the diagrams in this figure have been used for many years and are of widespread value.

(a) The complement fixation test works on the basis that complement is sequestered by antigen–antibody complexes. 'Sensitized' antibody-coated red blood cells, known amounts of complement, a virus antigen and the serum to be tested are added to the wells of a multi-well plate. In the absence of antibodies to the virus antigen, free complement is present and this causes lysis of the sensitized red blood cells (haemolysis). If, however, the test serum contains a sufficiently high titre of anti-virus antibodies, no free complement remains and haemolysis does not occur. Titrating the test serum by means of serial dilutions allows a quantitative measurement of the amount of anti-virus antibody present to be made.

(b) Immunofluorescence is performed using derivatized antibodies containing a covalently linked fluorescent molecule which emits a characteristically coloured light when illuminated by light of a different wavelength, e.g. rhodamine (red) or fluorescein (green). In direct immunofluorescence, the anti-virus antibody itself is conjugated to the fluorescent marker, whereas in indirect immunofluorescence, a second antibody reactive to the anti-virus antibody carries the marker. Immunofluorescence can be used not only to identify virus-infected cells in populations of cells or in tissue sections, but also to determine the subcellular localization of particular virus proteins, e.g. in the nucleus or in the cytoplasm.

(c) Enzyme-linked immunosorbent assays (ELISAs) are a rapid and sensitive means of identifying or quantifying small amounts of virus antigens or anti-virus antibodies. Either an antigen (in the case of an ELISA to detect antibodies) or antibody (in the case of an antigen ELISA) are bound to the surface of a multi-well plate. An antibody specific for the test antigen, which has been conjugated with an enzyme molecule (such as alkaline phosphatase or horseradish peroxidase), is then added. As with immunofluorescence, ELISA assays may rely on direct or indirect detection of the test antigen. During a short incubation, a colourless substrate for the enzyme is converted to a coloured product, thus amplifying the signal produced by a very small amount of antigen. The intensity of the product can easily be measured in a specialized spectrophotometer (a 'plate reader'). ELISA assays can be mechanized and are therefore suitable for routine tests on large numbers of clinical samples.

(d) Western blotting is used to analyse a specific virus protein from a complex mixture of antigens. Virus antigen-containing preparations (particles, infected cells or clinical materials) are subjected to electrophoresis on a polyacrylamide gel. Proteins from the gel are then transferred to a nitrocellulose or nylon membrane and immobilized in their relative positions from the gel. Specific antigens are detected by allowing the membrane to react with antibodies directed against the antigen of interest. By the use of samples containing proteins of known sizes in known amounts, the apparent molecular weight and relative amounts of antigen in the test samples can be determined.

ULTRASTRUCTURAL STUDIES

These can be considered under three areas: physical methods, chemical methods and electron microscopy. Physical measurements of virus particles began in the 1930s with the earliest determinations of their proportions by filtration through colloidal membranes of various pore sizes. Experiments of this sort led to the first (rather inaccurate) estimates of the size of virus particles. The accuracy of these was improved greatly by studies of the sedimentation properties of viruses in ultracentrifuges in the 1960s (Figure 1.4). Differential centrifugation proved to be of great

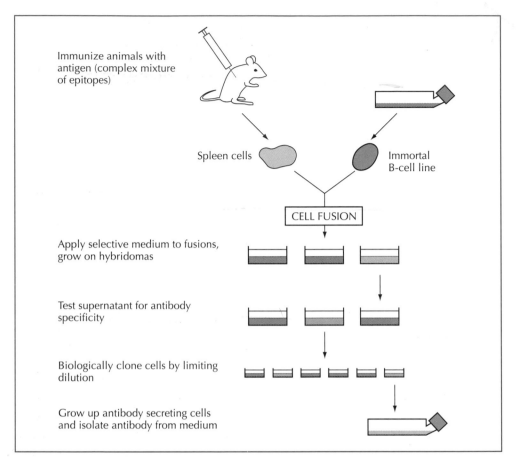

Immunize animals with antigen (complex mixture of epitopes)

Spleen cells

Immortal B-cell line

CELL FUSION

Apply selective medium to fusions, grow on hybridomas

Test supernatant for antibody specificity

Biologically clone cells by limiting dilution

Grow up antibody secreting cells and isolate antibody from medium

Figure 1.3 Monoclonal antibodies are produced by immunization of an animal with an antigen which usually contains a complex mixture of epitopes. Immature B cells are later prepared from the spleen of the animal and these are fused with a myeloma cell line, resulting in the formation of transformed cells continuously secreting antibodies. A small proportion of these will make a single type of antibody (a monoclonal antibody) against the desired epitope. Recently, *in vitro* molecular techniques have been developed to speed up the selection of monoclonal antibodies, although these have not yet replaced the original approach shown here.

use in obtaining purified and highly concentrated preparations of many different viruses, free of contamination from host cell components, which can be subjected to chemical analysis. The relative density of virus particles, measured in solutions of sucrose or caesium chloride (CsCl), is also a characteristic feature, revealing information about the proportions of nucleic acid and protein in the particles.

The physical properties of viruses can be determined by spectroscopy, using either ultraviolet light to examine the nucleic acid content of the particle or visible

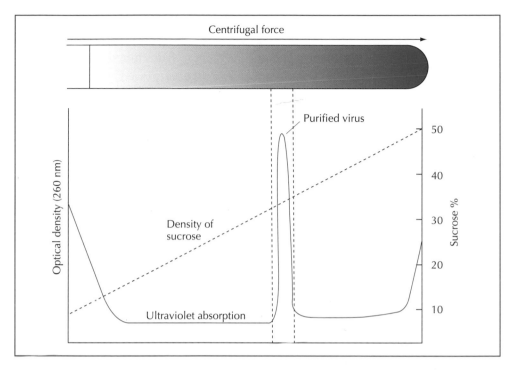

Figure 1.4 A number of different sedimentation techniques can be used to study viruses. In rate zonal centrifugation (shown here), virus particles are applied to the top of a preformed density gradient, i.e. a sucrose or salt solution of increasing density from the top to the bottom of the tube (top of figure). After a period of time in an ultracentrifuge, the gradient is separated into a number of fractions, which are analysed for the presence of virus particles. In the figure, the nucleic acid of the virus genome is detected by its absorption of ultraviolet light (below). This method can be used both to purify virus particles or nucleic acids or to determine their sedimentation characteristics. In equilibrium or isopycnic centrifugation, the sample is present in a homologous mixture containing a dense salt such as caesium chloride. A density gradient forms in the tube during centrifugation and the sample forms a band at a position in the tube equivalent to its own density. This method can thus be used to determine the density of virus particles and is commonly used to purify plasmid DNA.

light to determine its light–scattering properties. Electrophoresis of intact virus particles has yielded some limited information, but electrophoretic analysis of individual **virion** proteins by gel electrophoresis, and particularly also of nucleic acid **genomes** (Chapter 3), has been far more valuable. However, by far the most important method for the elucidation of virus structures has been the use of X–ray diffraction by crystalline forms of purified virus. This technique permits determination of the structure of virions at an atomic level.

The complete structures of many viruses, representative of many of the major groups, have now been determined at a resolution of a few angstroms (Å) (see Chapter 2, ✐). This has advanced our understanding of the functions of the virus particle considerably. However, a number of viruses have proved to be resistant to investigation by X-ray crystallography, a fact which highlights some of the problems inherent in this otherwise powerful technique. One problem is that the virus must first be purified to a high degree, otherwise specific information on the virus cannot be gathered. This presupposes that adequate quantities of the virus can be propagated in culture or obtained from infected tissues or patients and that a method is available to purify virus particles without loss of structural integrity. In a number of important cases, this requirement rules out further study (e.g. *Hepatitis C virus*). The purified virus must also be able to form paracrystalline arrays large enough to cause significant diffraction of the radiation source. For some viruses, this is relatively straightforward and crystals big enough to see with the naked eye and which diffract strongly are easily formed. This is particularly true for a number of plant viruses, such as *Tobacco mosaic virus* (TMV) (which was first crystallized by Wendell Stanley in 1935) and *Turnip yellow mosaic virus* (TYMV), the structures of which were among the first to be determined during the 1950s.

It is significant that these two viruses represent the two fundamental types of virus particle: **helical** in the case of TMV and **icosahedral** for TYMV (see Chapter 2). In many cases, however, only microscopic crystals can be prepared. A partial answer to this problem is to use ever more powerful radiation sources which enable good data to be collected from small crystals. Powerful synchotron sources which generate intense beams of radiation have been built during the last few decades and are now used extensively for this purpose. However, there is a limit beyond which this brute force approach fails to yield further benefit. A number of important viruses steadfastly refuse to crystallize – this is a particularly common problem with irregularly shaped viruses, for example those which have an outer lipid **envelope**, and to date, no complete high-resolution atomic structure has yet been determined for many viruses of this type (e.g. HIV). Modifications of the basic diffraction technique (such as electron scattering by membrane-associated protein arrays and cryoelectron microscopy) may help to provide more information in the future, but it is unlikely that these variations will solve this problem completely. One further limitation is that some of the largest virus particles, such as poxviruses, contain hundreds of different proteins and are at present too complex to be analysed using these techniques.

Nuclear magnetic resonance (NMR) is increasingly being used to determine the atomic structure of all kinds of molecules, including proteins and nucleic acids. The limitation of this method is that only relatively small molecules can be analysed before the signals obtained become so confusing that they are impossible to decipher with present technology. At present, the upper size limit for this technique restricts its use to molecules with a molecular weight of less than about

30 000–40 000 – considerably less than even the smallest virus particles. Nevertheless, this method may well prove to be of value in the future, certainly for examining isolated virus proteins, if not for intact **virions**

Chemical investigation can be used to determine not only the overall composition of viruses and the nature of the nucleic acid which comprises the virus **genome**, but also the construction of the particle and the way in which individual components relate to each other in the **capsid**. Many classic studies of virus structure have been based on gradual, stepwise disruption of particles by slow alteration of pH, or gradual addition of protein-denaturing agents such as urea, phenol or detergents. Under these conditions, valuable information can sometimes be obtained from relatively simple experiments. For example, as urea is gradually added to prep-arations of purified adenovirus particles, they break down in an ordered, stepwise fashion which releases subvirus protein assemblies, revealing how the particles are made up. In the case of TMV, similar studies of capsid organization have been performed by renaturation of the capsid protein under various conditions (Figure 1.5). In simple terms, the reagents used to denature virus capsids can indicate the basis of the stable interactions between its components. Proteins bound together by electrostatic interactions can be eluted by addition of ionic salts or alteration of pH, those bound by non-ionic, hydrophobic interactions can be eluted by reagents such as urea, and

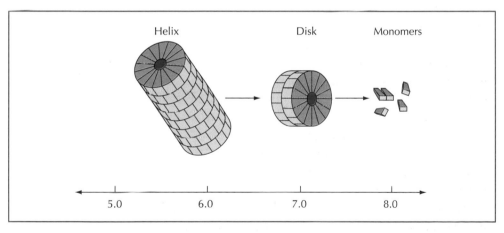

Figure 1.5 The structure and stability of virus particles can be examined by progressive denaturation or renaturation studies. At any particular ionic strength, the purified capsid protein of *Tobacco mosaic virus* (TMV) spontaneously assembles into different structures, dependent on the pH of the solution. At a pH of around 6.0, the particles formed have a helical structure very similar to that of infectious virus particles. As the pH is increased to about 7.0, disk-like structures are formed. At even higher pH values, individual capsid monomers fail to assemble into more complex structures.

proteins which interact with lipid components can be eluted by non-ionic detergents or organic solvents.

In addition to determining fundamental structure, progressive denaturation can also be used to observe alteration or loss of antigenic sites on the surface of particles and in this way, a picture of the physical state of the particle can be built up. Proteins exposed on the surface of viruses can be labelled with various compounds (e.g. iodine) to indicate which parts of the protein are exposed and which are protected inside the particle or by lipid membranes. Cross-linking reagents, such as psoralens, or newer synthetic reagents with side-arms of specific lengths are used to determine the spatial relationship of proteins and nucleic acids in intact viruses.

Electron microscopes, developed in the 1930s, overcome the fundamental limitation of light microscopes, i.e. the inability to resolve individual virus particles owing to physical constraints caused by the wavelength of visible light illumination and the optics of the instruments. The first electron micrograph of a virus (TMV) was published in 1939. During subsequent years, techniques were developed which allowed the direct examination of viruses at magnifications of over 100 000 times. There are two fundamental types of electron microscope, the transmission electron microscope (TEM) and the scanning electron microscope (SEM) (Figure 1.6). Although beautiful images with the appearance of three dimensions are produced by the SEM, for practical investigations of virus structure, the higher magnifications achievable with the TEM have proved to be of most value. Two fundamental types of information can be obtained by electron microscopy of viruses: the absolute number of virus particles present in any preparation (total count) and the appearance and structure of the **virions** (see below). Electron microscopy can provide a rapid method of virus detection and diagnosis, but in itself, may give misleading information. Many cellular components, for example ribosomes, can resemble 'virus-like particles,' particularly in crude preparations. This difficulty can be overcome by using antisera specific for particular virus antigens conjugated to electron-dense markers such as the iron-containing protein ferritin, or colloidal gold suspensions. This highly specific technique, known as immunoelectron microscopy, is gaining ground as a rapid method for diagnosis.

Developments in electron microscopy have allowed investigation of the structure of fragile viruses which cannot be determined by X-ray crystallography. These technologies include cryoelectron microscopy, in which the virus particles are maintained at very low temperatures on cooled specimen stages; examination of particles embedded in vitreous ice, which does not disrupt the particles by the formation of ice crystals; low-irradiation electron microscopy, reducing the destructive bombardment of the specimen with electrons; and sophisticated image-analysis and image-reconstruction techniques which permit accurate, three-dimensional images to be formed from multiple images that individually would appear as very poor quality. Conventional electron microscopy can resolve structures down to 50–70 Å in size (a typical atomic diameter is 2–3 Å, a protein α-helix 10 Å and a DNA

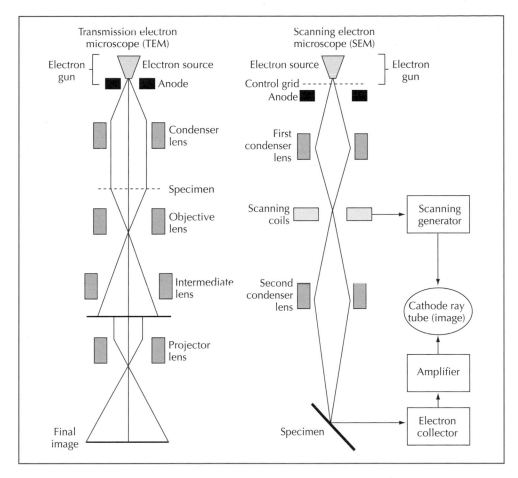

Figure 1.6 Working principles of transmission and scanning electron microscopes.

double helix 20 Å). Using these newer techniques it is possible to resolve structures of 25   30 Å.

In the late 1950s, Sidney Brenner and Robert Horne (among others) developed sophisticated techniques which enabled them to use electron microscopy to reveal many of the fine details of the structure of virus particles. One of the most valuable techniques proved to be the use of electron-dense dyes such as phosphotungstic acid or uranyl acetate to examine virus particles by negative staining. The small metal ions in such dyes are able to penetrate the minute crevices between the protein subunits in a virus **capsid** to reveal the fine structure of the particle. Using such data, Francis Crick and James Watson (1956) were the first to suggest that virus capsids are composed of numerous identical protein subunits arranged either in helical or cubic (**icosahedral**) symmetry. In 1962, Donald Caspar and Aaron Klug extended these observations and elucidated the fundamental principles of symmetry which allow repeated protomers to form virus capsids, based on the principle of **quasi–equivalence** (see Chapter 2). This combined theoretical and practical approach has resulted in our present understanding of the structure of virus particles.

'MOLECULAR BIOLOGY'

All the above techniques of investigation are themselves 'molecular biology' in the original sense of the term. However, the term 'molecular biology' ('genetic engineering' or 'genetic manipulation') has taken on a new and different meaning. These new techniques for manipulating nucleic acids *in vitro* (that is, outside living cells or organisms) do not comprise a new discipline, but are an outgrowth of earlier developments in biochemistry and cell biology over the previous 50 years. Nevertheless, this powerful new technology has revolutionized virology and, to a large extent, has shifted the focus of attention away from the virus particle onto the virus **genome** Again, this book is not the place to discuss in detail the technical aspects of these methods, and readers are referred to one of the many texts such as those given at the end of this chapter.

Virus infection has long been used to probe the working of 'normal' (i.e. uninfected) cells, for example, to look at macromolecular synthesis. This is true, for example, of the applications of **bacteriophages** in bacterial genetics, and in many instances the study of eukaryotic viruses has revealed fundamental information about the cell biology and genomic organization of higher organisms. In 1970, John Kates first observed that *Vaccinia virus* mRNAs were polyadenylated at their 3' ends. In the same year, Howard Temin and David Baltimore jointly identified the enzyme reverse transcriptase (RNA-dependent DNA polymerase) in retrovirus-infected cells. This shattered the so-called 'central dogma' of biology, i.e. that there is a one-way flow of information from DNA through RNA into protein, and revealed the plasticity of the **eukaryote** genome. Subsequently, the purification of this enzyme from retrovirus particles permitted cDNA cloning, which greatly accelerated the study of viruses with RNA genomes – a good illustration of the catalytic nature of scientific advances. In 1977 Richard Roberts, and independently Phillip Sharp, recognized that adenovirus mRNAs were spliced to remove intervening sequences, indicating the similarities between virus and cellular genomes.

Initially at least, the effect of this new technology was to shift the emphasis of investigation from proteins to nucleic acids. As the power of the techniques developed, it quickly became possible to determine the nucleotide sequences of entire virus **genomes**, beginning with the smallest **bacteriophages** in the mid-1970s and working up to the largest of all virus genomes, those of the herpesviruses and poxviruses, many of which have now been determined.

This nucleic acid-centred technology, in addition to its 'ultimate' achievement of nucleotide sequencing and the artificial manipulation of virus genomes, also offered significant advances in detection of viruses and virus infections involving nucleic acid hybridization techniques. There are many variants of this basic idea, but essentially, a hybridization probe, labelled in some fashion to facilitate detection, is allowed to react with a crude mixture of nucleic acids. The specific interaction of the probe sequence with complementary virus-encoded sequences, to which it binds by hydrogen bond formation between the complementary base pairs, reveals the presence of the virus genetic material (Figure 1.7). This approach has been taken a stage further by the development of various *in vitro* nucleic acid amplification procedures, such as the polymerase chain reaction (PCR). This is an even more sensitive technique, capable of detecting just a single molecule of virus nucleic acid (Figure 1.8).

More recently, there has also been renewed interest in virus proteins based on a new biology which is itself dependent on the manipulation of nucleic acids *in vitro* and advances in protein detection arising from immunology. Methods for the *in vitro* synthesis and expression of proteins from molecularly cloned DNA have advanced rapidly, and many new analytical techniques are now available. Studies of protein-nucleic acid interactions are proving to be particularly valuable in understanding virus structure and gene expression.

Molecular biologists have one further trick up their sleeves. Because of the repetitive, digitized nature of nucleotide sequences, computers are the ideal means of storing and processing this mass of information. 'Bioinformatics' is a broad term coined in the 1980s to encompass any application of computers to biology. This can imply anything from artificial intelligence and robotics to genome analysis. More specifically, the term applies to computer manipulation of biological sequence data, including protein structural analysis. Bioinformatics permits the inference of function from the linear sequence, and is thus central to all areas of modern biology. As the flood of sequence information continues, computers are being used increasingly to make predictions based on nucleotide sequences (Figure 1.9). These include detecting the presence of open reading frames (**ORFs**), the amino acid sequences of the proteins encoded by them, control regions of genes such as **promoters** and splice signals and the secondary structure of proteins and nucleic acids. However (particularly in the case of RNA), the secondary structure assumed by molecules is almost as important as the primary nucleotide sequence in determining the biological reactions which the molecule may undergo. Caution is needed in interpreting such predicted rather than factual information, and the validity of such predictions should not be accepted without question unless confirmed by biochemical and/or genetic data. However, once the structure of a protein has been determined by X-ray crystallography or NMR, the shape can be accurately modelled and explored in three dimensions on computers (Figure 1.10).

Vast international databases of nucleotide and protein sequence information have now been compiled, and these can rapidly be consulted by computers to compare newly determined sequences with those whose function may have been studied in great detail. At the time of publication, the complete genome sequences of some 500

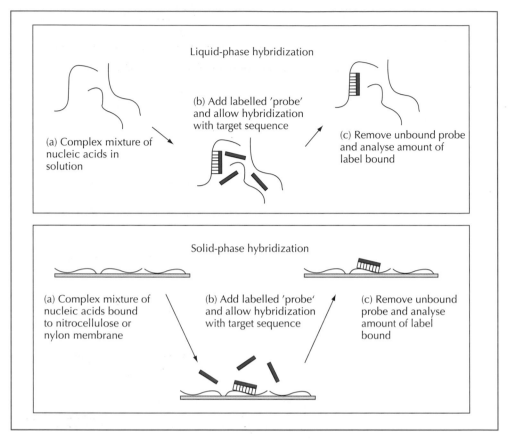

Figure 1.7 Nucleic acid hybridization relies on the specificity of base-pairing which allows a labelled nucleic acid probe to pick out a complementary target sequence from a complex mixture of sequences in the test sample. The label used to identify the probe may be a radioisotope or a non–isotopic label such as an enzyme or chemiluminescent system. Hybridization may be performed with both the probe and test sequences in the liquid phase (top of figure) or with the test sequences bound to a solid phase, usually a nitrocellulose or nylon membrane (below). Both methods may be used to quantify the amount of the test sequence present, but solid–phase hybridization is also used to locate the position of sequences immobilized on the membrane. Plaque and colony hybridization are used to locate recombinant molecules directly from a mixture of bacterial colonies or **bacteriophage** plaques on an agar plate. 'Northern' and 'Southern' blotting are used to detect RNA and DNA respectively after transfer of these molecules from gels following separation by electrophoresis (cf. 'western' blotting, Figure 1.2).

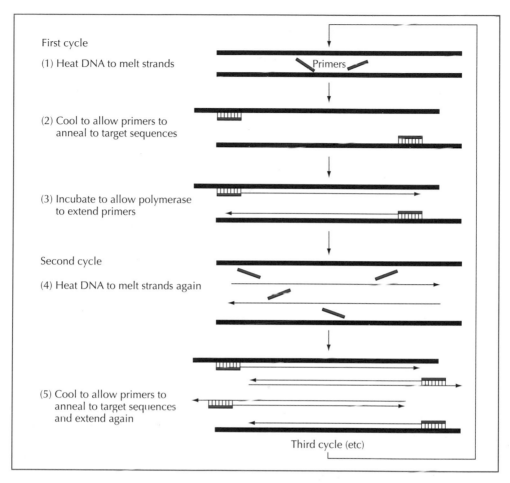

First cycle

(1) Heat DNA to melt strands

Primers

(2) Cool to allow primers to
    anneal to target sequences

(3) Incubate to allow polymerase
    to extend primers

Second cycle

(4) Heat DNA to melt strands again

(5) Cool to allow primers to
    anneal to target sequences
    and extend again

Third cycle (etc)

Figure 1.8 The polymerase chain reaction (PCR) relies on the specificity of base-pairing between short synthetic oligonucleotide probes and complementary sequences in a complex mixture of nucleic acids to prime DNA synthesis using a thermostable DNA polymerase. Multiple cycles of primer annealing, extension and thermal denaturation are carried out in an automated process, resulting in a massive amplification (2^n-fold increase after n cycles of amplification) of the target sequence located between the two primers.

different viruses had been published, with more appearing almost weekly (see 'Virology Online' ✐).

Thus we have, in a sense, come full circle in our investigations of viruses – from particles via **genomes** back to proteins again – and have emerged with a far more profound understanding of these organisms. However, the present pace of research in virology tells us that there is still far more that we need to know.

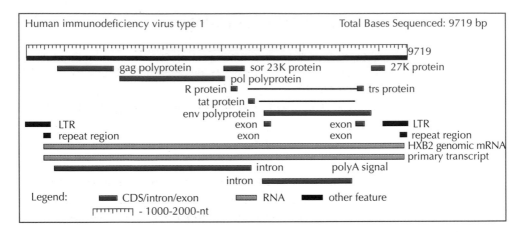

Figure 1.9 An example of the use of a computer to store and process 'digitized' information from a nucleic acid sequence. This figure shows an analysis of all of the open reading frames (**ORFs**) present in an HIV-1 **provirus**. The ORFs present in the three main retrovirus genes, *gag*, *pol* and *env*, can be seen. This complex analysis took only a few seconds to perform using an ordinary personal computer. Manually, the same task would have taken several days.

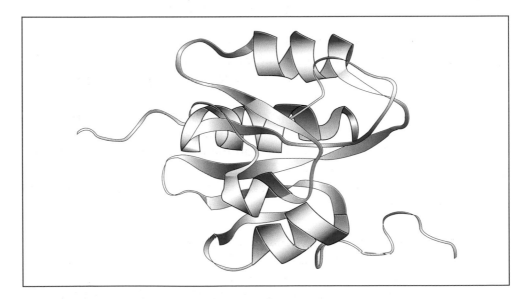

Figure 1.10 Three-dimensional structure of the DNA-binding domain of SV40 T-antigen reconstructed from NMR data using a computer.

FURTHER READING

Alberts, B., Bray, D., Johnson, A., Lewis, J., Walter, P. , Roberts, K. and Raff, M. (Eds) (1997). *Essential Cell Biology: An Introduction to the Molecular Biology of the Cell.* Garland, New York. ISBN 0815320450.

Attwood, T.K. and Parry-Smith, D.J. (1999). *Introduction to Bioinformatics.* Addison Wesley Longman, Harlow, Essex. ISBN 0582327881.

Cann, A.J. (1999). *Virus Culture: A Practical Approach.* Oxford University Press, Oxford. ISBN 0199637148.

Chisari, F.V. and Oldstone, M.B.A. (Eds) (1996). Transgenic models of human viral and immunological disease. *Current Topics in Microbiology and Immunology,* Vol. 206.

Glick, B.R. and Pasternak, J.J. (1998). *Molecular Biotechnology.* American Society for Microbiology, Washington, DC. ISBN 1555811361.

Goldsby, R.A., Kindt, T.J. and Osborne, B.A. (2000). *Kuby: Immunology* (4th edn). W.H. Freeman, New York. ISBN 0716733315.

Watt, I.M. (1997). *The Principles and Practice of Electron Microscopy* (2nd edn). Cambridge University Press, Cambridge. ISBN 0521435919.

SELF-ASSESSMENT QUESTIONS

(1.1) Are the following statements true or false?

T (a)   Viruses are submicroscopic, obligate intracellular parasites.

F (b)   Virus particles increase by the integrated sum of their components and reproduce by division.

T (c)   Viruses lack the genetic information which encodes apparatus necessary for the generation of metabolic energy.

T (d)   Viruses lack the genetic information which encodes apparatus necessary for protein synthesis (ribosomes).

F (e)   Prions are infectious agents believed to consist of a single nucleic acid component.

(1.2) Are the following statements true or false?

F (a)   Antony van Leeuwenhoek (1632–1723) was the first person to see virus particles under the microscope.

T (b)   Edward Jenner first vaccinated a patient against smallpox on 14 May 1796.

F (c)   Louis Pasteur invented the term 'virus' in the 1890s.

T (d)   Dimitri Iwanowski showed that viruses could pass through filters fine enough to retain the smallest known bacteria.

F (e)   Viruses which infect bacteria are called bacteriophiles.

(1.3) These are Koch's postulates (true or false?):

T (a)   The agent must be present in every case of the disease.
T (b)   The agent must be isolated from the host and grown *in vitro*.
T (c)   The disease must be reproduced when a pure culture of the agent is inoculated into a healthy susceptible host.
T (d)   The same agent must be recovered once again from the experimentally infected host.

(1.4) The following are immunological methods of studying viruses (true or false?):

T (a)   Complement fixation
F (b)   Northern blot — RNA
F (c)   Southern blot — DNA
T (d)   Western blot
F (e)   PCR   amplifying small quantities of NUCLEIC ACID.

(1.5) Are the following statements true or false?

F (a)   Electron microscopes allow direct examination of viruses at magnifications of up to 1000 times.   100. 000
T (b)   X-ray diffraction by crystalline forms of purified virus can be used to determine their structure.
F (c)   The atomic structures of all known viruses have now been determined.
F (d)   Viruses are believed to originate by spontaneous generation.
F (e)   Nuclear magnetic resonance is used to determine the structure of virus particles.

Answers to Self-Assessment Questions are given in Appendix 4.

PARTICLES

On completing this chapter, you should be able to:
- Understand the reasons why viruses encode the proteins to make particles
- Identify the main structural types of virus particle
- Explain how the virus capsid interacts with both the host cell and virus genome during replication.

THE FUNCTION AND FORMATION OF VIRUS PARTICLES

Much of the information about virus structures is highly visual in nature and is difficult to represent adequately in print. It is highly recommended that you view the virus structure resources on the accompanying CD ⊘.

Why bother to form a virus particle to contain the **genome**? Indeed, some infectious agents, such as **viroids**, do not (see Chapter 8). However, the fact that viruses struggle with the genetic and biochemical burden entailed in encoding and assembling the components of a particle indicates that there must be positive benefits to this strategy. At the simplest level, the function of the outer shells of a virus particle is to protect the fragile nucleic acid genome from physical, chemical or enzymatic damage. After leaving the host cell, the virus enters a hostile environment which would quickly inactivate the unprotected genome. Nucleic acids are susceptible to physical damage such as shearing by mechanical forces and to chemical modification by ultraviolet light (from sunlight). The natural environment is heavily laden with nucleases either derived from dead or leaky cells or deliberately secreted by vertebrates as defence against infection. In viruses with single-stranded genomes, the breaking of a single phosphodiester bond or chemical modification of one nucleotide is sufficient to inactivate that virus particle, making replication of the genome impossible. How is protection against this achieved? The protein subunits in a virus **capsid** are multiply redundant, i.e. present in many copies per particle. Damage to one or more subunits may render that particular subunit non-functional, but rarely does limited damage destroy the infectivity of the whole particle. This makes the capsid an effective barrier.

The outer surface of the virus is also responsible for recognition of and the first interaction with the host cell. Initially, this takes the form of binding of a specific **virus–attachment protein** to a cellular **receptor** molecule. However, the capsid also has a role to play in initiating infection by delivering the **genome** in a form in which it can interact with the host cell. In some cases this is a simple process which consists only of dumping the genome into the cytoplasm of the cell. In other cases this stage is much more complex; for example, retroviruses carry out extensive modifications to the virus genome while it is still inside the particle, converting two molecules of single-stranded RNA to one molecule of double-stranded DNA before delivering it to the cell nucleus. Hence, the role of the capsid is vital in allowing viruses to establish an infection.

To form infectious particles, viruses must overcome two fundamental problems. First, they must assemble the particle utilizing the information available from the components which make up the particle itself. Second, virus particles form regular geometric shapes, even though the proteins from which they are made are irregularly shaped. How do these simple organisms solve these difficulties? The solutions to both problems lie in the rules of symmetry.

CAPSID SYMMETRY AND VIRUS ARCHITECTURE

It is possible to imagine a virus particle, the outer shell of which (the **capsid**) consists of a single, hollow protein molecule, which as it folds to assume its mature conformation traps the virus **genome** inside. In practice, this arrangement cannot occur for the following reason. The triplet nature of the genetic code means that three nucleotides (or base pairs in the case of viruses with double-stranded genomes) are necessary to encode one amino acid. Viruses cannot, of course, utilize an alternative, more economical, genetic code because this could not be deciphered by the host cell. Since the approximate molecular weight of a nucleotide triplet is 1000 and the average molecular weight of a single amino acid is 150, a nucleic acid can only encode a protein that is at most 15% of its own weight. Therefore, virus capsids must be made up of multiple protein molecules (subunit construction) and viruses must overcome the problem of how these subunits are arranged.

In 1957, Heinz Fraenkel-Conrat and R.C. Williams showed that when mixtures of purified *Tobacco mosaic virus* (TMV) RNA and coat protein were incubated together, virus particles formed. The discovery that virus particles could form spontaneously from purified subunits without any extraneous information indicated that the particle was in the free energy minimum state and was therefore the favoured structure of the components. This stability is an important feature of the virus particle. Although some viruses are very fragile and unable to survive outside the protected host cell environment, many are able to persist for long periods, in some cases for years.

The forces which drive the assembly of virus particles include hydrophobic and electrostatic interactions – only rarely are covalent bonds involved in holding together the multiple subunits. In biological terms, this means that protein–protein, protein–nucleic acid and protein–lipid interactions are used. It would be fair to say that the subtlety of these interactions is not fully understood for the majority of virus structures, but we now have a good understanding of general principles and repeated structural motifs which appear to govern the construction of diverse, unrelated viruses. These are discussed below under the two main classes of virus structures: **helical** and **icosahedral** symmetry.

Helical capsids

Tobacco mosaic virus (TMV) is representative of one of the two major structural classes seen in viruses, those with helical symmetry. The simplest way to arrange multiple, identical protein subunits is to use rotational symmetry and to arrange the irregularly shaped proteins around the circumference of a circle to form a disk. Multiple disks can then be stacked on top of one another to form a cylinder, with the virus **genome** coated by the protein shell or contained in the hollow centre of the cylinder. Denaturation and phase-transition studies of TMV suggest that this is the form the particle takes (see Chapter 1).

Closer examination of the TMV particle by X-ray crystallography reveals that the structure of the **capsid** actually consists of a **helix** rather than a pile of stacked disks. A helix can be defined mathematically by two parameters: its amplitude (diameter) and pitch (the distance covered by each complete turn of the helix) (Figure 2.1). Helices are rather simple structures formed by stacking repeated components with a constant relationship (amplitude and pitch) to one another. Note that if this simple constraint is broken, a spiral forms rather than a helix and this is quite unsuitable for containing a virus genome. In terms of individual protein subunits, helices are described by the number of subunits per turn of the helix, m, and the axial rise per subunit, p. The pitch of the helix, P, is therefore equal to:

$$P = \mu \times p$$

For TMV, $\mu = 16.3$, that is, there are 16.3 coat protein molecules per helix turn, and $p = 0.14$ nm. Therefore, the pitch of the TMV helix is $16.3 \times 0.14 = 2.28$ nm. TMV particles are rigid, rod-like structures, but some helical viruses demonstrate considerable flexibility and longer helical virus particles are often curved or bent. Flexibility is

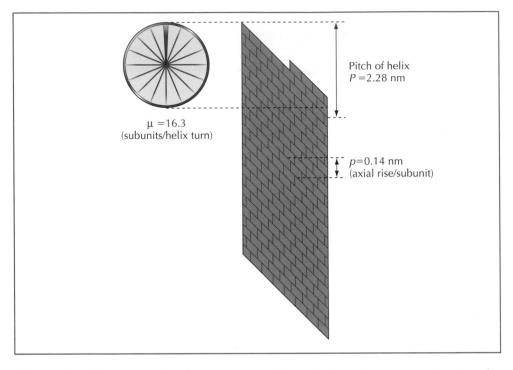

Figure 2.1 *Tobacco mosaic virus* has a capsid consisting of many molecules of a single coat protein arranged in a constant relationship, forming a helix with a pitch of 22.8 Å.

probably an important attribute. Long helical particles are likely to be subject to shear forces and the ability to bend reduces the likelihood of breakage or damage.

That **helical** symmetry is a useful way of arranging a single protein subunit to form a particle is confirmed by the large number of different types of virus which have evolved with this capsid arrangement. Among the simplest helical capsids are those of the well-known **bacteriophages** of the family *Inoviridae*, such as M13 and fd. These phages are about 900 nm long and 9 nm diameter and the particles contain five proteins (Figure 2.2). The major coat protein is the product of **phage** gene 8 (g8p) and there are 2700–3000 copies of this protein per particle, together with approximately five copies each of four minor capsid proteins, g3p, g6p, g7p and g9p, located at the ends of the filamentous particle. The primary structure of the major coat protein g8p explains many of the properties of the particle. Mature molecules of g8p consist of approximately 50 amino acid residues (a signal sequence of 23 amino acids is cleaved from the precursor protein during its translocation into the outer membrane of the host bacterium), and is almost entirely α-helical in structure so that the molecule forms a short rod. There are three distinct domains within this rod. At the amino-terminus there is a negatively charged region containing acidic amino acid residues which forms the outer, hydrophilic surface of the virus particle,

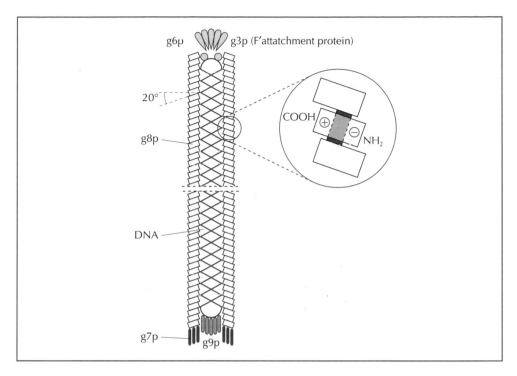

Figure 2.2 Schematic representation of the *Enterobacteria phage M13* particle (*Inoviridae*). Major coat protein g8p is arranged helically, the subunits overlapping 'like the scales of a fish'. Other capsid proteins required for the biological activity of the virion are located at either end of the particle. Inset shows the hydrophobic interactions between the g8p monomers (shaded region).

and at the carboxy-terminus there is a basic, positively charged region which lines the inside of the protein cylinder adjacent to the negatively charged DNA **genome**. Between these two, there is a hydrophobic region which is responsible for interactions between the g8p subunits that allow the formation of and stabilize the phage particle (Figure 2.2). *Inovirus* particles are held together by hydrophobic interactions between the coat protein subunits, as is demonstrated by the fact that the particles fall apart in the presence of chloroform, even though they do not contain any lipid component. The g8p subunits in successive turns of the helix interlock with the subunits in the turn below and are tilted at an angle of approximately 20° to the long axis of the particle, overlapping one another like the scales of a fish. The value of μ (number of protein subunits per complete helix turn) is 4.5 and p (axial rise per subunit) = 1.5 nm.

Because the **phage** DNA is packaged inside the core of the helical particle, the length of the particle is dependent on the length of the **genome**. In all *Inovirus* preparations, 'polyphage' (containing more than one genome length of DNA), 'miniphage' (deleted forms containing 0.2–0.5 phage genomes length of DNA), and 'maxiphage' (genetically defective forms but containing more than one phage genome length of

DNA) occur. This plastic property of these filamentous particles has been exploited by molecular biologists to develop the M13 genome as a cloning vector. Insertion of foreign DNA into the genome results in recombinant phage particles which are longer than the wild-type filaments. Unlike most viruses, there is no sharp cut-off genome length at which the genome can no longer be packaged into the particle. However, as M13 genome size increases, the efficiency of replication declines. While recombinant phage genomes 1–10% longer than the wild-type do not appear to be significantly disadvantaged, those 10–50% longer than the wild-type replicate significantly more slowly. Above a 50% increase over the normal genome length it becomes progressively more difficult to isolate recombinant phage.

The structure of the *Inovirus* capsid also explains the events which occur on infection of suitable bacterial host cells. *Inovirus* phages are 'male-specific', i.e. they require the F pilus on the surface of *Escherichia coli* for infection. The first event in infection is an interaction between g3p located at one end of the filament together with g6p, and the end of the F pilus. This interaction causes a conformational change in g8p. Initially, its structure changes from 100% α-helix to 85% α-helix, causing the filament to shorten. The end of the particle attached to the F pilus flares open, exposing the phage DNA. Subsequently, a second conformational change in the g8p subunits reduces its α-helical content from 85% to 50%, causing the phage particle to form a hollow spheroid about 40 nm in diameter and expelling the phage DNA, thus initiating the infection of the host cell.

Many plant viruses show helical symmetry (Appendix 2, ✐). These particles vary from approximately 100 nm (*Tobravirus*) to approximately 1000 nm (*Closterovirus*) in length. The best-studied example is, as stated above, TMV from the *Tobamovirus* group. Quite why so many groups of plant virus have evolved this structure is not clear, but it may be related either to the biology of the host plant cell or to the way in which they are transmitted between hosts.

Helical, naked (i.e. non-enveloped) animal viruses do not exist. Once again, this probably reflects aspects of host cell biology and virus transmission, but the reasons are not clear. There are a large number of animal viruses based on helical symmetry, but all have the addition of an outer lipid **envelope** (see below). There are too many viruses with this structure to list individually, but this category includes many of the best known human pathogens, such as influenza virus (*Orthomyxoviridae*), mumps and measles viruses (*Paramyxoviridae*) and *Rabies virus* (*Rhabdoviridae*). All possess single-stranded, **negative-sense RNA genomes** (see Chapter 3). The molecular design of all of these viruses is similar. The virus nucleic acid and a basic, nucleic acid-binding protein condense together in the infected cell to form a helical **nucleocapsid**. This protein–RNA complex serves to protect the fragile virus genome from physical and chemical damage and in some instances also provides other functions associated with virus replication. The envelope and its associated proteins are derived from the membranes of the host cell and are added to the nucleocapsid core of the virus during replication (see Chapter 4).

Some of these helical, **enveloped** animal viruses are relatively simple in structure, for example, rabies virus and the closely related *Vesicular stomatitis virus* (VSV) (Figure 2.3). These viruses are built up around the negative-sense RNA **genome**, which in rhabdoviruses is about 11 000 nucleotides (11 kilobases, 11 kb) long. The RNA genome and basic nucleocapsid (N) protein interact to form a helical structure with a pitch of approximately 5 nm, which, together with two non-structural proteins, L and NS (which form the virus polymerase: see Chapter 4), makes up the core of the virus particle. There are 30–35 turns of the nucleoprotein helix in the core, which is about 180 nm long and 80 nm in diameter. The individual N protein monomers are approximately $9 \times 5 \times 3$ nm and each covers about nine nucleotides of the RNA genome. As in the case of the filamentous **phage** particles described above, the role of the N protein is to stabilize the RNA genome and protect it from chemical, physical and enzymatic damage. In common with most enveloped viruses, the nucleocapsid is surrounded by an amorphous layer which interacts with both the core and the overlying lipid envelope linking them together. This is known as the matrix. The matrix (M) protein is usually the most abundant protein in the virus particle; for example, there are approximately 1800

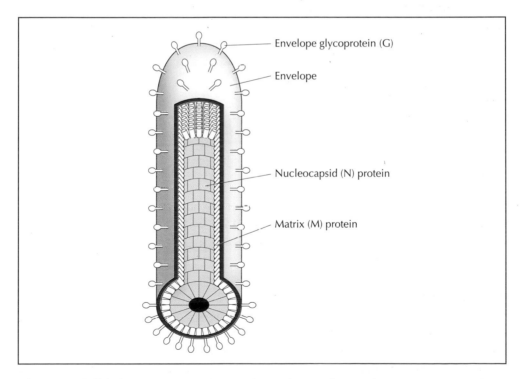

Figure 2.3 Rhabdovirus particles, such as those of *Vesicular stomatitis virus*, have an inner helical nucleocapsid surrounded by an outer lipid envelope and its associated glycoproteins.

copies of the M protein and approximately 1250 copies of the N protein in VSV particles. The lipid envelope and its associated proteins are discussed in more detail below.

It is clear that many different groups of viruses have evolved around helical symmetry. Simple viruses with small genomes use this architecture to provide protection for the genome without the need to encode multiple capsid proteins. More complex virus particles utilize this structure as the basis of the virus particle, but elaborate on it with additional layers of protein and lipid.

Icosahedral (isometric) capsids

An alternative way of building a virus capsid is to arrange protein subunits in the form of a hollow quasi-spherical structure, enclosing the **genome** within. The criteria for arranging subunits on the surface of a solid are a little more complex than those for building a helix. In theory, a number of solid shapes can be constructed from repeated subunits, e.g. a tetrahedron (four triangular faces), cube (six square faces), octahedron (eight triangular faces), dodecahedron (12 pentagonal faces) and an **icosahedron**, a solid shape consisting of 20 triangular faces arranged around the surface of a sphere (Figure 2.4).

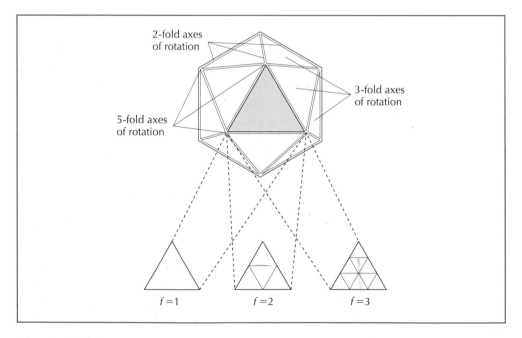

Figure 2.4 Illustration of the 2–3–5 symmetry of an icosahedron. More complex ('higher order') icosahedra can be defined by the triangulation number of the structure, $T = f^2 \times P$. Regular icosahedra have faces consisting of equilateral triangles and are formed when the value of P is 1 or 3. All other values of P give rise to more complex structures with either a left-hand or right-hand skew.

Early in the 1960s, direct examination of a number of small 'spherical' viruses by electron microscopy revealed that they appeared to have **icosahedral** symmetry. At first sight, it is not obvious why this pattern should have been 'chosen' by diverse virus groups. However, although in theory it is possible to construct virus **capsids** based on simpler symmetrical arrangements, such as tetrahedra or cubes, there are practical reasons why this does not occur. As described above, it is more economic in terms of genetic capacity to design a capsid based on a large number of identical, repeated protein subunits rather than fewer, larger subunits. It is unlikely that a simple tetrahedron consisting of four identical protein molecules would be large enough to contain even the smallest virus **genome**. If it were, it is probable that the gaps between the subunits would be so large that the particle would be leaky, and fail to carry out its primary function of protecting the virus genome.

In order to construct a capsid from repeated subunits, a virus must 'know the rules' which dictate how these are arranged. For an **icosahedron** the rules are based on the rotational symmetry of the solid, known as 2–3–5 symmetry, which has the following features (Figure 2.4):

- An axis of twofold rotational symmetry through the centre of each edge
- An axis of threefold rotational symmetry through the centre of each face
- An axis of fivefold rotational symmetry through the centre of each corner (vertex).

Since protein molecules are irregularly shaped and are not regular equilateral triangles, the simplest icosahedral capsids are built up by using three identical subunits to form each triangular face. This means that 60 identical subunits are required to form a complete capsid. A few simple virus particles are constructed in this way; for example, **bacteriophages** of the family *Microviridae*, such as φX174. An empty precursor particle called the procapsid is formed during assembly of this bacteriophage. Assembly of the procapsid requires the presence of the two scaffolding proteins which are structural components of the procapsid, but are not found in the mature virion.

In most cases, analysis reveals that icosahedral virus capsids contain more than 60 subunits, for the reasons of genetic economy given above. This presents a difficulty. A regular **icosahedron** composed of 60 identical subunits is a very stable structure because all the subunits are equivalently bonded, i.e. they show the same spacing relative to one another and each occupies the minimum free energy state. With more than 60 subunits it is impossible for them all to be arranged completely symmetrically with exactly equivalent bonds to all their neighbours, since a true regular icosahedron consists of only 20 subunits. To solve this problem, in 1962 Donald Caspar and Aaron Klug proposed the idea of **quasi-equivalence**. Their simple idea was that subunits in nearly the same local environment form nearly equivalent bonds with their neighbours, permitting self-assembly of icosahedral capsids from multiple subunits. In the case of these higher order icosahedra, the symmetry of the particle is defined by the **triangulation number** of the icosahedron (Figure 2.4). The triangulation number, *T*, is defined by:

$$T = f^2 \times P$$

where f is the number of subdivisions of each side of the triangular face; f^2 is there-fore the number of subtriangles on each face; and $P = h^2 + hk + k^2$, where h and k are any distinct, non-negative integers. This means that values of T fall into the series 1, 3, 4, 7, 9, 12, 13, 16, 19, 21, 25, 27, 28, etc. When $P = 1$ or 3, a regular icosahedron is formed. All other values of P give rise to icosahedra of the 'skew' class, where the subtriangles making up the icosahedron are not symmetrically arranged with respect to the edge of each face (Figure 2.5). Detailed structures of icosahedral virus par-ticles with $T = 1$ (*Microviridae*, e.g. φX174), $T = 3$ (many insect, plant and animal RNA viruses: see below), $T = 4$ (*Togaviridae*) and $T = 7$ (the heads of the tailed **bacteriophages** such as λ) have all been determined ⬦.

Virus particles with still larger triangulation numbers use different kinds of subunit assemblies for the faces and vertices of the icosahedron and have internal scaffolding proteins which act as a framework. These direct the assembly of the cap-sid, typically by bringing together pre-formed subassemblies of proteins (see dis-cussion of φX174 above). Variations on the theme of icosahedral symmetry occur over and over again in virus particles. For example, *Geminivirus* particles consist of a fused pair of $T = 1$ icosahedra joined where a pentamer is absent from each iosa-hedron (hence their name from the twins of Greek mythology, Castor and Pollux). *Geminivirus* particles consists of 110 capsid protein subunits and one molecule of single-stranded (+)sense DNA of ~2.7 kb (Chapter 3). Elements of icosahedral symmetry occur frequently as part of larger assemblies of proteins (see Complex Virus Structures).

The capsids of picornaviruses (*Picornaviridae*) provide a good illustration of the construction of icosahedral virus particles. In recent years, atomic structures of the capsids of a number of different picornaviruses have been determined. These include *Poliovirus* types 1 and 3 (PV1 and PV3), *Foot-and-mouth disease virus* (FMDV) and *Human rhinovirus 14* (HRV-14), and a number of others. In fact, the structure of these

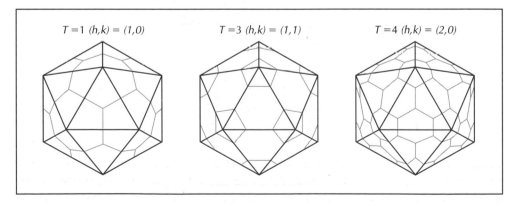

Figure 2.5 Icosahedra with triangulation numbers of 1, 3 and 4.

virus particles is remarkably similar to those of many other unrelated viruses, such as insect viruses of the family *Nodaviridae* and plant viruses from the *Comovirus* group. All these virus groups have icosahedral capsids approximately 30 nm diameter with **triangulation number** $T = 3$ (Figure 2.6). The capsid is composed of 60 repeated subassemblies of proteins, each containing three major subunits, VP1, VP2 and VP3. This means that there are $60 \times 3 = 180$ surface monomers in the whole picornavirus particle. All three proteins are based on a similar structure, consisting of 150–200 amino acid residues in what has been described as an '8-strand anti-parallel β-barrel' (Figure 2.7). This subunit structure has been found in all $T = 3$ icosahedral RNA virus capsids which have been examined so far (e.g. picornaviruses, comoviruses, nepoviruses), possibly reflecting distant evolutionary relationships between distinct virus families.

Knowledge of the structure of these $T = 3$ capsids also reveals information about the way in which they are assembled and the function of the mature capsid. Picornavirus capsids contain four structural proteins. In addition to the three major proteins VP1, VP2 and VP3 (above), there is a small fourth protein, VP4. VP4 is located predominantly on the inside of the capsid and is not exposed at the surface of the particle. The way in which the four capsid proteins are processed from the initial **polyprotein** (see Chapter 5) has long been known from biochemical studies of picornavirus-infected cells (Figure 2.8). VP4 is formed from cleavage of

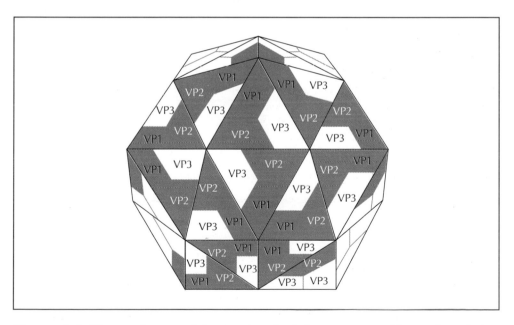

Figure 2.6 Picornavirus particles are icosahedral structures with a triangulation number $T = 3$. Three virus proteins, VP1, VP2 and VP3, comprise the surface of the particle. A fourth protein, VP4, is not exposed on the surface of the virion but is present in each of the 60 repeated units which make up the capsid.

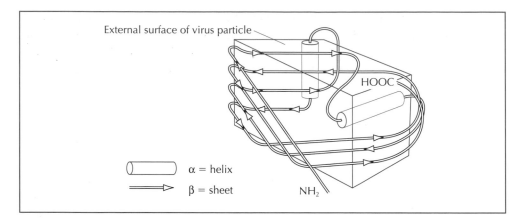

Figure 2.7 The '8-strand anti-parallel β-barrel' subunit structure found in all $T = 3$ icosahedral RNA virus capsids.

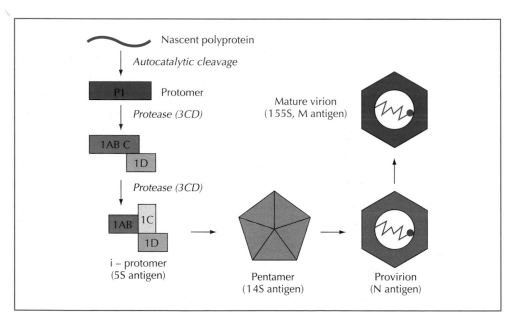

Figure 2.8 Proteolytic processing of picornavirus capsid proteins.

the VP0 precursor into VP2+VP4 late in assembly and is myristylated at its amino-terminus, i.e. it is modified after translation by the covalent attachment of myristic acid, a 14-carbon unsaturated fatty acid. Five VP4 monomers form a hydrophobic micelle, driving the assembly of a pentameric subassembly. There is biochemical evidence that these pentamers, which form the vertices of the mature capsid, are a major precursor in the assembly of the particle. Hence, the chemistry, structure and symmetry of the proteins which make up the picornavirus capsid reveal how assembly is driven.

Because they are the cause of a number of important human diseases, picorna-viruses have been studied intensively by virologists. This interest has resulted in an outpouring of knowledge about these structurally simple viruses. Detailed knowledge of the structure and surface geometry of rhinoviruses has revealed much about their interaction with host cells and with the immune system. In recent years, much has been learned not only about these viruses, but also about the identity of their cellular **receptor**, ICAM-1 (see below and Chapter 4). In addition, the immunological structure of a number of picornavirus particles has also been elucidated.

Several studies have been published using panels of monoclonal antibodies whose binding sites have been 'mapped' to the primary amino acid sequence of the virus by examining their reactivity towards mutant viruses or by using synthetic peptides to block binding. The information from these experiments has been used to identify a number of discrete antibody-neutralization sites on the surface of the virus particle. Some of these correspond to contiguous linear regions of the pri-mary amino acid sequence of the capsid proteins; others, known as conformational sites, result from the bringing together of separated stretches of amino acids in the mature virus. With the elucidation of detailed picornavirus capsid structures, these regions have now been physically identified on the surface of the particle. They correspond mostly to hydrophilic, exposed loops of amino acid sequence, readily accessible to antibody binding, which are repeated on each of the pentameric sub-assemblies of the capsid. Now that the physical constraints on these sites are known, this type of information is being used to artificially manipulate them, even to build 'antigenic chimeras' with the structural properties of one virus but expressing cru-cial antigenic sites from another. With the application of the rational, computer-aided design tools now available, it is probable that the efficiency with which this type of chimera can be designed and built should increase. Indeed, these compound viruses may prove to be the **vaccines** of the future.

ENVELOPED VIRUSES

So far, this chapter has concentrated on the structure of 'naked' virus particles, i.e. those in which the **capsid** proteins are exposed to the external environment. Such viruses are produced from infected cells at the end of the replicative cycle when the cell dies, breaks down and lyses, releasing the **virions** which have been built up internally. This simple strategy has drawbacks. In some circumstances it is wasteful, resulting in the premature death of the cell. It also reduces the possibilities for per-sistent or latent infections. Therefore, many viruses have devised strategies to effect an exit from the infected cell without its total destruction. The difficulty this presents is that all living cells are covered by a membrane composed of a lipid bilayer. The via-bility of the cell depends on the integrity of this membrane. Viruses leaving the cell must, therefore, allow this membrane to remain intact. This is achieved by extrusion (**budding**) of the particle through the membrane, during which process the particle becomes coated in a lipid **envelope** derived from the host cell membrane and with a similar composition (Figure 2.9).

Viruses have also turned this necessity into an advantage. The structure underlying the envelope may be based on helical or icosahedral symmetry and may be formed

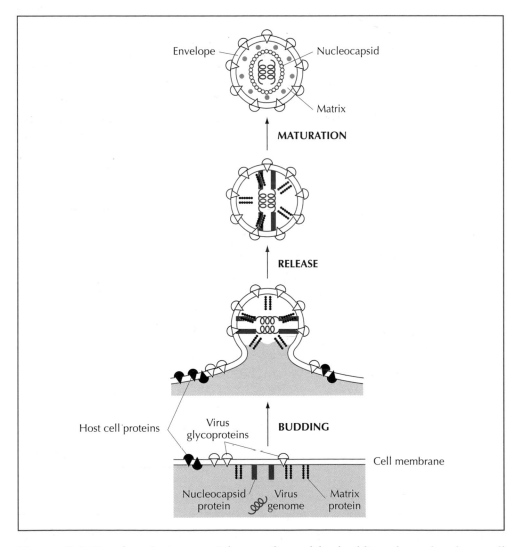

Figure 2.9 Enveloped virus particles are formed by budding through a host cell membrane, during which the particle becomes coated with a lipid bilayer derived from the cell membrane. For some viruses, assembly of the structure of the particle and budding occur simultaneously, whereas in others a preformed core pushes out through the membrane.

before or as the virus leaves the cell. In the majority of cases, enveloped viruses use cellular membranes as sites allowing them to direct assembly. The formation of the particle inside the cell, **maturation** and **release** are in many cases a continuous process. The site of assembly varies for different viruses. Not all use the cell surface membrane; many use cytoplasmic membranes such as the Golgi apparatus, others, such as herpesviruses, which replicate in the nucleus may utilize the nuclear membrane. In these cases, the virus is usually extruded into some form of vacuole, in which it is transported to the cell surface and subsequently released. These points are discussed in more detail in Chapter 4.

If the virus particle became covered in a smooth, unbroken lipid bilayer, this would be its undoing. Such a coating is effectively inert, and although effective as a protective layer preventing desiccation of or enzymatic damage to the particle, it would not permit recognition of **receptor** molecules on the host cell. Therefore, viruses modify their lipid envelopes by the synthesis of several classes of proteins which are associated in one of three ways with the envelope (Figure 2.10). These can be summarized as follows:

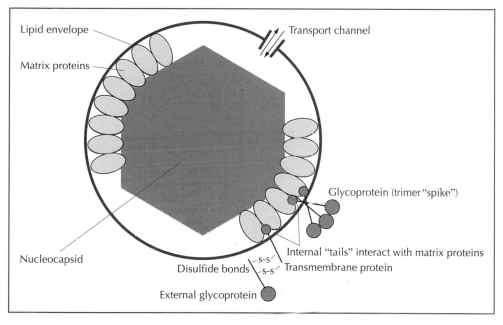

Figure 2.10 Several classes of proteins are associated with virus envelopes. Matrix proteins link the envelope to the core of the particle. Virus-encoded glycoproteins inserted into the envelope serve several functions. External glycoproteins are responsible for receptor recognition and binding, while transmembrane proteins act as transport channels across the envelope. Host-cell derived proteins are also sometimes found to be associated with the envelope, usually in small amounts.

■ *Matrix proteins*: These are internal **virion** proteins whose function is effectively to link the internal **nucleocapsid** assembly to the envelope. Such proteins are not usually glycosylated and are often very abundant, for example, in retroviruses they comprise approximately 30% of the total weight of the virion. Some matrix proteins contain transmembrane anchor domains, others are associated with the membrane by hydrophobic patches on their surface or by protein–protein interactions with envelope glycoproteins.

■ *Glycoproteins*: These are transmembrane proteins anchored to the membrane by a hydrophobic domain, and can be subdivided into two types by their function:

(a) *External glycoproteins* are anchored in the envelope by a single transmembrane domain. Most of the structure of the protein is on the outside of the membrane, with a relatively short internal tail. Often, individual monomers associate to form the 'spikes' visible in electron micrographs on the surface of many enveloped viruses. Such proteins are the major antigens of enveloped viruses. The glycosylation is either *N*- or *O*-linked, and many of these proteins are heavily glycosylated; up to 75% of the protein by weight may consist of sugar groups added post-translationally. These proteins are usually the major antigens of enveloped viruses and provide contact with the external environment, frequently serving a number of important functions; for example, influenza virus haemagglutinin is required for receptor binding, membrane **fusion** and **haemagglutination**.

(b) *Transport channel proteins* contain multiple hydrophobic transmembrane domains, forming a protein-lined channel through the envelope. This enables the virus to alter the permeability of the membrane (e.g. ion channels). Such proteins are often important in modifying the internal environment of the **virion**, permitting or even driving biochemical changes necessary for **maturation** of the particle and the development of infectivity (e.g. influenza virus M_2 protein).

While there are many enveloped vertebrate viruses, there are only a few enveloped plant viruses. Most of these belong to the *Rhabdoviridae*, whose structure has already been discussed (see Helical Capsids). Except for plant rhabdoviruses, only a few bunyaviruses which infect plants and the members of the *Tospovirus* genus have outer lipid envelopes. This relative paucity of enveloped plant viruses probably reflects aspects of host cell biology, in particular the mechanism of **release** of the virus from the infected cell, which requires a breach in the rigid cell wall. This constraint does not apply to viruses of **prokaryotic** organisms, where there are a number of enveloped virus families (e.g. the *Cystoviridae*, *Fuselloviridae*, *Lipothrixviridae* and *Plasmaviridae*).

COMPLEX VIRUS STRUCTURES

The majority of viruses can be fitted into one of the three structural classes outlined above, i.e. those with **helical** symmetry, **icosahedral** symmetry, or **enveloped** viruses. However, there are many viruses whose structure is more complex. In these cases, although the general principles of symmetry already described are often used to build part of the virus shell (this term being appropriate here since such viruses often consist of several layers of protein and lipid), the larger and more complex viruses cannot be simply defined by a mathematical equation as can a simple helix or icosahedron. Because of the complexity of some of these viruses, they have defied attempts to determine detailed atomic structures using the techniques described in Chapter 1.

An example of such a group is the *Poxviridae*. These viruses have oval or 'brick-shaped' particles 200–400 nm long. In fact, these particles are so large that they were first observed in **vaccine** lymph using high-resolution optical microscopes in 1886, and thought at that time to be 'the spores of micrococci'. The external surface of the **virion** is ridged in parallel rows, sometimes arranged helically. The particles are extremely complex and have been shown to contain more than 100 different proteins (Figure 2.11). During replication, two forms of particle are observed: extracellular forms, which contain two membranes, and intracellular particles, which only have an inner membrane. Poxviruses and other viruses with complex structures (such as *African swine fever virus*) obtain their membranes in a different way from 'simple' enveloped viruses such as retroviruses or influenza virus. Rather than budding at the cell surface or into an intracellular compartment, thus acquiring a single membrane, these complex viruses are wrapped by the endoplasmic reticulum, acquiring two layers of membrane (Figure 2.12).

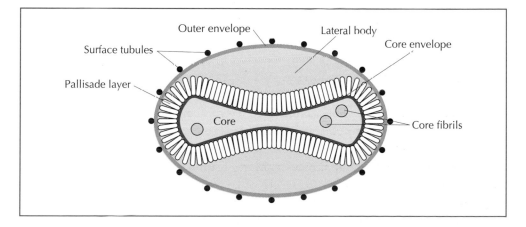

Figure 2.11 Poxvirus particles are the most complex virions known and contain more than 100 virus-encoded proteins, arranged in a variety of internal and external structures.

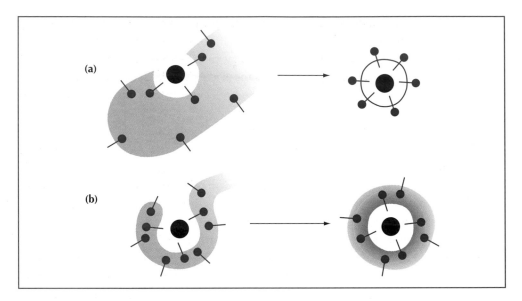

Figure 2.12 (a) 'Simple' enveloped viruses acquire a single-layer envelope by budding at the cell surface or into intracellular compartments. (b) 'Complex' enveloped viruses acquire multiple membrane layers by being wrapped by the endoplasmic reticulum or other cellular membranes.

Under the electron microscope, thin sections of poxviruses reveal that the outer surface of the virion is composed of lipid and protein. This surrounds the core, which is biconcave (dumbbell-shaped), and two 'lateral bodies' whose function is unknown. The core is composed of a tightly compressed nucleoprotein and the double-stranded DNA **genome** is wound around it. Antigenically, poxviruses are very complex, inducing both specific and cross-reacting antibodies – hence the possibility of vaccinating against one disease with another virus (e.g. the use of *Vaccinia virus* to immunize against smallpox (variola) virus). Poxviruses and a number of other complex viruses also emphasize the true complexity of some viruses – there are at least 10 enzymes present in poxvirus particles, mostly involved in nucleic acid metabolism/genome replication.

Poxviruses form the most complex particles known and even though the complete nucleotide sequence of the **genome** of several representatives of this family has now been determined (see Chapter 3), a complete elucidation of the structure of these particles has not yet been achieved. This is an extreme case in virology, included here as a counterbalance to the description of some of the simplest viruses given above. In other cases, the particle structure of complex viruses has been much more completely investigated. One of the prime examples of such a group are the tailed phages of enterobacteria. The order *Caudovirales*, comprising the families *Myoviridae*, *Siphoviridae* and *Podoviridae*, has been extensively studied for excellent reasons – these viruses are easy to propagate in bacterial cells, can be obtained in high **titres**, and are easily purified, facilitating biochemical and structural studies. The head of the particles consists essentially of an icosahedral shell with $T = 7$ symmetry, attached by a collar to a contractile, helical tail. At the end of the tail is a plate which functions in attachment to the bacterial host and also in **penetration** of the bacterial cell wall by virtue of lysozyme-like enzymes associated with the plate. In addition to these structures, thin protein fibres are attached to the plate, which, along with the tail plate, are involved in binding to the **receptor** molecules in the wall of the host cell. The structure of these phages is actually rather more complex than this simple picture; for example, there are several internal proteins and polyamines associated with the genomic DNA in the head and an internal tube structure inside the outer sheath of the helical tail. In the infected bacterial cell, there are separate assembly pathways for the head and tail sections of the particle, which come together at a late stage to make up the **virion** (Figure 2.13). Therefore, these viruses illustrate how complex particles can be built up from the simple principles outlined above.

An even clearer example of this phenomenon is provided by the structure of *Geminivirus* particles, which consist of two twinned $T = 1$ icosahedra. Each icosahedron has one morphological subunit missing and the icosahedra are joined at the point such that the mature particle contains 110 protein monomers arranged in 22 morphological subunits.

Members of the reovirus genus have non-enveloped, icosahedral $T = 13$ **capsids** composed of a double protein shell with a complex structure (Figure 2.14). The structure of the transcriptionally active *Bluetongue virus* core was recently reported and represents the largest structure yet determined to atomic resolution (3.5 Å). The outer shell of this virus is approximately 80 nm in diameter and the inner shell (core) about 60 nm. The structure of the outer shell is complex and has not yet been determined at atomic resolution, but has been analysed at a lesser resolution of 3 nm by the alternative structural investigation techniques of electron cryo-microscopy and image-processing. Although these methods can only give structural resolution about 10-fold less than X-ray diffraction, these techniques are useful for complex or fragile structures which cannot be crystallized. The double-stranded RNA **genome** of the virus is packed tightly inside the core, surrounding transcription complexes at the apices of the particle. These genome segments maintain their order during transcription. Twelve 'spikes' protrude from the core through the outer shell. The overall composition of bluetongue particles is shown in Table 2.1.

After many years of study and the isolation of a very large number of mutants, there is now probably more detail known about the structure–function relationships of the reovirus capsid than that of any other virus, with the possible exception of the picornaviruses. These particles are very stable in the environment – this is notably the case with the rotaviruses, which are commonly spread through contaminated drinking water. *Rotavirus* particles in faecal material stored at room temperature are able to retain their infectivity for 7 months and are not very susceptible to chlorine-containing disinfectants, thus demonstrating the efficiency with which these complex particles protect the fragile RNA genome.

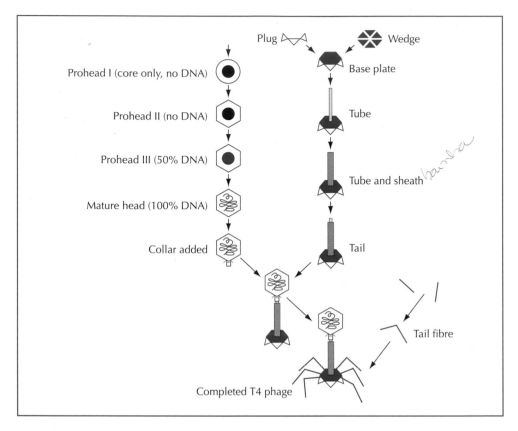

Figure 2.13 Simplified version of the assembly of *Enterobacteria phage T4* particles (*Myoviridae*). The head and tail sections are assembled separately and are brought together at a relatively late stage. This complex process was painstakingly worked out by the isolation of phage mutants in each of the virus genes involved. In addition to the major structural proteins, a number of minor 'scaffolding' proteins are involved in guiding the formation of the complex particle.

The final example of complex virus structure to be considered is the *Baculoviridae* (Figure 2.15). In recent years, these viruses have attracted much interest for a number of reasons. They are natural pathogens of arthropods and naturally occurring as well as genetically manipulated baculoviruses are under active investigation as biological control agents for insect pests. In addition, occluded baculoviruses (see below) are increasingly being used as expression vectors to produce large amounts of recombinant proteins. These complex viruses contain 12–30 structural proteins, and consist of a rod-like (hence 'baculo') **nucleocapsid** 30–60 nm diameter and 250–300 nm long which contains the 88–160 kbp double-stranded DNA genome. The nucleocapsid is surrounded by an **envelope**, outside which there may or may not be a crystalline protein matrix. If this outer protein shell is present, the whole assemblage is referred to as an 'occlusion body' and the virus is said to be occluded (Figure 2.15). There are

Table 2.1 The proteins of bluetongue virus and related orbiviruses

Genome segment (bp)	Protein	Location	Copy number / Particle	Properties and functions
1 (3954)	VP1 (Pol)	Subcore, at 5-fold axis	11	RNA dependent RNA polymerase
2 (2926)	VP2	Outer capsid	180	Serotype-specific antigen, cell attachment protein
3 (2770)	VP3 (T2)	Subcore capsid layer	120	RNA binding protein, interacts with internal minor proteins, physical organization of genome
4 (2011)	VP4 (Cap)	Subcore, at 5-fold axis	?	Capping enzyme, guanylyl-transferase
5 (1769)	NS1 (TuP)	Cytoplasm, forms tubules	0	Forms tubules of unknown function in the cell cytoplasm
6 (1638)	VP5	Inner layer of the outer capsid	360	Antigenic glycoprotein
7 (1156)	VP7 (T13)	Outer core (T=13 symmetry)	780	Immunodominant major serogroup specific antigen
8 (1124)	NS2 (ViP)	Cytoplasm, viral inclusion bodies	0	Phosphorylated inclusion body matrix protein, ssRNA binding
9 (1046)	VP6 (Hel)	Subcore, at 5-fold axis	72	ssRNA and dsRNA binding, helicase, NTPase
10 (822)	NS3, NS3a	Cell membranes	0	Glycosylated membrane proteins involved in cell exit, cytotoxic, can disrupt cell membranes

Table compiled by Peter Mertens and Dennis Bamford, Institute of Animal Health, UK:
http://www.iah.bbsrc.ac.uk/virus/Reoviridae/orbivirus/btvproteins.htm

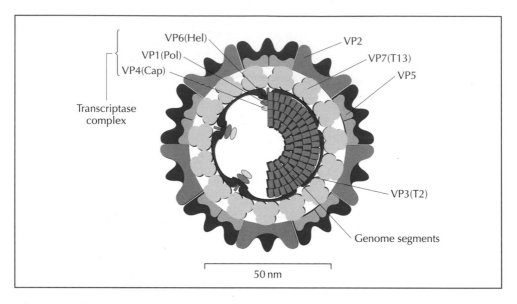

Figure 2.14 Reovirus particles consist of an icosahedral, double–shell arrangement of proteins surrounding the core. This diagram represents the known structural information about the *Bluetongue virus* particle. (Information generously supplied by Peter Mertens, Institute for Animal Health, UK.)

two genera of occluded baculoviruses: the *Nucleopolyhedrovirus* genus with polyhedral occlusions 1000–15 000 nm in diameter, which may contain multiple nucleocapsids within the envelope (e.g. *Autographa californica nucleopolyhedrovirus*), and the *Granulovirus* genus with ellipsoidal occlusions 200–500 nm in diameter (e.g. *Cydia pomonella granulovirus*). The function of these enormous occlusion bodies is to confer resistance to adverse environmental conditions, which enables the virus to persist in soil or on plant materials for extended periods of time waiting to be ingested by a new host.

The effectiveness of this strategy is such that these viruses can be regarded as being literally armour-plated. Interestingly, the strategy of producing occluded particles appears to have evolved independently in at least three groups of insect viruses. In addition to the baculoviruses, occluded particles are also produced by insect reoviruses (cytoplasmic polyhedrosis viruses) and poxviruses (entomopoxviruses). However, this resistant coating would be the undoing of the virus if it were not removed at an appropriate time to allow replication to proceed. This is achieved by virtue of the fact that the occlusion body is alkali-labile and dissolves in the high pH environment of the insect midgut, releasing the nucleocapsid and allowing it to infect the host. Although the structure of the whole particle has not been completely determined, it is known that the occlusion body is composed of many copies of a single protein of approximately 245 amino acids, polyhedrin. To form the occlusion body, this single gene product is hyperexpressed late in infection by a very strong

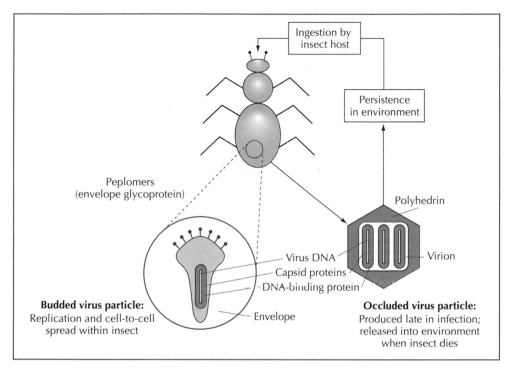

Figure 2.15 Some baculovirus particles exist in two forms: a relatively simple 'budded' form found within the host insect and a crystalline, protein–occluded form responsible for environmental persistence.

transcriptional **promoter**. Cloned foreign genes can be expressed by the polyhedrin promoter, hence baculoviruses have been manipulated as expression vectors.

PROTEIN–NUCLEIC ACID INTERACTIONS AND GENOME PACKAGING

The primary function of the virus particle is to contain and protect the **genome** before delivering it to the appropriate host cell. Therefore, it is clear that the proteins of the **capsid** must interact with the nucleic acid genome. Once again the physical constraints of incorporating a relatively large nucleic acid molecule into a relatively small capsid present considerable problems which must be overcome. In most cases, the linear virus genome when stretched out in solution is at least an order of magnitude longer than the diameter of the capsid. Merely folding the genome in order to stuff it into such a confined space is quite a feat of topology in itself, but is compounded by the fact that repulsion by the cumulative negative electrostatic charges on the phosphate groups of the nucleotide backbone mean that the genome resists being crammed into a small space. Viruses overcome this difficulty by packaging along with the genome a number of positively charged molecules to counteract this negative charge repulsion. These include small, positively charged ions (Na, Mg, K, etc.), polyamines and various nucleic acid-binding proteins. Some of these latter proteins are virus-encoded and contain amino acids with basic side-chains such as arginine and lysine which interact with the genome. There are many examples of such proteins, for example, retrovirus NC and rhabdovirus N (**nucleocapsid**) proteins, and influenza virus NP protein (nucleoprotein).

Many viruses with double-stranded DNA genomes have basic histone-like molecules closely associated with the DNA. Again, some of these are virus-encoded, e.g. adenovirus polypeptide VII. In other cases, however, the virus may utilize cellular proteins; for example, the polyomavirus genome assumes a **chromatin**-like structure in association with four cellular histone proteins, H2A, H2B, H3 and H4, similar to those of the host cell genome.

The second problem the virus must overcome is how to achieve the specificity required to select and encapsidate the virus **genome** from the large background of cellular nucleic acids. In most cases, by the late stages of virus infection when assembly of virus particles occurs (see Chapter 4), transcription of cellular genes has been reduced and a large pool of virus genomes have accumulated. The overproduction of virus nucleic acids eases but does not eliminate the problem of specific genome packaging. Therefore, a specific virus-encoded capsid or nucleocapsid protein is required to achieve this end and many viruses, even those with relatively short, compact genomes such as retroviruses and rhabdoviruses, encode this type of protein.

Viruses with segmented **genomes** (see Chapter 3) face further problems: they must not only encapsidate only virus nucleic acid and exclude host cell molecules, but they must also attempt to package one of each of the required genome segments. It is important to realize that during assembly, viruses frequently make mistakes. These can be physically measured by particle : infectivity ratios, i.e. the ratio of the total number of particles in a virus preparation (counted by electron microscopy) to the number of particles able to give rise to infectious progeny (measured by **plaque** or limiting dilution assays). This value is in some cases found to be several thousand particles to each infectious **virion** and only rarely approaches a ratio of 1 : 1. However, a few simple calculations show that viruses such as influenza have far lower particle : infectivity ratios than could be achieved by random packaging of eight distinct genome segments. It is now believed that each influenza virus particle contains more than eight RNA segments. This redundancy may be sufficient to ensure that a reasonable proportion of virus particles in the population will contain at least one of each of the eight segments and will thus be infectious. However, it is not certain that this is the case and it is possible that influenza virus has a mechanism not yet discovered, e.g. incorporation of ribonucleoprotein complexes during morphogenesis, that ensures a complete genetic complement in the majority of particles.

On the other side of the packaging equation are the specific nucleotide sequences in the **genome** (the **packaging signal**) which permit the virus to select genomic nucleic acids from the cellular background. The packaging signal from a number of virus genomes has been identified. Examples are the Ψ ('psi') signal in murine retrovirus genomes which has been used to package synthetic 'retrovirus vector' genomes into a virus particle, and the sequences responsible for packaging the genomes of several DNA virus genomes (some adenoviruses and herpesviruses) which have been clearly and unambiguously defined. However, it is clear from a number of different approaches that accurate and efficient genome packaging requires information (not only from the linear nucleotide sequence of the genome, but also from regions of secondary structure formed by the folding of the genomic nucleic acid into complex forms. In many cases, attempts to find a unique, linear packaging signal in virus genomes have failed. The probable reason for this is that the key to the specificity of genome packaging in most viruses lies in the secondary structure of the genome.

Like many other aspects of virus assembly, the way in which packaging is controlled is, in many cases, not well understood. However, the key must lie in the specific molecular interactions between the **genome** and the **capsid**. Until recently, the physical structure of virus genomes within virus particles has been poorly studied, although the genetics of packaging have been extensively investigated in recent years. This is a pity, because it is unlikely that we will be able fully to appreciate this important aspect of virus replication without this information, but is understandable because the techniques used to determine the structure of virus capsids (e.g. X-ray diffraction) only rarely reveal any information about the state of the genome within its protein shell. However, there are some cases where detailed knowledge about the mechanism and specificity of genome encapsidation is now available. These include both viruses with helical symmetry and some with icosahedral symmetry.

Undoubtedly the best understood packaging mechanism is that of a (+)sense RNA helical plant virus, *Tobacco mosaic virus* (TMV). This is due to the relative simplicity of this virus, which only has a single major coat protein, and will spontaneously assemble from its purified RNA and protein components *in vitro*. In the case of TMV, particle assembly is initiated by association of preformed aggregates of coat protein molecules ('discs') with residues 5444-5518 in the 6.4 kb RNA **genome**, known as the origin of assembly sequence (OAS) (Figure 2.16). The flat discs have 17 subunits per ring, close to the 16.34 subunits per turn found in the mature virus particle. In fact, the discs are not completely symmetrical, they have a pronounced polarity. Assembly begins when a disc interacts with the OAS in genomic RNA. This converts the discs to a helical 'locked washer' structure, each of which contains $3'$ coat protein subunits. Further discs add to this structure, switching to the 'locked washer' conformation. RNA is drawn into the assembling structure in what is known as a 'travelling loop', which gives the common name to this mechanism of particle formation. The vRNA is trapped and subsequently buried in the middle of the disc as the helix grows. Extension of the helical structure occurs in both directions but at unequal rates. Growth in the $5'$ direction is rapid because a disc can add straight to the protein filament and the travelling loop of RNA is drawn up through it. Growth

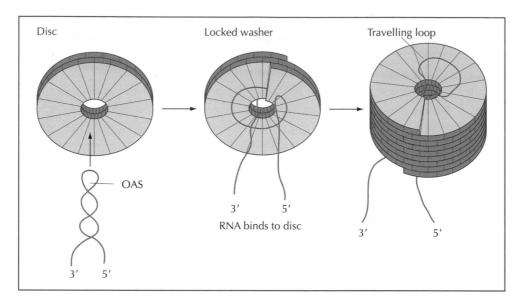

Figure 2.16 Assembly of *Tobacco mosaic virus* (TMV) particles.

in the 3′ direction is slower because the RNA has to be threaded through the disc before it can add to the structure.

Enterobacteria phage M13 is another helical virus where protein–nucleic acid interactions in the virus particle are relatively simple to understand (Figure 2.2). The primary sequence of the g8p molecule determines the orientation of the protein in the **capsid**. In simple terms, the inner surface of the rod-like **phage** capsid is positively charged and interacts with the negatively charged **genome**, while the outer surface of the cylindrical capsid is negatively charged. However, the way in which the capsid protein and genome are brought together is a little more complex than this. During replication, the genomic DNA is associated with a non-structural DNA-binding protein, g5p. This is the most abundant of all virus proteins in the infected *E. coli* cell, and coats the newly replicated single-stranded phage DNA, forming an intracellular rod-like structure similar to the mature phage particle, but somewhat longer and thicker (1100 × 16 nm). The function of this protein is to protect the genome from host cell nucleases and to interrupt genome replication, sequestering newly formed strands as substrates for encapsidation. Newly synthesized coat protein monomers (g8p) are associated with the inner (cytoplasmic) membrane of the cell and it is at this site that assembly of the virus particle occurs. The g5p coating is stripped off as the particle passes out through the membrane and is essentially exchanged for the mature g8p coat (plus the accessory proteins). The forces which drive this process are not fully understood, but the protein–nucleic acid interactions which occur appear to be rather simple and involve opposing electrostatic charges and the stacking of the DNA bases between the planar side-chains of the proteins. This is confirmed by the plasticity of the M13 genome and its ability to freely encapsidate extra genetic material.

Protein–nucleic acid interactions in other helical viruses, such as rhabdoviruses, are rather more complex. In most **enveloped** helical viruses, a nucleoprotein core forms first and this is then coated by matrix proteins, the envelope and its associated glycoproteins (Figure 2.3). The fine structure of the core has not been determined, but appears to show cross-striations 4.5–5.0 nm apart, each of these presumably equating to one turn of the protein–RNA complex (rather like TMV). The matrix protein shows an apparently hexagonal pattern and it is not clear how this is related to the structure of the underlying **nucleocapsid**, or how the rounded end of the virus particle is formed.

Rather less is known about the arrangement of the **genome** inside virus particles with icosahedral symmetry. There are, however, some exceptions to this statement. These are the $T = 3$ icosahedral RNA viruses whose subunits consist largely of the '8-strand anti-parallel β-barrel' structural motif discussed earlier. In these viruses, positively charged inward-projecting arms of the capsid proteins interact with the RNA in the centre of the particle. In *Bean pod mottle virus* (BPMV), a $T = 3$ *Comovirus* with a bipartite genome, X-ray crystallography has shown that the RNA is folded in such a way that it assumes icosahedral symmetry, corresponding to that of the capsid surrounding it. The regions which contact the capsid proteins are single-stranded and appear to interact by electrostatic forces rather than covalent bonds. The atomic structure of φX174 also shows that a portion of the DNA genome interacts with arginine residues exposed on the inner surface of the capsid in a manner similar to BPMV.

Therefore, a consensus about the physical state of nucleic acids within icosahedral virus capsids appears to be emerging. Just as the icosahedral capsids of many genetically unrelated viruses are based on monomers with a common '8-strand anti-parallel β-barrel' structural motif, the genomes inside also appear to display icosahedral symmetry, the vertices of which interact with basic amino acid residues on the inner surface of the capsid. Thus, these common structural motifs may in time explain how viruses selectively package the required genomic nucleic acids and may even offer opportunities to design specific drugs to inhibit these interactions.

VIRUS RECEPTORS – RECOGNITION AND BINDING

Cellular **receptor** molecules used by a number of different viruses from diverse taxonomic groups have now been identified. The interaction of the outer surface of a virus with a cellular receptor is a major event in determining the subsequent events in replication and the outcome of infections. It is this binding event which activates inert extracellular virus particles and initiates the replication cycle. Receptor binding is considered in detail in Chapter 4.

OTHER INTERACTIONS OF THE VIRUS CAPSID WITH THE HOST CELL

As stated at the beginning of this chapter, the function of the virus **capsid** is not only to protect the **genome**, but also to deliver it to a suitable host cell and, more specifically, the appropriate compartment of the host cell (in the case of **eukaryote** hosts) to allow replication to proceed. One example is the **nucleocapsid** proteins of viruses which replicate in the nucleus of the host cell. These molecules contain within their primary amino acid sequences 'nuclear localization signals' which are responsible for the migration of the virus genome plus its associated proteins into the nucleus where replication can occur. Again, these events are discussed in Chapter 4.

Virions are not inert structures. Many virus particles contain one or more enzymatic activities, although in most cases these are not active outside the biochemical environment of the host cell. All viruses with negative-sense RNA **genomes** must carry with them a virus-specific RNA–dependent RNA polymerase because most **eukaryotic** cells have no mechanism for RNA-dependent RNA polymerization and, therefore, genome replication could not occur if this enzyme were not included in the virus particle. Reverse transcription of retrovirus genomes occurs inside a particulate complex and not free in solution. The more complex DNA viruses (e.g. herpesviruses and poxviruses) carry a multiplicity of enzymes, mostly concerned with some aspect of nucleic acid metabolism.

SUMMARY

This chapter is not intended to be a complete list of all the virus structures that are now known, but attempts to illustrate with examples some of the principles that control the assembly of viruses and the difficulties of studying these minute structures. Readers must refer to scientific articles and databases for the fine detail of known virus structures and for the many which continuously appear. Nevertheless, there are a number of repeated structural motifs found in many different virus groups. The most obvious is the division of many virus structures into those based on **helical** or **icosahedral** symmetry. More subtly, common protein structures such as the '8-strand anti-parallel β-barrel' structural motif found in many $T = 3$ icosahedral virus capsids and the icosahedral folded RNA **genome** present inside some of these viruses are beginning to emerge. Virus particles are not inert. Many are armed with a variety of enzymes which carry out a range of complex reactions, most frequently involved in the replication of the genome.

FURTHER READING

Ackerman, H-W. and Berthiaume, L. (Eds) (1995). *Atlas of Virus Diagrams*. CRC Press, Boca Raton. ISBN 0849324572.

Chiu, W. and Burnett, R.M. (Eds) (1997). *Structural Biology of Viruses*. Oxford University Press, Oxford. ISBN 0195118502.

Dokland, T., Bernal, R.A, Burch, A., Pletnev, S., Fane, B.A. and Rossmann, M.G. (1999). The role of scaffolding proteins in the assembly of the small, single-stranded DNA virus φX174. *Journal of Molecular Biology* 288: 595–608.

Gouet, P. , Diprose, J.M., Grimes, J.M., Malby, R., Burroughs, J.N., Zientara, S., Stuart, D.I. and Mertens, P. P. (1999). The highly ordered double-stranded RNA genome of *Bluetongue virus* revealed by crystallography. *Cell* 97: 481–490.

Grimes, J.M., Burroughs, J.N., Gouet, P., Diprose, J.M., Malby, R., Zientara, S., Mertens, P. P. and Stuart, D.I. (1998). The atomic structure of the *Bluetongue virus* core. *Nature* 395: 470–478.

McKenna, R., Xia, D., Willingmann, P. , Ilag, L.L., Krishnaswamy, S., Rossmann, M.G., Olson, N.H., Baker, T.S. and Incardona, N.L. (1992). Atomic structure of single-stranded DNA bacteriophage φX174 and its functional implications. *Nature* 355: 137–143.

Prasad, B.V., Yamaguchi, S. and Roy, P. (1992). Three-dimensional structure of single-shelled *Bluetongue virus*. *Journal of Virology* 66: 2135–2142.

Rasched, I. and Oberer, E. (1986). Ff coliphages: structural and functional relationships. *Microbiological Reviews* 50: 401–427.

SELF-ASSESSMENT QUESTIONS

(2.1) Are the following statements true or false?

F (a) Nucleic acids are resistant to physical damage such as shearing by mechanical forces and to chemical modification.

T (b) The protein subunits in a virus capsid are multiply redundant, i.e. present in many copies per particle.

T (c) The forces which drive the assembly of virus particles include hydrophobic and electrostatic interactions.

F (d) The protein subunits in virus capsids are held *RARELY* together by covalent bonds.

F (e) The only function of the outer shells of a virus particle is to protect the fragile genome from physical, chemical or enzymatic damage.

(2.2) Are the following statements true or false?

T (a) A helix can be constructed by stacking repeated components with a constant relationship to one another.

T (b)   A helix can be defined by two parameters: amplitude and pitch.
F (c)   A helix can be defined mathematically by the equation: $P = \mu \times p^2$
T (d)   The 'amplitude' of a helix is its diameter.
F (e)   Bacteriophage M13 particles are 270 nm long.

(2.3) Are the following statements true or false?
F (a)   The particles of all known plant viruses have helical symmetry.
T (b)   There are no known non-enveloped helical viruses of animals.
T (c)   Rhabdovirus particles have a helical nucleocapsid.
T (d)   Bacteriophage M13 is a member of the *Inovirus* genus.
T (e)   Bacteriophage M13 requires CD4 on the surface of *Escherichia coli*
         for infection.   *I pilus*

(2.4) Are the following statements true or false?
F (a)   An icosahedron is a solid shape consisting of 30 triangular faces
         arranged around the surface of a sphere.   20
F (b)   An icosahedron has an axis of threefold rotational symmetry through
         the centre of each edge. *face*
F (c)   An icosahedron has an axis of fivefold rotational symmetry through
         the centre of each face. *vertix /corner*
F (d)   An icosahedron has an axis of twofold rotational symmetry through
         the centre of each corner. *edge*
F (e)   Most icosahedral virus capsids contain only 60 subunits.
                                                   or more

**(2.5) All the following virus groups have icosahedral symmetry
(true or false?):**
F (a)   Orthomyxoviruses
F (b)   Paramyxoviruses
→T (c)   Picornaviruses
F (d)   Rhabdoviruses
F (e)   Tobamoviruses

(2.6) Are the following statements true or false?
F (a)   The lipid composition of a virus envelope is distinct from that of
         the host cell.   *similar*
T (b)   Virus envelopes are acquired during extrusion (budding) of the parti-
         cle through the host cell membrane.
F (c)   Budding can only occur from the host cell surface membrane.
F (d)   All enveloped viruses have underlying helical symmetry.
F (e)   All virus envelope proteins are encoded by the host cell.

(2.7)   All the following virus groups possess lipid envelopes (true or false?):

T (a)   Orthomyxoviruses
T (b)   Paramyxoviruses
F (c)   Picornaviruses
T (d)   Rhabdoviruses
F (e)   Tobamoviruses

(2.8)   Are the following statements true or false?

T (a)   Matrix proteins are internal virion proteins that link the internal nucleocapsid assembly to the envelope.
T (b)   Matrix proteins are often very abundant in the virus particle.
T (c)   External glycoproteins are usually the major antigens of enveloped viruses.
T (d)   External glycoproteins are usually the virus attachment proteins of enveloped viruses.
T (e)   The influenza virus M_2 peptide is a transmembrane protein.

(2.9)   Are the following statements true or false?

F (a)   Poxvirus particles have overall helical symmetry.
T (b)   Poxvirus particles contain more than 100 different proteins
F (c)   The tailed phages of E. coli are released from the host cell by bud- LYSIS
         ding.
T (d)   The tailed phages of E. coli have separate assembly pathways for the head and tail sections of the particle.
T (e)   Reovirus capsids are composed of a double protein shell.

(2.10) Genome packaging (true or false?):

F (a)   is completely specific for virus nucleic acids. virus make mistakes!
T (b)   requires interaction with a specific virus-encoded capsid or nucleo-capsid protein.
T (c)   requires specific nucleotide sequences in the virus genome.
T (d)   requires positively charged groups to overcome negative electrostat-ic charges on the genome.
T (e)   in TMV is initiated by the OAS region of the genome.

Answers to Self-Assessment Questions are given in Appendix 4.

CHAPTER 3

GENOMES

Learning Objectives

On completing this chapter, you should be able to:
- Recognize the possible structures and compositions which comprise the range of virus genomes
- Understand the major genetic mechanisms which affect viruses
- Describe several representative virus genomes.

THE STRUCTURE AND COMPLEXITY OF VIRUS GENOMES

The compositions and structures of virus **genomes** are more varied than any of those seen in the entire bacterial, plant or animal kingdoms. The nucleic acid comprising the genome may be single-stranded or double-stranded, and in a linear, circular or segmented configuration. Single-stranded virus genomes may be either positive (+)sense, i.e. of the same polarity (nucleotide sequence) as **mRNA**, negative (−)sense, or **ambisense** – a mixture of the two. Virus genomes range in size from approximately 3500 nucleotides (nt) (e.g. **bacteriophages** of the family *Leviviridae* such as MS2 and Qβ) to approximately 380 000 bp (760 000 nt) members of the *Phycodnaviridae*. Unlike the genomes of all cells, which are composed of DNA, virus genomes may contain their genetic information encoded in either DNA or RNA.

Whatever the particular composition of a virus genome, all must conform to one condition. Since viruses are obligate intracellular parasites only able to replicate inside the appropriate host cells, the genome must contain information encoded in a form which can be recognized and decoded by the particular type of cell parasitized.

The genetic code employed by the virus must match or at least be recognized by the host organism. Similarly, the control signals which direct the expression of virus genes must be appropriate to the host. Chapter 4 describes the means by which virus genomes are replicated and Chapter 5 deals in more detail with the mechanisms that regulate the expression of virus genetic information. The purpose of this chapter is to describe the diversity of virus genomes and to examine how and why this variation may have arisen.

Although molecular biology has developed many techniques for the manipulation of proteins, the power of this technology has concentrated in the main on nucleic acids. There has been a strong and synergistic relationship between advances in virology dependent on this new technology and the opportunities which viruses themselves have afforded to develop new techniques of investigation. Thus, the first complete genome to be sequenced (in 1977) was that of a virus, the bacteriophage φX174. This virus was chosen for a number of reasons. First, it has one of the smallest genomes (5386 nt). Second, large amounts of the **phage** could be propagated in *Escherichia coli*, easily purified and the genomic DNA extracted. Third, the genome of this phage consists of single-stranded DNA which could be directly sequenced by chain-termination methods. Although methods of sequencing double-stranded DNA were also being developed at this time, φX174 proved the utility of bacteriophages with single-stranded genomes as cloning vectors for DNA sequencing and phages such as M13 have subsequently been highly developed for this purpose.

Virus genome structures and nucleotide sequences have been intensively studied in recent years because the power of recombinant DNA technology has focused much attention in this area. It would be wrong to present molecular biology as the only means of addressing unanswered problems in virology, but it would be equally foolish to ignore the opportunities which it offers and the explosion of knowledge which has resulted from it in recent decades.

Some of the simpler **bacteriophages** have been cited above as examples of the smallest and least complex genomes known. At the other end of the scale, the genomes of the largest double-stranded DNA viruses such as herpesviruses and poxviruses are sufficiently complex to have escaped complete functional analysis to date (even though the complete nucleotide sequences of the genomes of a growing number of examples are now known). Many of the DNA viruses of **eukaryotes** closely resemble their host cells in terms of the biology of their genomes:

- Some DNA virus genomes are complexed with cellular histones to form a **chromatin**-like structure inside the virus particle. Once inside the nucleus of the host cell, these genomes behave like miniature satellite chromosomes, following the dictates of cellular enzymes and the cell cycle.
- *Vaccinia virus* mRNAs were found to be polyadenylated at their 3' ends by John Kates in 1970 – the first observation of this phenomenon.

- Split genes containing non-coding **introns**, protein coding **exons** and spliced mRNAs were first discovered in adenoviruses by Richard Roberts and Phillip Sharp in 1977.

Introns in prokaryotes were first discovered in the genome of bacteriophage T4 in 1984. Several examples of this phenomenon have now been discovered in T4 and in other phages. All are similar, being of the class I 'self-splicing' type. However, this observation raises an important point. The conventional view is that prokaryote genomes are smaller and replicate faster than those of **eukaryotes**, and hence can be regarded as 'streamlined'. The genome of phage T4 consists of 160 kbp of double-stranded DNA and is highly compressed; for example, **promoters** and translation control sequences are nested within the coding regions of overlapping upstream genes. The presence of introns in **bacteriophage** genomes, which are under constant ruthless pressure to exclude 'junk sequences', indicates that these genetic elements must have evolved mechanisms to escape or neutralize this pressure and to persist as parasites within parasites.

All virus genomes experience pressure to minimize their size. For example, viruses with **prokaryotic** hosts must be able to replicate sufficiently quickly to keep up with their host cells and this is reflected in the compact nature of many (but not all) bacteriophages. Overlapping genes are common and the maximum genetic capacity is compressed into the minimum genome size. In viruses with **eukaryotic** hosts there is also pressure on genome size. Here, however, the pressure is mainly from the 'packaging size' of the virus particle, i.e. the amount of nucleic acid which can be incorporated into the **virion**. Therefore, these viruses commonly show tremendous compression of genetic information when compared with the low density of information in the genomes of eukaryotic cells.

As already stated, there are exceptions to this simple 'rule'. Some bacteriophages (e.g. the family *Myoviridae*, such as T4) have relatively large genomes, up to 170 kbp. The largest virus genomes presently known are those of the *Phycodnaviridae* at up to 380 000 bp. Among viruses of eukaryotes, herpesviruses and poxviruses also have large genomes, up to 235 000 bp. It is notable that these virus genomes contain many genes involved in their own replication, particularly enzymes concerned with nucleic acid metabolism. Therefore, these viruses partially escape the restrictions of the biochemistry of the host cell by encoding additional biochemical apparatus. The penalty is that they have to encode all the information necessary for a large and complex particle to package the genome – also an upward pressure on genome size.

Later sections of this chapter contain detailed descriptions of both small compact and large complex virus genomes.

MOLECULAR GENETICS

As already described, the new techniques of molecular biology have had a major influence in concentrating attention on the virus genome. It is beyond the scope of this book to give detailed accounts of this technology. Indeed, it is assumed that readers already have a firm grasp of the principles behind these techniques, as well as the jargon involved! However, it is perhaps worth taking some time here to illustrate how some of these techniques have been applied to virology, remembering that these newer techniques are complementary to and do not replace the classical techniques of virology. Initially, any investigation of a virus genome will usually include questions about the following:

- Composition – DNA or RNA, single-stranded or double-stranded, linear, or circular
- Size and number of segments
- Terminal structures
- Nucleotide sequence
- Coding capacity – open reading frames
- Regulatory signals – transcription **enhancers**, **promoters** and terminators.

It is possible to separate the molecular analysis of virus genomes into two types of approach: physical analysis of structure and nucleotide sequence, essentially performed *in vitro*, and a more biological approach to examine the structure–function relationships of intact virus genomes and individual genetic elements, usually involving analysis of the virus phenotype *in vivo*.

The conventional starting point for the physical analysis of virus genomes has been the isolation of nucleic acids from virus preparations of varying degrees of purity. To some extent, this is still true of molecular biology, although the emphasis on extensive purification has declined as techniques of molecular cloning have become more advanced. DNA virus genomes can be analysed directly by restriction endonuclease digestion without resort to molecular cloning and this was achieved for the first time with SV40 DNA in 1971. The first pieces of DNA to be molecularly cloned were restriction fragments of bacteriophage λ DNA, which were cloned into the DNA genome of SV40 by Paul Berg and colleagues in 1972. Thus virus genomes were both the first cloning vectors and the first nucleic acids to be analysed by these techniques! As already mentioned, the genome of φX174 was the first **replicon** to be completely sequenced.

Subsequently, phage genomes such as M13 were highly modified for use as vectors in DNA sequencing. The enzymology of RNA-specific nucleases was comparatively advanced at this time, such that a spectrum of enzymes with specific cleavage sites could be used to analyse and even determine the sequence of RNA virus genomes (the first short nucleotide sequences of tRNAs having been determined in the mid-1960s). However, direct analysis of RNA by these methods was laborious and notoriously difficult. RNA sequence analysis did not begin to advance rapidly until the widespread use of reverse transcriptase (isolated from avian myeloblastosis virus) to convert RNA into cDNA in the 1970s. Since the 1980s, the polymerase chain reaction (PCR) has further accelerated the investigation of virus genomes (Chapter 1).

In addition to molecular cloning, other techniques of molecular analysis have also been of great value in virology. Direct analysis by electron microscopy, if calibrated with known standards, can be used to estimate the size of nucleic acid molecules. Perhaps the most important single technique has been gel electrophoresis (Figure 3.1). The earliest gel matrix employed for separating molecules was based on starch and gave relatively poor resolution. It is now most common to use agarose gels to separate large nucleic acid molecules (which may be very large indeed – several

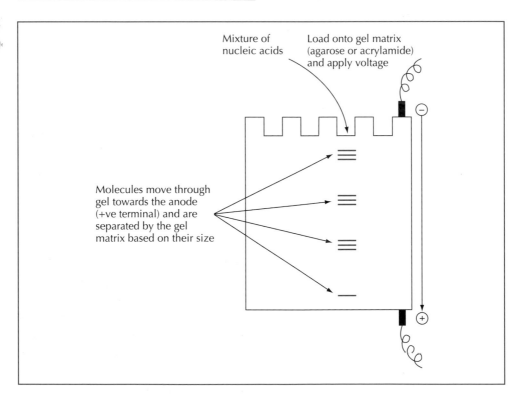

Figure 3.1 In gel electrophoresis, a mixture of nucleic acids (or proteins) are applied to a gel and move through the gel matrix when an electric field is applied. The net negative charge due to the phosphate groups in the backbone of nucleic acid molecules results in their movement away from the cathode and towards the anode. Smaller molecules are able to slip though the gel matrix more easily and thus migrate further than larger molecules, which are retarded, resulting in a net separation based on the size of the molecules.

megabases (million base pairs) in the case of techniques such as pulsed-field gel electrophoresis (PFGE)) and polyacrylamide gel electrophoresis (PAGE) to separate
smaller pieces (down to sizes of a few nucleotides). Apart from the fact that sequencing depends on the ability to separate molecules that differ from each other by only
one nucleotide in length, gel electrophoresis has been of great value in analysing
intact virus genomes, and particularly the analysis of viruses with segmented
genomes (below). Hybridization of complementary nucleotide sequences can also be
used in a number of ways to analyse virus genomes (Chapter 1).

Phenotypic analysis of virus populations has long been a standard technique of
virology. Examination of variant viruses and naturally occurring spontaneous
mutants has been a longstanding method of determining the function of virus genes.
Molecular biology has added to this the ability to design and create specific mutations, deletions and recombinants *in vitro*; it is a very powerful tool indeed. Although
coding capacity and to some extent protein properties can be determined *in vitro* by
the use of cell-free extracts to translate **mRNAs**, complete functional analysis of
virus genomes can only be performed on intact viruses. Fortunately, the relative simplicity of virus genomes (compared with even the simplest cell) offers a major advantage here – the ability to 'rescue' infectious virus from purified or cloned nucleic
acids. Infection of cells caused by nucleic acid alone is referred to as **transfection**.

Virus genomes which consist of (+)sense RNA are infectious when the purified
RNA (vRNA) is applied to cells in the absence of any virus proteins. This is because
(+)sense vRNA is essentially mRNA and the first event in a normally infected cell
is to translate the vRNA to make the virus proteins responsible for genome replication. In this case, direct introduction of RNA into cells circumvents the earliest stages
of the replicative cycle (Chapter 4). Virus genomes which are composed of double-
stranded DNA are also infectious. The events which occur here are a little more
complex, since the virus genome must first be transcribed by host polymerases to
produce mRNA. This is relatively simple for phage genomes introduced into
prokaryotes, but for viruses which replicate in the nucleus of **eukaryotic** cells, such
as herpesviruses, the DNA must first find its way to the appropriate cellular compartment. Most of the DNA which is introduced into cells by transfection is degraded by cellular nucleases. However, irrespective of its sequence, a small proportion
of the newly introduced DNA finds its way into the nucleus, where it is transcribed
by cellular polymerases.

Unexpectedly, cloned cDNA genomes of (+)sense RNA viruses (e.g. picornaviruses), are also infectious, although less efficient at infecting cells than the vRNA.
This is presumably because the DNA is transcribed by cellular enzymes to make
RNA – RNA transcribed *in vitro* from the cDNA template of the genome is more
efficient at initiating infection. Using these techniques, virus can be rescued from
cloned genomes, including those which have been manipulated *in vitro*.

Until recently, this type of approach was not possible for analysis of viruses with
(−)sense genomes. This is because such virus particles all contain a virus-specific

polymerase. The first event when these virus genomes enter the cell is that the (−)sense genome is copied by the polymerase, forming either (+)sense transcripts which are used directly as **mRNA**, or a double-stranded molecule, known either as the replicative intermediate (RI) or replicative form (RF), which serves as a template for further rounds of mRNA synthesis. Therefore, since purified (−)sense genomes cannot be directly translated and are not replicated in the absence of the virus polymerase, these genomes are inherently non-infectious. Systems have recently been developed which permit the rescue of viruses with (−)sense genomes from purified or cloned nucleic acids. Such experiments are frequently referred to as 'reverse genetics', i.e. the manipulation of a (−)sense RNA genome via a DNA intermediate. All such systems rely on a ribonucleoprotein complex which can serve as a template for genome replication by RNA-dependent RNA polymerase, but there are two different approaches:

- In vitro *complex formation*: Virus proteins purified from infected cells are mixed with RNA transcribed from cloned cDNAs to form complexes which are then introduced into susceptible cells to initiate an infection. This method has been used for paramyxoviruses, rhabdoviruses and bunyaviruses.
- In vivo *complex formation*: Ribonucleoprotein complexes formed *in vitro* are introduced into cells infected with a 'helper' virus strain. This method has been used for influenza virus, bunyaviruses and double-stranded RNA viruses such as reoviruses and birnaviruses.

   Such developments open up possibilities for genetic investigation of negative- and double-stranded RNA viruses that have not previously existed.

VIRUS GENETICS

Conventional genetic analysis of animal viruses is based largely on isolation and analysis of mutants, usually achieved using plaque purification ('biological cloning'). In the case of viruses for which no such systems exist (either because they are not cytopathic or do not replicate in culture), little genetic analysis was possible before the development of molecular genetics. However, certain tricks make it possible to extend standard genetic techniques to non-cytopathic viruses:

- *Biochemical analysis*: The use of metabolic inhibitors to construct genetic 'maps'. Inhibitors of translation (such as puromycin and cycloheximide) and transcription (actinomycin D) can be used to decipher genetic regulatory mechanisms.
- *Focal immunoassays*: Replication of non-cytopathic viruses can be visualized by immune-staining to produce visual foci (e.g. *Human immunodeficiency virus*).
- *Molecular biology*: e.g. nucleotide sequencing.

- *Physical analysis*: The use of high-resolution electrophoresis to identify genetic polymorphisms of virus proteins or nucleic acids.
- *Transformed foci*: Production of transformed 'foci' of cells by non-cytopathic 'focus-forming' viruses (e.g. DNA and RNA tumour viruses).

Various types of genetic map can be derived:

- *Recombination maps*: These are an ordered sequence of mutations derived from the probability of **recombination** between two genetic markers, which is proportional to the distance between them – a classical genetic technique. This method works for viruses with non-segmented genomes (DNA or RNA).
- *Reassortment maps (or groups)*: In viruses with segmented genomes, the assignment of mutations to particular genome segments results in the identification of genetically linked reassortment groups equivalent to individual genome segments.

Other types of map which can be constructed include the following:

- *Physical maps*: Mutations or other features can be assigned to physical locations on a virus genome using the 'rescue' of mutant genomes by small pieces of the wild-type genome (e.g. heteroduplex formation between mutant and wild-type DNA), after **transfection** of susceptible cells. Alternatively, cells can be co-transfected with the mutant genome plus individual restriction fragments to localize the mutation. Similarly, various polymorphisms (such as electrophoretic mobility of proteins) can be used to determine the genetic structure of a virus.
- *Restriction maps*: Site-specific cleavage of DNA by restriction endonucleases can be used to determine the structure of virus genomes. RNA genomes can be analysed in this way after cDNA cloning.
- *Transcription maps*: Maps of regions encoding various mRNAs can be determined by hybridization of mRNA species to specific genome fragments (e.g. restriction fragments). The precise start/finish of mRNAs can be determined by single strand-specific nuclease digestion of radiolabelled probes. Proteins encoded by individual mRNAs can be determined by translation *in vitro*. Ultraviolet (UV) irradiation of RNA virus genomes can also be used to determine the position of open reading frames because those farthest from the translation start are the least likely to be expressed by *in vitro* translation after partial degradation of the virus RNA by UV light.
- *Translation maps*: Pactamycin (which inhibits the initiation of translation) has been used to map protein-coding regions of enteroviruses. Pulse labelling results in incorporation of radioactivity only into proteins initiated before addition of the drug. Proteins nearest the 3' end of the genome are the most heavily labelled, those at the 5' end of the genome the least.

VIRUS MUTANTS

'Mutant', 'strain', 'type', 'variant' and even 'isolate' are all terms used rather loosely by virologists to differentiate particular viruses from each other and from the original 'parental', 'wild-type' or 'street' isolates of that virus. More accurately, these terms are generally applied as follows:

- *Strain*: Different lines or isolates of the same virus, e.g. from different geographical locations or patients
- *Type*: Different serotypes of the same virus (e.g. various antibody neutralization phenotypes)
- *Variant*: A virus whose phenotype differs from the original wild-type strain but where the genetic basis for the difference is not known.

The origin of mutant viruses

Spontaneous mutations

In some viruses, mutation rates may be as high as 10^{-3}–10^{-4} per incorporated nucleotide (e.g. in retroviruses such as HIV), whereas in others, they may be as low as 10^{-8}–10^{-11} (e.g. in herpesviruses), which is equivalent to the mutation rates seen in cellular DNA. These differences are due to the mechanism of genome replication, with error rates in RNA-dependent RNA polymerases generally being higher than those in DNA-dependent DNA polymerases. Some RNA virus polymerases do have proofreading functions, but in general, mutation rates are considerably higher in most RNA viruses than in DNA viruses. For a virus, mutations are a mixed blessing. The ability to generate antigenic variants which can escape the immune response is a clear advantage, but mutation also results in many defective particles, since most mutations are deleterious. In the most extreme cases, e.g. HIV, the error rate is 10^{-3}–10^{-4} per nucleotide incorporated. The HIV genome is approximately 9.7 kb long; therefore, there will be 0.9–9.7 mutations in every genome copied. Hence in this case, the 'wild-type' virus actually consists of a fleeting majority type which dominates the dynamic equilibrium (i.e. the population of genomes) present in all cultures of the virus. These mixtures of molecular variants are known as **quasi-species** and also occur in other RNA viruses, e.g. picornaviruses. However, the majority of these types will be non-infectious or seriously disadvantaged and are therefore rapidly weeded out of a replicating population. This mechanism is an important force in virus evolution (see Evolution and Epidemiology).

Induced mutations

Historically, most genetic analysis of viruses has been performed on virus mutants isolated from mutagen-treated populations. Mutagens can be divided into two types:

1 In vitro *mutagens*: These chemically modify nucleic acids and do not require replication for their activity. Examples include nitrous acid, hydroxylamine and alkylating agents (e.g. nitrosoguanidine).

2 In vivo *mutagens*: These require metabolically active, i.e. replicating, nucleic acid for their activity. They are incorporated into newly replicated nucleic acids and cause mutations to be introduced during subsequent rounds of replication. Examples include base analogues such as 5-bromouracil, which result in erroneous base pairing; intercalating agents (e.g. acridine dyes), which stack between bases, causing insertions or deletions; UV irradiation, which causes the formation of pyrimidine dimers which are excised from DNA by repair mechanisms that are much more error-prone than the usual enzymes used in DNA replication.

Experiments involving chemical mutagens suffer from a number of drawbacks:

- *Safety*: Mutagens are usually carcinogens and are also frequently highly toxic. They are very unpleasant compounds to work with.
- *Dosage*: The dose of mutagen used must be chosen carefully to give an average of 0.1 mutation per genome, otherwise the resultant viruses will contain multiple mutations which can complicate interpretation of the phenotype. If most of the viruses which result do not contain any mutations, it makes the process very inefficient since screening for mutants can be very laborious.
- *Control*: There is no control over where mutations occur and it is sometimes difficult or impossible to isolate mutations in a particular gene or region of interest.

For these reasons, site-specific molecular biological methods such as oligonucleotide-directed mutagenesis or PCR-based mutagenesis are now much more commonly used. Together with techniques such as enzyme digestion (to create deletions) and linker scanning (to create insertions), it is now possible to introduce almost any type of mutation precisely and safely at any specific site in a virus genome.

Types of mutant virus

The phenotype of a mutant virus depends on the type of mutation(s) it has and also upon the location of the mutation(s) within the genome. Each of the classes of mutations below can occur naturally in viruses or may be artificially induced for experimental purposes:

- *Biochemical markers*: This category includes drug resistance mutations; specific mutations which result in altered virulence; polymorphisms resulting in altered electrophoretic mobility of proteins or nucleic acids; and altered sensitivity to inactivating agents.

- *Deletions:* These are similar in some ways to nonsense mutants (below), but may include one or more virus genes and involve non-coding control regions of the genome (**promoters**, etc.). Spontaneous deletion mutants often accumulate in virus populations as **defective-interfering (D.I.) particles**. These non-infectious but not necessarily genetically inert genomes are thought to be important in establishing the course and pathogenesis of certain virus infections (see Chapter 6). Genetic deletions can only revert to wild-type by **recombination**, which usually occurs at comparatively low frequencies. Deletion mutants are very useful for assigning structure–function relationships to virus genomes, since they are easily mapped by physical analysis.
- *Host range:* This term can refer either to whole animal hosts or to permissive cell types *in vitro*. **Conditional mutants** of this class have been isolated using amber-suppressor cells (mostly for phages, but also for animal viruses using *in vitro* systems).
- *Nonsense:* These mutations result from alteration of coding sequence of a protein to one of three translation stop codons (UAG, amber; UAA, ochre; UGA, opal). Translation is terminated, resulting in the production of an amino-terminal fragment of the protein. The phenotype of these mutations can be suppressed by propagation of virus in a cell (bacterial or, more recently, animal) with altered suppressor tRNAs. Nonsense mutations are rarely 'leaky' (i.e. the normal function of the protein is completely obliterated) and can only revert to wild-type at the original site (see below). They therefore usually show a low reversion frequency.
- *Plaque morphology:* Mutants may be either large-plaque mutants which replicate more rapidly than the wild-type, or small-plaque mutants, which are the opposite. Plaque size is often related to a temperature-sensitive (t.s.) phenotype (see below). These mutants are often useful as unselected markers in multifactorial crosses.
- *Temperature-sensitive (t.s.):* This type of mutation is very useful as it allows the isolation of conditional-lethal mutations, a powerful means of examining virus genes which are essential for replication and whose function cannot otherwise be interrupted. Temperature-sensitive mutations usually result from mis-sense mutations in proteins (i.e. amino acid substitutions), resulting in proteins of full size with subtly altered conformation which can function at (permissive) low temperatures but not at (non-permissive) higher ones. Generally, the mutant proteins are immunologically unaltered, which is frequently a useful attribute. These mutations are usually 'leaky', i.e. some of the normal activity is retained even at non-permissive temperatures. Conversely, protein function is often impaired, even at the permissive temperature. Therefore, a high frequency of reversion is often a problem with this type of mutation, because the wild-type virus replicates faster than the mutant. In some viruses (e.g. reoviruses, influenza virus), very many t.s. mutants have been derived over the years for every virus gene, which permitted complete genetic analysis of these genomes before the advent of molecular biology.
- *Cold-sensitive (c.s.):* These mutants are the opposite of t.s. mutants and are very useful in bacteriophages and plant viruses whose host cells can be propagated at low

temperatures, but less useful for animal viruses because their host cells generally will not grow at significantly lower temperatures than normal.

■ *Revertants*: Reverse mutation is a valid type of mutation in its own right. Most of the above classes can undergo reverse mutations, which may be either simple 'back mutations' (i.e. correction of the original mutation) or second site 'compensatory mutations', which may be physically distant from the original mutation, and not even necessarily in the same gene as the original mutation.

Suppression

Suppression is the inhibition of a mutant phenotype by a second suppressor mutation, which may be either in the virus genome or in the host cell genome. It is important to point out that this mechanism of suppression is not the same as the suppression of chain-terminating amber mutations by host-encoded suppressor tRNAs (above), which could be called 'informational suppression'. Genetic suppression results in an apparently wild-type phenotype from a virus which is still genetically mutant – a **pseudorevertant**. This phenomenon has been best characterized in **prokaryotic** systems. More recently, some examples have been discovered in animal viruses, for example, reoviruses, vaccinia, influenza (where it has been observed in an attenuated vaccine, leading to an apparently virulent virus – this could therefore be medically important). Suppression may also be important biologically, in allowing viruses to overcome the deleterious effects of mutations, and would therefore be positively selected. Mutant viruses can therefore appear to revert to their original phenotype by three pathways:

1 Back mutation of the original mutation to give a wild-type genotype/phenotype (true reversion).
2 A second, compensatory mutation may occur in the same gene as the original mutation, correcting it, e.g. a second frameshift mutation restoring the original reading frame (intragenic suppression).
3 A suppressor mutation in a different virus gene or a host gene (extragenic suppression).

GENETIC INTERACTIONS BETWEEN VIRUSES

Genetic interactions between viruses often occur naturally, since host organisms are frequently infected with more than one virus. However, these situations are generally too complicated to be analysed successfully. Experimentally, genetic interactions can be analysed by mixed infection (**superinfection**) of cells in culture. Two types of information can be obtained from such experiments:

1   The assignment of mutants to functional groups known as **complementation** groups
2   The ordering of mutants into a linear genetic map by analysis of **recombination** frequencies.

Complementation

Complementation results from the interaction(s) of virus gene products during superinfection which results in production of one or both of the parental viruses being increased while both viruses remain unchanged genetically. In this situation, one of the viruses in a mixed infection provides a functional gene product for another virus which is defective for that function (Figure 3.2). If both mutants are defective in the same function, enhancement of replication does not occur and the two mutants are said to be in the same complementation group. The importance of this test is that it allows functional analysis of unknown mutations, if the biochemical basis of any one of the mutations in a particular complementation group is known. In theory, the number of complementation groups is equal to the number of genes

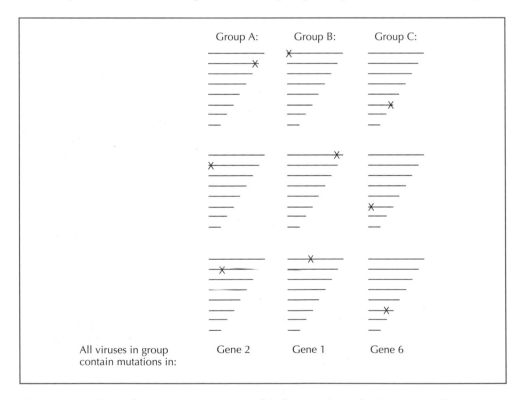

Figure 3.2 Complementation groups of influenza (or other) viruses all contain a mutation in the same virus gene, preventing the rescue of another mutant virus genome from the same complementation group.

in the virus genome. In practice, there are usually fewer complementation groups than genes, since mutations in some genes are always lethal and other genes are non-essential and therefore cannot be scored in this type of test. There are two possible types of complementation:

- Allelic (intragenic) complementation occurs where different mutants have complementing defects in the same protein, e.g. in different functional domains, or in different subunits of a multimeric protein (although this is rare).
- Non-allelic (intergenic) complementation results from mutants with defects in different genes. This is the more common type.

Complementation can be asymmetric, i.e. only one of the (mutant) parental viruses will replicate. This can be an absolute or a partial restriction. When complementation occurs naturally, it is usually the case that a replication-competent wild-type virus 'rescues' a replication-defective mutant. In these cases, the wild-type is referred to as a 'helper virus', for example, as in the case of defective transforming retroviruses containing **oncogenes** (Figure 3.3, see also Chapter 7).

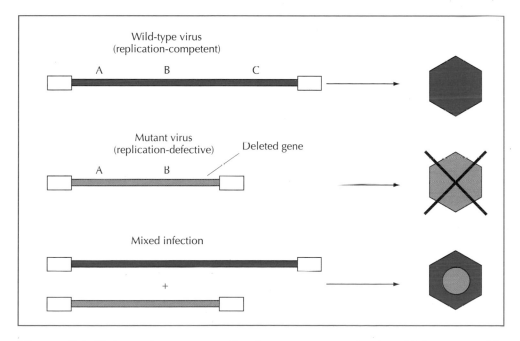

Figure 3.3 Helper viruses are replication-competent viruses which are capable of rescuing replication-defective genomes in a mixed infection, permitting their multiplication and spread.

Recombination

Recombination is the physical interaction of virus genomes during superinfection, resulting in gene combinations not present in either parent. There are three mechanisms by which this can occur, depending on the organization of the virus genome:

1 *Intramolecular recombination by strand breakage and re-ligation*: This process occurs in all DNA viruses and RNA viruses which replicate via a DNA intermediate. It is believed to be mediated by cellular enzymes, since no virus mutants with specific recombination defects have been isolated.

2 *Intramolecular recombination by 'copy-choice'*: This process occurs in RNA viruses (it has been known in picornaviruses since the 1960s, but has been recognized in other virus groups, such as coronaviruses, only recently), probably by a mechanism in which the virus polymerase switches template strands during genome synthesis. The molecular details of this process are not well understood. There are cellular enzymes which could be involved (e.g. **splicing** enzymes), but this is unlikely and the process is thought to occur essentially as a random event. **Defective interfering (D.I.) particles** in RNA virus infections are frequently generated in this way (see Chapter 6).

3 *Reassortment*: In viruses with segmented genomes, the genome segments can be randomly shuffled during **superinfection**. Progeny viruses receive (at least) one of each of the genome segments, but probably not from a single parent. For example, influenza virus has eight genome segments, therefore in a mixed infection, there could be $2^8 = 256$ possible progeny viruses. Packaging mechanisms in these viruses are not understood (see Chapter 2) but may be involved in generating reassortants.

In intramolecular recombination, the probability that breakage-reunion or strand-switching will occur between two markers (resulting in recombination) is proportional to the physical distance between them. Therefore, pairs of markers can be arranged on a linear genetic map, with distances measured in 'map units', i.e. percentage recombination frequency. In reassortment, the frequency of recombination between two markers is either very high (indicating that the markers are on two different genome segments) or comparatively low (which means that they are on the same segment). This is because the frequency of reassortment usually swamps the lower background frequency which is due to intermolecular recombination between strands.

Reactivation is the generation of infectious (recombinant) progeny from non-infectious parental virus genomes. This process has been demonstrated *in vitro* and may be important *in vivo*. For example, it has been suggested that the rescue of defective, long-dormant HIV **proviruses** during the long clinical course of AIDS may result in increased antigenic diversity and contribute to the pathogenesis of the disease.

Recombination occurs frequently in nature, e.g. influenza virus reassortment has resulted in worldwide epidemics (pandemics) which have killed millions of people (Chapter 6). This makes these genetic interactions of considerable practical interest and not merely a dry academic matter.

NON-GENETIC INTERACTIONS BETWEEN VIRUSES

A number of non-genetic interactions between viruses occur which can affect the outcome and interpretation of the results of genetic crosses. **Eukaryotic** cells have a diploid genome with two copies of each chromosome, each bearing its own allele of the same gene. The two chromosomes may differ in allelic markers at many loci. Among viruses, only retroviruses are truly diploid with two complete copies of the entire genome, but some DNA viruses, such as herpesviruses, have repeated sequences and are therefore partially heterozygous. In a few (mostly **enveloped**) viruses, aberrant packaging of multiple genomes may occasionally result in multiploid particles which are heterozygous (e.g. up to 10% of *Newcastle disease virus* particles). This process is known as **heterozygosis** and can contribute to the genetic complexity of virus populations.

Another non-genetic interaction which is commonly seen between viruses is interference. This process results from the resistance to **superinfection** by a virus seen in cells already infected by another virus. Homologous interference (i.e. against the same virus) often results from the presence of D.I. particles which compete for essential cell components and block replication. However, interference can also result from other types of mutation (e.g. dominant t.s. mutations) or by sequestration of virus **receptors** due to the production of **virus–attachment proteins** by viruses already present within the cell (e.g. in the case of avian retroviruses).

Phenotypic mixing can vary from extreme cases, where the genome of one virus is completely enclosed within the **capsid** or **envelope** of another (**pseudo-typing**), to more subtle cases where the capsid/envelope of the progeny contains a mixture of proteins from both viruses. This mixing gives the progeny virus the phenotypic properties (e.g. cell **tropism**) dependent on the proteins incorporated into the particle, without any genetic change. Subsequent generations of viruses inherit and display the original parental phenotypes. This process can occur easily in viruses with naked capsids (non-enveloped) which are closely related (e.g. different strains of enteroviruses), or in enveloped viruses which need not be related to one another (Figure 3.4). In this latter case, the phenomenon is due to the non-specific incorporation of different virus glycoproteins into the envelope, resulting in a mixed phenotype. Rescue of replication-defective transforming retroviruses by helper virus is a form of pseudotyping. Phenotypic mixing has proved to be a very useful tool to examine biological properties of viruses. *Vesicular stomatitis virus* readily forms pseudotypes containing retrovirus envelope glycoproteins, giving a

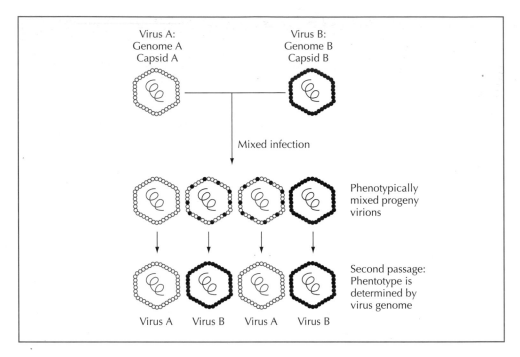

Figure 3.4 Phenotypic mixing occurs in mixed infections, resulting in genetically unaltered virus particles which have some of the properties of the other parental type.

plaque-forming virus with the properties of VSV but with the cell tropism of the retrovirus. This trick has been used to study the cell tropism of HIV and other retroviruses.

'LARGE' DNA GENOMES

There are a number of virus groups which have double-stranded DNA genomes of considerable size and complexity. In many respects, these viruses are genetically very similar to the host cells which they infect. Two examples are the members of the *Adenoviridae* and *Herpesviridae* families.

Herpesviridae

Herpesviridae is a large family containing more than 100 different members, at least one for most animal species examined to date. There are eight human herpesviruses, all of which share a common overall genome structure, but which differ in the fine details of genome organization and at the level of nucleotide sequence. The family is divided into three subfamilies, based on their biological properties (Table 3.1) (Appendix 2, ✐).

Table 3.1 Herpesviruses		
Alphaherpesvirinae: Latent infections in sensory ganglia; genome size 120–180 kbp		
Simplexvirus	*Human herpesvirus 1, 2* (HSV-1, HSV-2)	
Varicellovirus	*Human herpesvirus 3* (VZV)	
Betaherpesvirinae: Restricted host range; genome size 140–235 kbp		
Cytomegalovirus	*Human herpesvirus 5* (HCMV)	
Muromegalovirus	Mouse cytomegalovirus 1	
Roseolovirus	*Human herpesvirus 6, 7* (HHV-6, HHV-7)	
Gammaherpesvirinae: Infection of lymphoblastoid cells; genome size 105–175 kbp		
Lymphocryptovirus	*Human herpesvirus 4* (EBV)	
Rhadinovirus	*Human herpesvirus 8* (HHV-8)	

Herpesviruses have very large genomes composed of up to 235 kbp of linear, double-stranded DNA and correspondingly large and complex virus particles containing about 35 virion polypeptides. All encode a variety of enzymes involved in nucleic acid metabolism, DNA synthesis and protein processing (e.g. protein kinases). The different members of the family are widely separated in terms of genomic sequence and proteins, but all are similar in terms of structure and genome organization (Figure 3.5a). Some but not all herpesvirus genomes consist of two covalently joined sections, a unique long (U_L) and a unique short (U_S) region, each

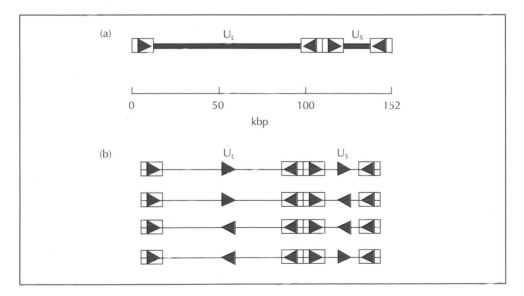

Figure 3.5 (a) Some herpesvirus genomes (e.g. herpes simplex virus) consist of two covalently joined sections, U_L and U_S, each bounded by inverted repeats. (b) This organization permits the formation of four different isomeric forms of the genome.

bounded by inverted repeats. The repeats allow structural rearrangements of the unique regions and, therefore, these genomes exist as a mixture of four isomers, all of which are functionally equivalent (Figure 3.5b). Herpesvirus genomes also contain multiple repeated sequences and, depending on the number of these, the genome size of various isolates of a particular virus can vary by up to 10 kbp.

The prototype member of the family is *Herpes simplex virus* (HSV), whose genome consists of approximately 152 kbp of double-stranded DNA, the complete nucleotide sequence of which has now been determined. This virus contains about 80 genes, densely packed and with overlapping reading frames. However, each gene is expressed from its own **promoter** (cf. adenoviruses below). Most of the eight human herpesvirus genomes have now been completely sequenced. Nucleotide sequences are increasingly used as a major criterion in classification of herpesviruses, e.g. in the case of the recently discovered *Human herpesvirus 8* (HHV-8, see Chapter 8). Before the development of nucleotide sequencing, the HSV genome had already been extensively mapped by 'conventional' genetic analysis, including the study of a very large number of t.s. mutants. HSV is perhaps the most intensively studied complex virus genome.

Adenoviridae

In contrast to herpesviruses, the genomes of adenoviruses consist of linear, double-stranded DNA of 30–38 kbp, the precise size of which varies between groups. These virus genomes contain 30–40 genes (Figure 3.6). The terminal sequence of each DNA strand is an inverted repeat of 100–140 bp and, therefore, the denatured single strands can form 'pan-handle' structures. These structures are important in DNA replication, as is a 55 kDa protein, known as the terminal protein, covalently attached to the 5′ end of each strand. During genome replication, this protein acts as a primer, initiating the synthesis of new DNA strands. Although adenovirus genomes are considerably smaller than those of herpesviruses, the expression of the genetic information is rather more

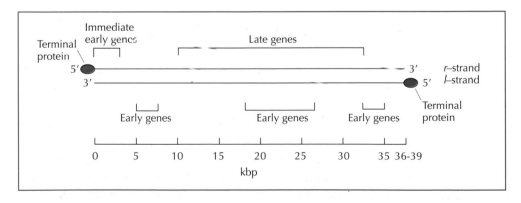

Figure 3.6 Organization of the *Adenovirus* genome.

complex. Clusters of genes are expressed from a limited number of shared **promoters**. Multiply spliced mRNAs and alternative **splicing** patterns are used to express a variety of polypeptides from each promoter (see Chapter 5).

'SMALL' DNA GENOMES

Enterobacteria phage M13 has already been mentioned in Chapter 2. The genome of this phage consists of 6.4 kb of single-stranded, (+)sense, circular DNA and encodes 10 genes. Unlike most **icosahedral** virions, the filamentous M13 **capsid** can be expanded by the addition of further protein subunits. Hence the genome size can also be increased by the addition of extra sequences in the non-essential intergenic region without becoming incapable of being packaged into the capsid. In other bacteriophages, the packaging constraints are much more rigid; for example, in phage λ, only DNA of between approximately 95 and 110% (approximately 46–54 kbp) of the normal genome size (49 kbp) can be packaged into the virus particle. Not all bacteriophages have such simple genomes as M13; for example, the genome of phage λ is approximately 49 kbp and that of phage T4 is about 160 kbp double-stranded DNA. These last two bacteriophages also illustrate another common feature of linear virus genomes – the importance of the sequences present at the ends of the genome.

In the case of phage λ, the substrate which is packaged into the phage heads during assembly consists of long concatemers of phage DNA which are produced during the later stages of vegetative replication. The DNA is apparently 'reeled in' by the phage head and when a complete genome has been incorporated, the DNA is cleaved at a specific sequence by a phage-coded endonuclease (Figure 3.7). This enzyme leaves a 12 bp 5′ overhang on the end of each of the cleaved strands, known as the *cos* site. Hydrogen bond formation between these 'sticky ends' can result in the formation of a circular molecule. In a newly infected cell, the gaps on either side of the *cos* site are closed by DNA ligase and it is this circular DNA which undergoes vegetative replication or integration into the bacterial chromosome.

Enterobacteria phage T4 illustrates another molecular feature of certain linear virus genomes – **terminal redundancy**. Replication of the T4 genome also produces long concatemers of DNA. These are cleaved by a specific endonuclease, but unlike the λ genome, the lengths of DNA incorporated into the particle are somewhat longer than a complete genome length (Figure 3.8). Therefore, some genes are repeated at each end of the genome, and the DNA packaged into the phage particles contains reiterated information. Bacteriophage genomes are neither necessarily small nor simple!

As further examples of small DNA genomes, consider those of two groups of animal viruses, the parvoviruses and polyomaviruses. *Parvovirus* genomes are linear, non-segmented, single-stranded DNA of about 5 kb. Most of the strands packaged into **virions** are (−)sense, but some parvoviruses package equal amounts of (+) and

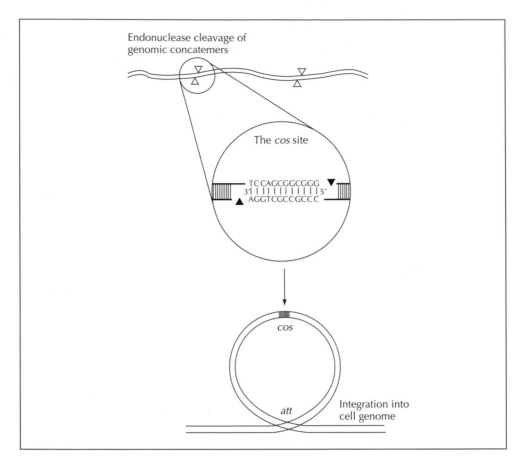

Figure 3.7 The cohesive 'sticky-ends' of the *cos* site in the bacteriophage λ genome are ligated together in newly infected cells, forming a circular molecule. Integration of this circular form into the *Escherichia coli* chromosome occurs by specific recognition and cleavage of the *att* site in the phage genome.

(−) strands, and all appear to package at least a proportion of (+)sense strands. These are very small genomes, and even the replication-competent parvoviruses contain only two genes: *rep*, which encodes proteins involved in transcription, and *cap*, which encodes the coat proteins. However, the expression of these genes is rather complex, resembling the pattern seen in adenoviruses, with multiple **splicing** patterns seen for each gene (Chapter 5). The ends of the genome have palindromic sequences of about 115 nt, which form 'hairpins' (Figure 3.9). These structures are essential for the initiation of genome replication, again emphasizing the importance of the sequences at the ends of the genome.

The genomes of polyomaviruses consist of double-stranded, circular DNA molecules of approximately 5 kbp. The architecture of the *Polyomavirus* genome (i.e. number and arrangement of genes and function of the regulatory signals and systems) has

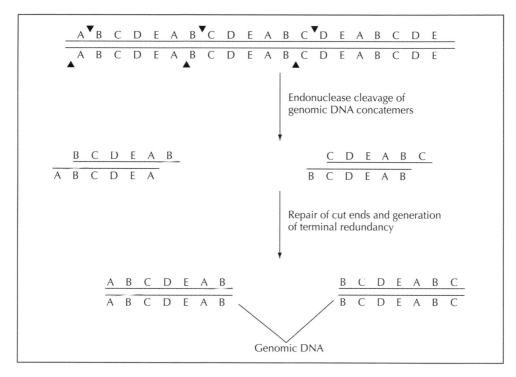

Figure 3.8 Terminal redundancy in the bacteriophage T4 genome results in the reiteration of some genetic information.

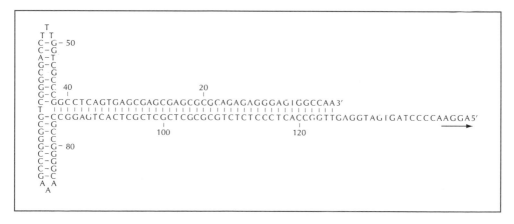

Figure 3.9 Palindromic sequences at the ends of *Parvovirus* genomes result in the formation of hairpin structures involved in the initiation of replication.

been studied in great detail at a molecular level. Within the particles, the virus DNA assumes a supercoiled form and is associated with four cellular histones called H2A, H2B, H3 and H4 (see Chapter 2). The genomic organization of these viruses has evolved to pack the maximum information (six genes) into minimal space (5 kbp).

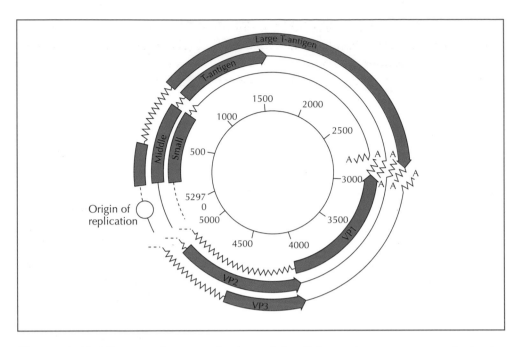

Figure 3.10 The complex organization of the *Polyomavirus* genome results in the compression of much genetic information into a relatively short sequence.

This has been achieved by use of both strands of the genome DNA and overlapping genes (Figure 3.10). VP1 is encoded by a dedicated open reading frame (**ORF**), but the VP2 and VP3 genes overlap so that VP3 is contained within VP2. The origin of replication is surrounded by non-coding regions which control transcription. Polyomaviruses also encode 'T-antigens', which are proteins that can be detected by sera from animals bearing polyomavirus-induced tumours. These proteins bind to the origin of replication and show complex activities, in that they are involved both in DNA replication and in the transcription of virus genes. This is discussed further in Chapter 7.

POSITIVE-STRAND RNA VIRUSES

The ultimate size of single-stranded RNA genomes is limited by the fragility of RNA and the tendency of long strands to break. In addition, RNA genomes tend to have higher mutation rates than those composed of DNA because they are copied less accurately. This has also tended to drive RNA viruses towards smaller genomes. Single-stranded RNA genomes vary in size from those of coronaviruses, which are approximately 30 kb long, to those of bacteriophages such as MS2 and Qβ, at about 3.5 kb. Although members of distinct families, most (+)sense RNA viruses of vertebrates share common features in terms of the biology of their genomes. In particular, purified (+)sense virus RNA is directly infectious when applied to susceptible host cells in the absence of any virus proteins (although it is about one million times less infectious than virus particles). On examining the features of these families, although the details of genomic organization vary, repeated themes emerge (Figure 3.11).

Picornaviruses

The *Picornavirus* genome consists of one single-stranded, (+)sense RNA molecule of between 7.2 kb in human rhinoviruses (HRV) to 8.5 kb in foot-and-mouth disease viruses (FMDV), containing a number of features conserved in all picornaviruses:

- There is a long (600–1200 nt) untranslated region (UTR) at the 5′ end which is important in translation, virulence, and possibly encapsidation and a shorter 3′ untranslated region (50–100 nt) necessary for (−)strand synthesis during replication.
- The 5′ UTR contains a 'clover-leaf' secondary structure known as the **IRES** (internal ribosome entry site) (Chapter 5).
- The rest of the genome encodes a single **polyprotein** of between 2100 and 2400 amino acids.

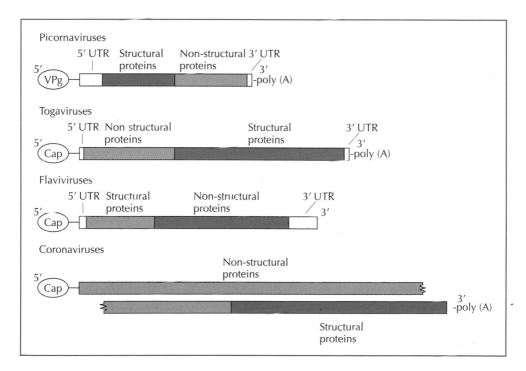

Figure 3.11 Genomic organization of positive-stranded RNA viruses.

- Both ends of the genome are modified, the 5' end by a covalently attached small, basic protein VPg (23 amino acids), and the 3' end by polyadenylation.

Togaviruses

The *Togavirus* genome comprises single-stranded, (+)sense, non-segmented RNA of approximately 11.7 kb. It has the following features:

- It resembles cellular mRNAs in that it has a 5' methylated cap and 3' poly(A) sequences.
- Expression is achieved by two rounds of translation, producing first non-structural proteins encoded in the 5' part of the genome and later structural proteins from the 3' part.

Flaviviruses

The *Flavivirus* genome comprises one single-stranded, (+)sense RNA molecule of about 10.5 kb with the following features:

- It has a 5' methylated cap but in most cases the RNA is not polyadenylated at the 3' end.
- Genetic organization differs from that of the togaviruses (above) in that the structural proteins are encoded in the 5' part of the genome and non-structural proteins in the 3' part.
- Expression is similar to that of the picornaviruses, involving the production of a **polyprotein**

Coronaviruses

The *Coronavirus* genome consists of non-segmented, single-stranded, (+)sense RNA, approximately 27–30 kb long, which is the longest of any RNA virus. It also has the following features:

- It has a 5' methylated cap and 3' poly(A) and the vRNA functions directly as mRNA.
- The 5' 20 kb segment of the genome is translated first to produce a virus polymerase, which then produces a full-length (−)sense strand. This is used as a template to produce mRNA as a 'nested set' of transcripts, all with an identical 5' non-translated leader sequence of 72 nt and coincident 3' polyadenylated ends.
- Each mRNA is **monocistronic**, the genes at the 5' end being translated from the longest mRNA and so on. These unusual cytoplasmic structures are produced not by **splicing** (post-transcriptional modification) but by the polymerase during transcription.

Positive-sense RNA plant viruses

The majority (but not all) of plant virus families have (+)sense RNA genomes. The genome of the *Tobamovirus Tobacco mosaic virus* (TMV) is a well-studied example (Figure 3.12):

- The TMV genome is a 6.4 kb RNA molecule which encodes four genes.
- There is a 5′ methylated cap and the 3′ end of the genome contains extensive secondary structure, but no poly(A) sequences.
- Expression is somewhat reminiscent but distinct from that of togaviruses, producing non-structural proteins by direct translation of the open reading frame encoded in the 5′ part of the genome and the virus coat protein and further non-structural proteins from two subgenomic RNAs encoded by the 3′ part.

The similarities and differences between genomes in this class will be considered further in the discussion of virus evolution below and in Chapter 5.

NEGATIVE-STRAND RNA VIRUSES

Viruses with **negative-sense** RNA genomes are a little more diverse than the positive-stranded viruses discussed above. Possibly because of the difficulties of expression, they tend to have larger genomes encoding more genetic information. Because of this, segmentation is a common, although not universal, feature of such viruses (Figure 3.13). None of these genomes are infectious as purified RNA. Although a gene encoding an RNA-dependent RNA polymerase has recently

Figure 3.12 Organization of the TMV genome.

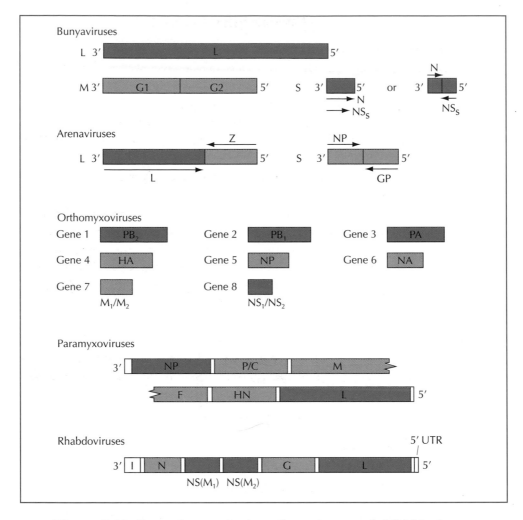

Figure 3.13 Genomic organization of negative-stranded RNA viruses.

been found in some eukaryotic cells, most uninfected cells do not contain enough RNA-dependent RNA polymerase activity to support virus replication, and since the (−)sense genome cannot be translated as mRNA without the virus polymerase packaged in each particle, these genomes are effectively inert. Some of the viruses described in this section are not strictly 'negative-sense' but **ambisense**, since they are part (−)sense and part (+)sense. Ambisense coding strategies occur in both plant (e.g. the *Tospovirus* genus of the bunyaviruses, and tenuiviruses such as *Rice stripe virus*) and animal viruses (the *Phlebovirus* genus of the bunyaviruses, and arenaviruses).

Bunyaviruses

Members of the *Bunyaviridae* have single-stranded, (−)sense, segmented RNA. The genome has the following features:

- The genome comprises three molecules: L (8.5 kb), M (5.7 kb) and S (0.9 kb).
- All three RNA species are linear, but in the **virion** they appear circular because the ends are held together by base-pairing. The three segments are not present in virus preparations in equimolar amounts.
- In common with all (−)sense RNAs, the 5′ ends are not capped and the 3′ ends are not polyadenylated.
- The members of the *Phlebovirus* and *Tospovirus* genera differ from the other three genera in the family (*Bunyavirus, Nairovirus* and *Hantavirus*) in that genome segment S is rather larger and the overall genome organization is different – **ambisense** (i.e. the 5′ end of each segment is (+)sense, but the 3′ end is (−)sense). The *Tospovirus* genus also has an ambisense coding strategy in the M segment of the genome.

Arenaviruses

Arenavirus genomes consist of linear, single-stranded RNA. There are two genome segments: L (5.7 kb) and S (2.8 kb). Both have an ambisense organization, as above.

Orthomyxoviruses

See discussion of segmented genomes (below).

Paramyxoviruses

Members of the *Paramyxoviridae* have non-segmented, (−)sense RNA of 15–16 kb. Typically, six genes are organized in a linear arrangement (3′-NP-P/C/V-M-F-I IN-L-5′) separated by repeated sequences: a polyadenylation signal at the end of the gene, an intergenic sequence (GAA), and a translation start signal at the beginning of the next gene.

Rhabdoviruses

Viruses of the *Rhabdoviridae* have non-segmented, (−)sense RNA of approximately 11 kb. There is a leader region of approximately 50 nt at the 3′ end of the genome and a 60 nt untranslated region (UTR) at the 5′ end of the vRNA. Overall, the genetic arrangement is similar to that of paramyxoviruses, with a conserved polyadenylation signal at the end of each gene and short intergenic regions between the five genes.

SEGMENTED AND MULTIPARTITE VIRUS GENOMES

There is often some confusion over these two categories of genome structure. Segmented virus genomes are those which are divided into two or more physically separate molecules of nucleic acid, all of which are then packaged into a single virus particle. In contrast, although multipartite genomes are also segmented, each genome segment is packaged into a separate virus particle. These discrete particles are structurally similar and may contain the same component proteins, but often differ in size depending on the length of the genome segment packaged. In one sense, multipartite genomes are, of course, segmented, but this is not the strict meaning of these terms as they will be used here.

Segmentation of the virus genome has a number of advantages and disadvantages. There is an upper limit to the size of a non-segmented virus genome which results from the physical properties of nucleic acids, particularly the tendency of long molecules to break due to shear forces (and for each particular virus, the length of nucleic acid which can be packaged into the **capsid**). The problem of strand breakage is particularly relevant for single-stranded RNA, which is much more chemically labile than double-stranded DNA. The longest single-stranded RNA genomes are those of the coronaviruses, at approximately 30 kb, but the longest double-stranded DNA virus genomes are considerably longer, e.g. Phycodnaviruses at up to 380 kbp. Physical breakage of the genome results in its biological inactivation, since it cannot be completely transcribed, translated or replicated. Segmentation means that the virus avoids 'having all its eggs in one basket' and also reduces the probability of breakages due to shearing, thus increasing the total potential coding capacity of the entire genome. However, the disadvantage of this strategy is that all the individual genome segments must be packaged into each virus particle, or the virus will be defective as a result of loss of genetic information. In general, it is not understood how this control of packaging is achieved.

Separating the genome segments into different particles (the multipartite strategy) removes the requirement for accurate sorting, but introduces a new problem in that all the discrete virus particles must be taken up by a single host cell to establish a **productive infection**. This is perhaps the reason multipartite viruses are only found in plants. Many of the sources of infection by plant viruses, such as inoculation by sap-sucking insects or after physical damage to tissues, result in a large inoculum of infectious virus particles, providing opportunities for infection of an initial cell by more than one particle.

The genetics of segmented genomes are essentially the same as those of non-segmented genomes, with the addition of the reassortment of segments, as discussed above. Reassortment can occur whether the segments are packaged into a single particle or are in a multipartite configuration. Reassortment is a powerful means of achieving rapid generation of genetic diversity; this could be another possible reason for its evolution. Segmentation of the genome also has implications for the partition of genetic information and the way in which it is expressed; this will be considered further in Chapter 5.

To understand the complexity of these genomes, consider the organization of a segmented virus genome (*Orthomyxovirus* – influenza virus) and a multipartite genome (*Geminivirus*). The influenza virus genome is composed of eight segments (in influenza A and B strains, seven in influenza C) of single-stranded, (−)sense RNA (Table 3.2). The identities of the proteins encoded by each genome segment were determined originally by genetic analysis of the electrophoretic mobility of the individual segments from reassortant viruses and by analysis of a large number of mutants covering all eight segments. The eight segments have common nucleotide sequences at the 5′ and 3′ ends (Figure 3.14) which are necessary for replication of the genome (Chapter 4). These sequences are complementary to one another and, inside the particle, the ends of the genome segments are held together by base-pairing, forming a 'pan-handle' structure, which again is believed to be involved in replication. The RNA genome segments are not packaged as naked nucleic acid, but in association with the gene 5 product, the nucleoprotein, and are visible in electron micrographs as **helical** structures. Here, there is a paradox. Biochemically and genetically, each genome segment behaves as an individual, discrete entity. However, in electron micrographs of influenza virus particles disrupted with non-ionic detergents, the **nucleocapsid** has the physical appearance of a single, long helix. Clearly, there is some interaction between the genome segments and it is this which explains the ability of influenza virus particles to select and package the genome segments within each particle with a surprisingly low error rate, considering the difficulty of the task (Chapter 2). The genome sequences and protein interaction which operate this subtle mechanism have not yet been defined.

Table 3.2 Influenza virus genome segments			
Segment	Size (nt)	Polypeptide(s)	Function (Location)
1	2341	PB_2	Transcriptase: cap binding
2	2341	PB_1	Transcriptase: elongation
3	2233	PA	Transcriptase: (?)
4	1778	HA	Haemagglutinin
5	1565	NP	Nucleoprotein: RNA binding; part of transcriptase complex
6	1413	NA	Neuraminidase
7	1027	M_1	Matrix protein: major component of virion
		M_2	Integral membrane protein – ion channel
8	890	NS_1	Non-structural (nucleus) function unknown
		NS_2	Non-structural (nucleus + cytoplasm) function unknown

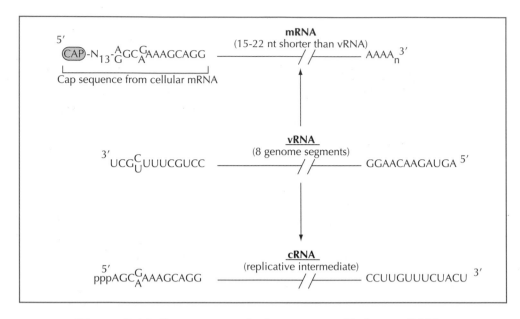

Figure 3.14 Common terminal sequences of influenza RNAs.

In many tropical and subtropical parts of the world, geminiviruses are important plant pathogens. Geminiviruses are divided into three genera based on their host plants (monocotyledons or dicotyledons) and insect vectors (leafhoppers or whiteflies). In the *Mastrevirus* and *Curtovirus* genera, the genome consists of a single-stranded DNA molecule of approximately 2.7 kb. The DNA packaged into these **virions** has been arbitrarily designated as (+)sense, although both the (+)sense and (−)sense strands found in infected cells contain protein coding sequences. The genome of geminiviruses in the genus *Begmovirus* is bipartite and consists of two circular, single-stranded DNA molecules, each of which is packaged into a discrete particle (Figure 3.15). Both of the strands comprising the genome are approximately 2.7 kb long and differ from one another completely in nucleotide sequence, except for a shared 200 nt non-coding sequence involved in DNA replication. The two genomic DNAs are packaged into entirely separate **capsids**. Because establishment of a **productive infection** requires both parts of the genome it is necessary for a minimum of two virus particles bearing one copy of each of the genome segments to infect a new host cell. Although geminiviruses do not multiply in the tissues of their insect vectors (**non-propagative transmission**), a sufficiently large amount of virus is ingested and subsequently deposited onto a new host plant to favour such **superinfections**.

Both of these examples show a high density of coding information. In influenza virus, genes 7 and 8 both encode two proteins in overlapping reading frames. In geminiviruses, both strands of the virus DNA found in infected cells contain coding information, some of which is present in overlapping reading frames. It is possible that this

Figure 3.15 Organization and protein-coding potential of a bipartite *Begmovirus* (*Geminiviridae*) genome. Proteins encoded by the (+)sense virion strand are named 'A' or 'B' according to the genome component on which they are located, plus 'V' or 'C' depending on whether they are encoded by the (+)sense virion strand or the (−)sense complementary strand.

high density of genetic information is the reason these viruses have resorted to divided genomes, in order to regulate the expression of this information (see Chapter 5).

REVERSE TRANSCRIPTION AND TRANSPOSITION

The first successes of molecular biology were the discovery of the double-helix structure of DNA and the elucidation of the language of the genetic code. The importance of these findings does not lie in the mere facts, but in their importance in allowing predictions to be made about the fundamental nature of living organisms. The confidence which flowed from these early triumphs resulted in the development of a grand universal theory, which was called the 'central dogma of molecular biology', namely that all cells (and hence viruses) worked on a simple organizing principle − the unidirectional flow of information from DNA, through RNA, into proteins. In the mid–1960s, there were rumblings that life might not be so simple.

In 1963, Howard Temin showed that the replication of retroviruses, whose particles contain RNA genomes, was inhibited by actinomycin D, an antibiotic which binds only to DNA. The replication of other RNA viruses is not inhibited by this drug. So pleased was the scientific community with an all-embracing dogma that these facts were largely ignored until 1970, when Temin and David Baltimore simultaneously published the observation that retrovirus particles contain an RNA-dependent DNA polymerase – reverse transcriptase. This finding alone was important enough, but like the earlier conclusions of molecular biology, has subsequently had reverberations for the genomes of all organisms, and not merely a few virus families. It is now known that **retrotransposons** with striking similarities to retrovirus genomes form a substantial part of the genomes of all higher organisms, including humans. Earlier ideas of genomes as constant, stable structures have been replaced with the realization that they are, in fact, dynamic and rather fluid entities.

The concept of transposable genetic elements – specific sequences that are able to move from one position in the genome to another – was put forward by Barbara McClintock in the 1940s. Such **transposons** fall into two groups:

1 Simple transposons, which do not undergo reverse transcription and are found in **prokaryotes** (e.g. the genome of *Enterobacteria phage Mu*).
2 Retrotransposons, which closely resemble retrovirus genomes and are bounded by long direct repeats (long terminal repeats, LTRs). These move by means of a transcription/reverse transcription/integration mechanism and are found in **eukaryotes** (the *Metaviridae* and *Pseudoviridae*).

Both types show a number of similar properties:

- They are believed to be responsible for a high proportion of apparently 'spontaneous' mutations.
- They promote a wide range of genetic rearrangements in host cell genomes, such as deletions, inversions, duplications and translocations of the neighbouring cellular DNA.
- The mechanism of insertion generates a short (3–13 bp) duplication of the DNA sequence on either side of the inserted element.
- The ends of the transposable element consist of inverted repeats, 2–50 bp long.
- Transposition is often accompanied by replication of the element – necessarily so in the case of **retrotransposons**, but this also often occurs with prokaryotic transposition.
- Transposons control their own transposition functions, encoding proteins which are either *cis*-**acting** (affecting the activity of contiguous sequences on the same

nucleic acid molecule) or *trans*-acting (encoding diffusible products that act on regulatory sites in any stretch of nucleic acid present in the cell).

Enterobacteria phage Mu infects *E. coli* and consists of a complex, tailed particle containing a linear, double-stranded DNA genome of about 40 kb, with host cell-derived sequences of between 0.5 and 3.0 kbp attached to the right-hand end of the genome (Figure 3.16). Mu is a **temperate bacteriophage** whose replication can proceed through two pathways; one involves integration of the genome into that of the host cell and results in **lysogeny**, and the other is **lytic** replication which results in the death of the cell (see Chapter 5). Integration of the phage genome into that of the host bacterium occurs at random sites in the cell genome. Integrated phage genomes are known as **prophage** and integration is essential for the establishment of lysogeny. At intervals in bacterial cells lysogenic for Mu, the prophage undergoes transposition to a different site in the host genome. The mechanism leading to transposition is different from that responsible for the initial integration of the phage genome (which is conservative, i.e. does not involve replication), and is a complex process requiring numerous phage-encoded and host cell proteins. Transposition is tightly linked to replication of the phage genome and results in the formation of a 'co-integrate', i.e. a duplicated copy of the phage genome flanking a target sequence in which insertion has occurred. The original Mu genome remains in the same location where it first integrated and is joined by a second integrated genome at another site. (N.B. Not all prokaryotic transposons use this process. Some, such as TN10, are not replicated during transposition but are excised from the original integration site and integrate elsewhere.) There are two consequences of such a transposition: first the phage genome is replicated during this process (advantageous for the virus) and second, the sequences flanked by the two phage genomes (which form repeated sequences) are at risk of secondary rearrangements, including deletions, inversions, duplications and translocations (possibly but not necessarily deleterious for the host cell).

Figure 3.16 Organization of the bacteriophage Mu genome.

The yeast Ty viruses are representative of a class of sequences found in yeast and other **eukaryotes** known as **retrotransposons**. Unlike *Enterobacteria phage Mu*, such elements are not true viruses, but do bear striking similarities to retroviruses. The genomes of most strains of *Saccharomyces cerevisiae* contain 30–35 copies of the Ty elements, which are around 6 kbp long and contain direct repeats of 245–371 bp at each end (Figure 3.17). Within this repeat sequence is a **promoter** which results in the transcription of a terminally redundant 5.6 kb mRNA. This contains two genes, *TyA*, which has homology to the *gag* gene of retroviruses, and *TyB*, which is homologous to the *pol* gene. The protein encoded by *TyA* is capable of forming a roughly spherical, 60 nm diameter 'virus-like particle' (VLP). The 5.6 kb RNA transcript can be incorporated into such particles, resulting in the formation of intracellular structures known as Ty-VLPs. Unlike true viruses, these particles are not infectious for yeast cells, but if accidentally taken up by a cell, can carry out reverse transcription of their RNA content to form a double-stranded DNA Ty element which can then integrate into the host cell genome (see below).

The most significant difference between retrotransposons such as Ty, *copia* (a similar element found in *Drosophila melanogaster*) and retroviruses proper is the presence of an additional gene in retroviruses, *env*, which encodes an **envelope** glycoprotein (see Chapter 2). The envelope protein is responsible for **receptor** binding and has allowed retroviruses to escape the intracellular lifestyle of retrotransposons, to form a true virus particle and propagate themselves widely by infection of other cells (Figure 3.17). Retrovirus genomes have four unique features:

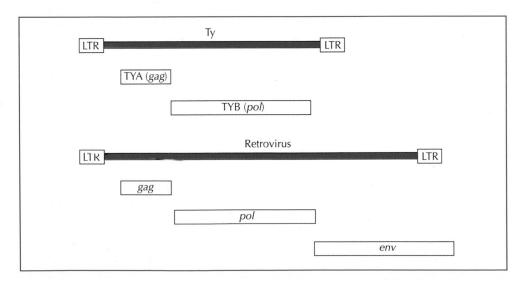

Figure 3.17 The genetic organization of retrotransposons such as Ty (above) and retrovirus genomes (below) shows a number of similarities, including the presence of direct long terminal repeats (LTRs) at either end.

1 They are the only viruses which are truly diploid.
2 They are the only RNA viruses whose genome is produced by cellular transcriptional machinery (without any participation by a virus-encoded polymerase).
3 They are the only viruses whose genome requires a specific cellular RNA (tRNA) for replication.
4 They are the only (+)sense RNA viruses whose genome does not serve directly as mRNA immediately after infection.

During the process of reverse transcription (Figure 3.18), the two single-stranded (+)sense RNA molecules which comprise the virus genome are converted into a double-stranded DNA molecule somewhat longer than the RNA templates owing to the duplication of direct repeat sequences at each end – the long terminal repeats (LTRs) (Figure 3.19). Some of the steps in reverse transcription have remained mysterious; for example, the apparent jumps which the polymerase makes from one end of the template strand to the other. In fact, these steps can be explained by the observation that complete conversion of retrovirus RNA into double-stranded DNA only occurs in a partially uncoated core particle and cannot be duplicated accurately *in vitro* with the reagents free in solution. This indicates that the conformation of the two RNAs inside the retrovirus **nucleocapsid** dictates the course of reverse transcription – the 'jumps' are nothing of the sort, since the ends of the strands are probably held adjacent to one another inside the core.

Reverse transcription has important consequences for retrovirus genetics. First, it is a highly error-prone process, because reverse transcriptase does not carry out the proofreading functions performed by cellular DNA-dependent DNA polymerases. This results in the introduction of many mutations into retrovirus genomes and, consequently, rapid genetic variation (see Spontaneous Mutations, above). In addition, the process of reverse transcription promotes genetic **recombination**. Since two RNAs are packaged into each **virion** and used as the template for reverse transcription, recombination can and does occur between the two strands. Although the mechanism responsible for this is not clear, if one of the RNA strands differs from the other, for example, by the presence of a mutation, and recombination occurs, then the resulting virus will be genetically distinct from either of the parental viruses.

After reverse transcription is complete, the double-stranded DNA migrates into the nucleus, still in association with virus proteins. The mature products of the *pol* gene are, in fact, a complex of polypeptides which include three distinct enzymatic activities: reverse transcriptase and RNAse H, which are involved in reverse transcription, and integrase, which catalyses integration of virus DNA into the host cell **chromatin**, following which it is known as the **provirus** (Figure 3.20). Three forms of double-stranded DNA are found in retrovirus-infected cells following reverse transcription: linear DNA and two circular forms which contain either one or two LTRs. From the structure at the ends of the provirus, it was previously believed that

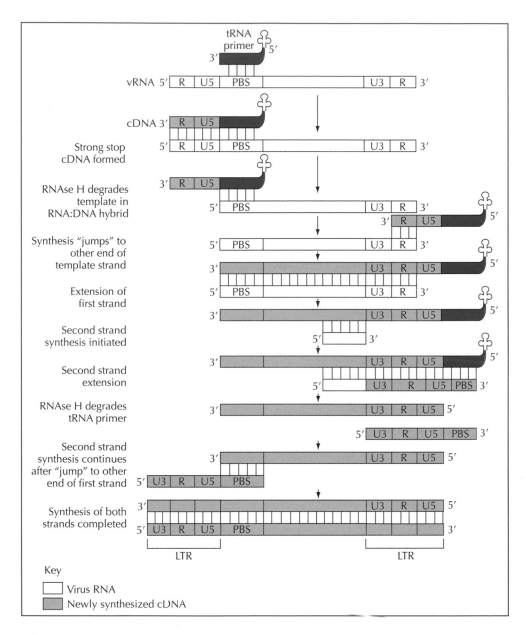

Figure 3.18 Mechanism of reverse transcription of retrovirus RNA genomes, in which two molecules of RNA are converted into a single (terminally redundant) double-stranded DNA provirus.

the two-LTR circle was the form used for integration. In recent years, systems which have been developed to study the integration of retrovirus DNA *in vitro* have shown that it is the linear form which integrates. This discrepancy can be resolved by a model in which the ends of the two LTRs are held in close proximity by the reverse transcriptase–integrase complex. The net result of integration is that 1–2 bp are lost from the end of each LTR and 4–6 bp of cellular DNA are duplicated on either side of the provirus. It is unclear whether there is any specificity regarding the site of integration into the cell genome. What is obvious is that there is no simple target sequence, but it is possible that there may be (numerous) regions or sites in the **eukaryotic** genome which are more likely to be integration sites than others.

Following integration, the DNA provirus genome becomes essentially a collection of cellular genes and is at the mercy of the cell for expression. There is no mechanism for the precise excision of integrated proviruses, some of which are known to have been 'fossilized' in primate genomes through millions of years of evolution, although proviruses may sometimes be lost or altered by modifications of the cell genome. The only way out for the virus is transcription, forming what is essentially a full-length mRNA (minus the terminally redundant sequences from the LTRs). This RNA is the vRNA and two copies are packaged into **virions** (Figure 3.19).

There are, however, two different genome strategies used by viruses which involve reverse transcription. It is at this point that the difference between them becomes obvious. One strategy, as used by retroviruses and described above, culminates in the packaging of RNA into virions as the virus genome. The other, used

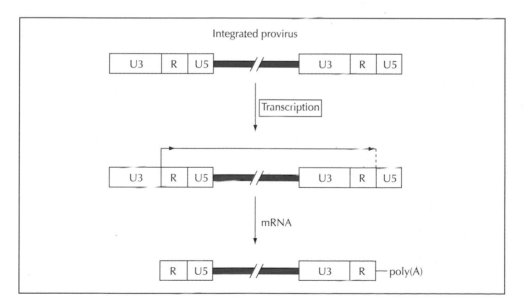

Figure 3.19 Generation of repeated information in retrovirus long terminal repeats. In addition to their role in reverse transcription, these sequences contain important control elements involved in the expression of the virus genome including a transcriptional promoter in the U3 region and polyadenylation signal in the R region.

by hepadnaviruses and caulimoviruses, switches the RNA and DNA phases of replication and results in DNA virus genomes. This is achieved by utilizing reverse transcription not as an early event in replication as retroviruses do, but as a late step during the formation of the virus particle.

Hepatitis B virus (HBV) is the prototype member of the family *Hepadnaviridae*. HBV **virions** are spherical, lipid-containing particles, 42–47 nm diameter, which contain a partially double-stranded ('gapped') DNA genome, plus an RNA-dependent DNA polymerase (i.e. reverse transcriptase) (Figure 3.21). Hepadnaviruses have very small genomes consisting of a (−)sense strand of 3.0–3.3 kb (varies between different hepadnaviruses) and a (+)sense strand of 1.7–2.8 kb (varies between different particles). On infection of cells, three major genome transcripts are produced: 3.5, 2.4 and 2.1 kb mRNAs. All have the same polarity (i.e. are transcribed from the same strand of the virus genome) and the same 3′ ends, but have different 5′ ends (i.e. initiation sites). These transcripts are heterogeneous in size and it is not completely clear which proteins each transcript encodes, but there are four known genes in the virus:

- C encodes the core protein
- P encodes the polymerase
- S encodes the three polypeptides of the surface antigen, pre-S1, pre-S2, and S (which are derived from alternative start sites)
- X encodes a transactivator of virus transcription (and possibly cellular genes?).

Closed circular DNA is found soon after infection in the nucleus of the cell and is probably the source of the above transcripts. This DNA is produced by repair of the gapped virus genome as follows:

1 Completion of the (+)sense strand.
2 Removal of a protein primer from the (−)sense strand and an oligoribonucleotide primer from the (+)sense strand.
3 Elimination of **terminal redundancy** at the ends of the (−)sense strand.
4 Ligation of the ends of the two strands.

It is not known how or by which proteins (virus or cellular) these events are carried out. The 3.5 kb RNA transcript, core antigen and polymerase form core particles and the polymerase converts the RNA to DNA in the particles as they form in the cytoplasm.

The genome structure and replication of *Cauliflower mosaic virus* (CaMV), the prototype member of the *Caulimovirus* genus, is reminiscent of that of hepadnaviruses, although there are differences between them. The CaMV genome consists of a gapped, circular double-stranded DNA molecule of about 8 kbp, one strand of which is known as the α strand and contains a single gap, and a complementary strand which contains two gaps (Figure 3.22). There are eight genes encoded in this

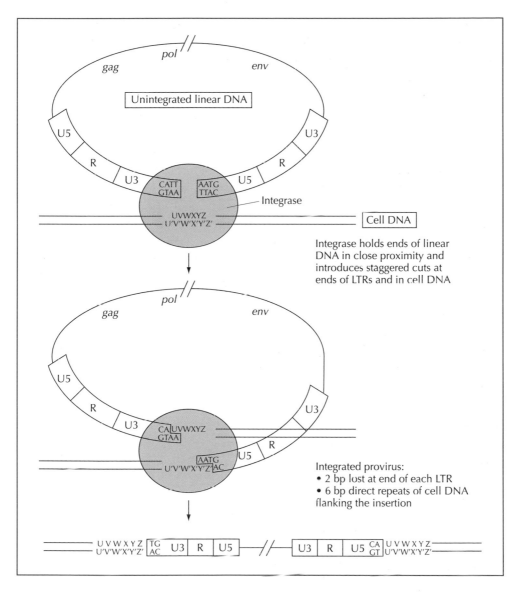

Figure 3.20 Mechanism of integration of retrovirus genomes into the host cell chromatin.

genome, although not all eight products have been detected in infected cells. Replication of the CaMV genome is similar to that of HBV. The first stage is the migration of the gapped virus DNA to the nucleus of the infected cell where it is repaired to form a covalently closed circle. This DNA is transcribed to produce two polyadenylated transcripts, one long (35S) and one shorter one (19S). In the cytoplasm, the 19S mRNA is translated to produce a protein which forms large **inclusion bodies** in the cytoplasm of infected cells and it is in these sites that

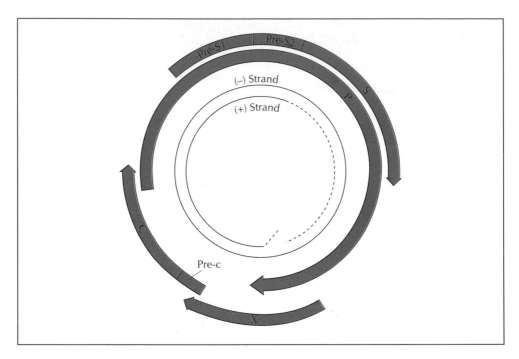

Figure 3.21 Structure, organization and protein–coding potential of the *Hepatitis B virus* genome.

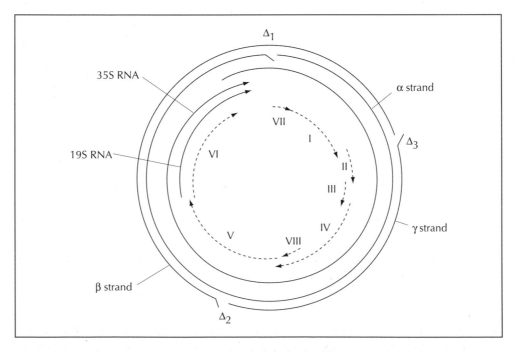

Figure 3.22 Structure, organization and protein–coding potential of the *Cauliflower mosaic virus* genome.

Table 3.3 Reverse transcription of virus genomes			
Features	**Caulimoviruses**	**Hepadnaviruses**	**Retroviruses**
Genome	DNA	DNA	RNA
Primer for (−)strand synthesis	tRNA	Protein	tRNA
Terminal repeats (LTRs)	No	No	Yes
Specific integration of virus genome	No	No	Yes

the second phase of replication occurs. In these replication complexes, some copies of the 35S mRNA are translated while others are reverse transcribed and packaged into **virions** as they form. The differences between reverse transcription of these virus genomes and those of retroviruses are summarized in Table 3.3.

EVOLUTION AND EPIDEMIOLOGY

Epidemiology is concerned with the distribution of disease and the derivation of strategies to reduce or prevent it. Virus infections present considerable difficulties for this process. Except for **epidemics** where acute symptoms are obvious, the major evidence of virus infection available to the epidemiologist is the presence of antivirus antibodies in patients. This information frequently provides an incomplete picture, and it is often difficult to assess whether a virus infection occurred recently or at some time in the past. Alternative techniques, such as the isolation of viruses in experimental plants or animals, are laborious and impossible to apply to large populations. Molecular biology provides sensitive, rapid and sophisticated techniques to detect and analyse the genetic information stored in virus genomes and has resulted in a new area of investigation, molecular epidemiology.

One drawback of molecular genetic analysis is that some knowledge of the nature of a virus genome is necessary before it can be investigated. However, it should be obvious from this chapter that we now possess a great amount of information about the structure and nucleotide sequences of at least a few representative members of most of the known virus groups. This information allows virologists to look in two directions: back to where viruses came from and forward to chart the course of future epidemics and diseases. Sensitive detection of nucleic acids by amplification techniques such as the polymerase chain reaction is already having a major impact on this type of epidemiological investigation.

There are (at least!) three theories which seek to explain the origin of viruses:

- *Regressive evolution*: This theory states that viruses are degenerate life-forms which have lost many functions that other organisms possess and have only retained the genetic information essential to their parasitic way of life.

- *Cellular origins*: In this theory viruses are thought to be subcellular, functional assemblies of macromolecules which have escaped their origins inside cells.
- *Independent entities*: This says that viruses evolved on a parallel course to cellular organisms from the self–replicating molecules believed to have existed in the primitive prebiotic 'RNA world'.

While each of these theories has its devotees and this subject provokes fierce disagreements, the fact is that viruses exist, and we are all infected with them. The practical importance of the origin of viruses is that this issue may have implications for virology here and now. Genetic and nucleotide sequence relationships between viruses can reveal the origins not only of individual viruses, but also of whole families and possible 'superfamilies' (Figure 3.23). In a number of groups of viruses previously thought to be unrelated, nucleotide sequencing has revealed that functional regions appear to be grouped together in a similar way. The extent to which there is any sequence similarity between these regions in different viruses varies, although clearly, the active sites of enzymes such as virus **replicases** are strongly conserved. The

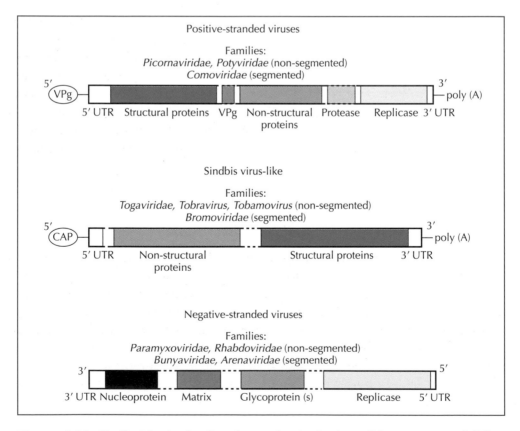

Figure 3.23 Similarities in the function and organization of the genomes of different virus families allow them to be grouped together as 'superfamilies'.

emphasis in these groupings is more on functional and organizational similarities. The original classification scheme for viruses did not recognize a higher level grouping than the 'family' (see Appendix 2 ✐). However, there arc now three groupings of related virus families equivalent to the 'orders' of formal biological nomenclature:

- *Mononegavirales*: Negative-sense RNA viruses with non-segmented genomes: *Bornaviridae, Filoviridae, Paramyxoviridae, Rhabdoviridae*.
- *Caudovirales*: Tailed bacteriophages: *Myoviridae, Podoviridae, Siphoviridae*.
- *Nidovirales*: 'Nested' viruses – because of their pattern of transcription: *Arteriviridae, Coronaviridae*.

Knowledge drawn from taxonomic relationships may allow us to predict the properties and behaviour of new viruses, or to develop new drugs based on what is already known about existing viruses. Whether these shared patterns suggest the descent of present-day viruses from a limited number of primitive ancestors or are evidence of convergent evolution between different virus families is uncertain. Although it is tempting to speculate on events that may have occurred before the origins of 'life' as it is presently recognized, it would be unwise to discount the pressures which might result in viruses with diverse origins assuming common genetic solutions to common problems of storing, replicating and expressing genetic information. This is particularly true now that we appreciate the plasticity of virus and cellular genomes and the mobility of genetic information from virus to virus, cell to virus, and virus to cell. There is no reason to believe that virus evolution has stopped, and it would be perilous to do so. The practical consequences of ongoing evolution and the concept of **emergent viruses** are described in Chapter 7.

SUMMARY

Molecular biology has put much emphasis on the structure and function of the virus genome. At first sight, this tends to emphasize the tremendous diversity of virus genomes. On closer examination, similarities and unifying themes become more apparent. Sequences and structures at the ends of virus genomes are in some ways functionally more significant than the unique coding regions within them. Common patterns of genetic organization seen in virus superfamilies suggest either that many viruses have evolved from common ancestors or that convergent evolution and exchange of genetic information between viruses has resulted in common solutions to common problems.

FURTHER READING

Cann, A.J. (1999). *DNA Viruses: A Practical Approach*. Oxford University Press, Oxford. ISBN 0199637199.

Cann, A.J. (2000). *RNA Viruses: A Practical Approach*. Oxford University Press, Oxford. ISBN 0199637172.

Conzelmann, K.K. (1998). Nonsegmented negative-strand RNA viruses: genetics and manipulation of viral genomes. *Annual Review of Genetics* 32: 123–162.

Domingo, E., Webster, R.G. and Holland, J.J. (2000). *Origin and Evolution of Viruses*. Academic Press, London. ISBN 0122203607.

Dreher, T.W. (1999). Functions of the 3′-untranslated regions of positive strand RNA viral genomes. *Annual Review of Phytopathology* 37: 151–174.

Haren, L., Ton-Hoang, B., and Chandler, M. (1999). Integrating DNA: transposases and retroviral integrases. *Annual Review of Microbiology* 53: 245–281.

Ramig, R.F. (1997) Genetics of the rotaviruses. *Annual Review of Microbiology* 51: 225–255.

Saedler, H. and Gierl, A. (Eds) (1996). Transposable elements. *Current Topics in Microbiology and Immunology*, Vol. 204.

Zaccomer, B., Haenni, A.L. and Macaya, G. (1995). The remarkable variety of plant RNA virus genomes. *Journal of General Virology* 76: 231–247.

SELF-ASSESSMENT QUESTIONS

(3.1) Are the following statements true or false?

(a) Virus genomes vary in size from 3500 nucleotides to approximately 380 kbp.

(b) The genetic code of a virus must be distinct from that of the host organism.

(c) Virus genomes consisting of (+)sense RNA are infectious when the purified vRNA is applied to cells in the absence of any virus proteins.

(d) 'Reverse genetics' makes possible the manipulation of (−)sense RNA virus genomes.

(e) Infection of cells caused by nucleic acid alone is referred to as transfection.

(3.2) Are the following statements true or false?

(a) 'Superinfection' is where two viruses produce more than one virus particle.

(b) The probability of recombination between two genetic markers is inversely proportional to the distance between them.

(c)   In viruses with segmented genomes, 'reassortment groups' are equiva-
        lent to the individual genome segments.
(d)   Populations of virus genomes consisting of mixtures of molecular
        variants are known as quasi-species.
(e)   Site-specific molecular biological methods are commonly used to
        mutagenize virus genomes.

(3.3) Are the following statements true or false?
(a)   Mutation rates in herpesvirus genomes may be as high as 10^3 to 10^4
        per nucleotide incorporated.
(b)   Mutation rates in retrovirus genomes may be as low as 10^8 to 10^{11} per
        nucleotide incorporated.
(c)   Every new HIV provirus formed contains, on average, at least one
        new mutation.
(d)   Temperature sensitive (t.s.) mutants are very stable and rarely revert to
        the original phenotype.
(e)   t.s. mutations usually result from mis-sense mutations in proteins.

(3.4) Are the following statements true or false?
(a)   Deletion mutants are very useful for assigning structure-function rela-
        tionships to virus genomes, because they are easily mapped by
        physical analysis.
(b)   Deletion mutants can only revert to wild-type by recombination,
        which only occurs at low frequencies.
(c)   Complementation may be asymmetric or symmetrical.
(d)   Phenotypic mixing is where individual progeny viruses from a mixed
        infection contain genes derived from both parental viruses.
(e)   Most virus genomes are diploid.

(3.5) Are the following statements true or false?
(a)   Herpesvirus genomes vary in size from 5 to 25 kbp.
(b)   Herpesvirus genomes consist of linear, double-stranded DNA.
(c)   In *Herpes simplex virus* (HSV), each gene is expressed from its own
        promoter.
(d)   The HSV genome is approximately 152 kbp.
(e)   The HSV genome contains about 80 genes, densely packed and with
        overlapping reading frames.

(3.6) Are the following statements true or false?
(a)   Parvovirus genomes consist of linear, non-segmented, single-stranded
        DNA.

(b)   The ends of parvovirus genomes are palindromic sequences of about
        115 nt required for replication.
(c)   Polyomaviruses are about 5 kbp and contain six genes.
(d)   In the virus particle, *Polyomavirus* DNA assumes a supercoiled form
        and is associated with cellular histones.
(e)   The *Polyomavirus* genome contains overlapping reading frames on
        both strands of the DNA.

(3.7)   (+)sense RNA virus genomes (true or false?):
(a)   can be up to 90 kbp in length.
(b)   are usually modified at the 5′ end.
(c)   are always polyadenylated at the 3′ end.
(d)   are all expressed as a polyprotein.
(e)   all require splicing for expression.

(3.8)   (−)sense RNA virus genomes (true or false?):
(a)   are sometimes segmented.
(b)   cannot have an ambisense coding strategy.
(c)   are never capped at the 5′ end.
(d)   are never polyadenylated at the 3′ end.
(e)   are always circular.

(3.9)   Retroviruses (true or false?):
(a)   are the only family of viruses to encode reverse transcriptase.
(b)   are the only RNA viruses whose genome is produced by cellular
        transcriptional machinery.
(c)   are the only (+)sense RNA viruses whose genome does not serve
        directly as mRNA immediately after infection.
(d)   have high mutation rates.
(e)   have a high rate of recombination.

(3.10) Are the following statements true or false?
(a)   Segmentation of virus genomes reduces the probability of breakage
        due to shearing.
(b)   Hepadnaviruses have large genomes of up to 55 kbp.
(c)   The *Cauliflower mosaic virus* (CaMV) genome consists of a gapped,
        circular double-stranded DNA molecule.
(d)   The *Cauliflower mosaic virus* (CaMV) genome is generated by reverse
        transcription.
(e)   Virus superfamilies prove that many viruses had a common ancestor.

Answers to Self-Assessment Questions are given in Appendix 4.

REPLICATION

On completing this chapter, you should be able to:
- Understand how the nature of a virus genome determines its pattern of replication
- Describe a typical, generalized replication cycle of a virus
- Compare the patterns of replication of each of the seven major virus groups.

OVERVIEW OF VIRUS REPLICATION

The way in which viruses are classified has altered as our perception of them has changed:

1 *Classification by disease*: Many early civilizations, such as those of ancient Egypt and Greece, were well aware of the pathogenic effects of many different viruses. From these times we have several surprisingly accurate descriptions of diseases of humans, animals and crops, although of course the nature of the agents responsible for these calamities was not realized at the time. Accurate though these descriptions were, a major problem with such a system of classification is that many diverse viruses cause similar symptoms; for example, respiratory infections with fever may be caused by many different viruses.

2 *Classification by morphology*: As increasing numbers of viruses were isolated and techniques of analysis were improved, it became possible during the 1930s-1950s to classify viruses based on the structure of virus particles. Although this is an improvement on the above scheme, there are still problems in distinguishing

between viruses that are morphologically similar but cause disparate clinical symptoms (e.g. the various picornaviruses). During this era, serology became an important aid in virus classification, and particle morphology continues to be an important strand in virus classification.

3 *Functional classification*: In recent years, more emphasis has been placed on the replication strategy of the virus. This is particularly true for the composition and structure of the virus **genome** and the constraints which this imposes on replication. This approach has accelerated since the development of molecular biology due to the central importance of the virus genome in this new technology. Molecular analysis of virus genomes permits rapid and unequivocal identification of individual virus strains, but is also predictive of the properties of a previously unknown or novel virus with a familiar genome structure. (The classification of viruses is described in Appendix 2 ⊘.)

In a teleological sense (i.e. crediting an inanimate organism such as a virus with a conscious purpose), the sole objective of a virus is to replicate its genetic information. The nature of the virus genome is therefore pre-eminent in determining what steps are necessary to achieve this aim. In reality, there is a surprising amount of variation that can occur in these processes, even for viruses with seemingly similar genome structures. The reason for this lies in compartmentalization, both of **eukaryotic** cells into nuclear and cytoplasmic compartments, and of genetic information and biochemical capacity between the virus genome and that of the host cell.

The type of cell infected by the virus has a profound effect on the process of replication. For viruses of **prokaryotes**, replication reflects to some extent the relative simplicity of their host cells. For viruses with eukaryotic hosts, matters are frequently more complex. There are many examples of animal viruses undergoing different replicative cycles in different cell types. However, the coding capacity of the **genome** forces all viruses to choose a strategy for replication. This might be one involving heavy reliance on the host cell, in which case the virus genome can be very compact and need only encode the essential information for a few proteins, e.g. parvoviruses. Alternatively, large and complex virus genomes, such as those of poxviruses, encode most of the information necessary for replication, and the virus is only reliant on the cell for the provision of energy and the apparatus for macromolecular synthesis, such as ribosomes (see Chapter 1). Viruses with an RNA lifestyle, i.e. an RNA genome plus messenger RNAs, have no apparent need to enter the nucleus, although during the course of replication, many do. 'DNA viruses', as might be expected, mostly replicate in the nucleus where host cell DNA is replicated and where the biochemical apparatus necessary for this process is located. However, some viruses with DNA genomes (e.g. poxviruses) have evolved to contain sufficient biochemical capacity to be able to replicate in the cytoplasm, with minimal requirement for host cell functions. Most of this chapter will examine the process of virus replication and will look at some of the variations on the basic theme.

INVESTIGATION OF VIRUS REPLICATION

Bacteriophages have long been used by virologists as models to understand the biology of viruses. This is particularly true of virus replication. Two particularly significant experiments which illustrated the fundamental nature of viruses were performed on bacteriophages. The first of these was accomplished by Emory Ellis and Max Delbruck in 1939 and is usually referred to as the 'single-burst' experiment or 'one-step growth curve' (Figure 4.1 ✐). This was the first experiment to show the three essential phases of virus replication:

1 Initiation of infection
2 Replication and expression of the virus genome
3 Release of mature **virions** from the infected cell.

In this experiment, bacteriophages were added to a culture of rapidly growing bacteria and after a period of a few minutes, the culture was diluted, effectively preventing further interaction between the **phage** particles and the cells. This simple step is the key to the entire experiment, since it effectively synchronizes the infection of the cells and allows the subsequent phases of replication in a population of individual cells and virus particles to be viewed as if it were a single interaction (in much the same way that molecular cloning of nucleic acids allows analysis of populations of nucleic acid molecules as single species). Repeated samples of the culture were taken at short intervals and analysed for bacterial cells by plating onto agar plates and for phage particles by plating onto lawns of bacteria. As can be seen in Figure 4.1, there is a stepwise increase in the concentration of phage particles with time, each increase in phage concentration representing one replicative cycle of the virus. However, the data from this experiment can also by analysed in a different way, by plotting the number of **plaque-forming units (p.f.u.)** per bacterial cell against time (Figure 4.2). In this type of assay, a plaque-forming unit can be either a single extracellular virus particle or an infected bacterial cell. These two can be distinguished by disruption of the bacteria with chloroform before plating, which releases any intracellular phage particles, giving the total virus count, i.e. intracellular plus extracellular particles.

Several additional features of virus replication are visible from the graph in Figure 4.2. Immediately after dilution of the culture, there is a phase of 10-15 minutes when no phage particles are detectable; this is known as the **eclipse period**. This represents a time when virus particles have broken down after penetrating cells, releasing their **genomes** as a prerequisite to replication. At this stage, they are no longer infectious and therefore cannot be detected by the plaque assay. The **latent period** is the time before the first new extracellular virus particles appear and is of the order of 20–25 minutes for most bacteriophages. About 40 minutes after the cells were infected, the curves for the total number of virus particles and for extracellular virus merge

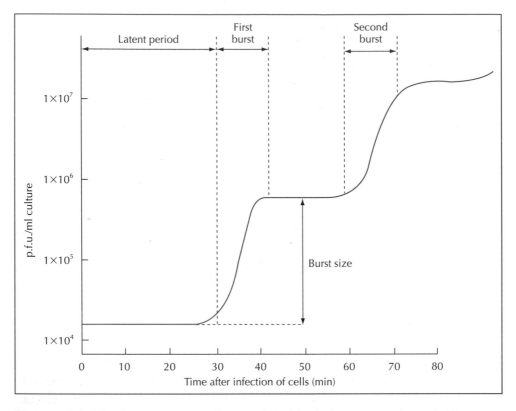

Figure 4.1 The 'one-step growth curve' or 'single-burst experiment'. First performed by Ellis and Delbruck in 1939, this classic experiment illustrates the true nature of virus replication. Details of the experiment are given in the text. Two bursts (crops of phage particles released from cells) are shown in this particular experiment.

because the infected cells have lysed and released any intracellular phage particles by this time. The yield (i.e. number) of particles produced per infected cell can be calculated from the overall rise in phage **titre**.

Following the development of **plaque** assays for animal viruses in the 1950s, 'single-burst' experiments have now been performed for many viruses of **eukaryotes**, with similar results (Figure 4.3). The major difference between these viruses and bacteriophages is the much longer time interval required for replication, which is measured in terms of hours and, in some cases, days, rather than minutes after infection. This difference reflects the much slower growth rate of eukaryotic cells, and in part, the complexity of virus replication in compartmentalized cells. Biochemical analysis of virus replication in eukaryotic cells has also been used to analyse the levels of virus and cellular protein and nucleic acid synthesis and to examine the intracellular events occurring during synchronous infections (Figure 4.4). The application of various metabolic inhibitors has also proved to be a valuable tool in such

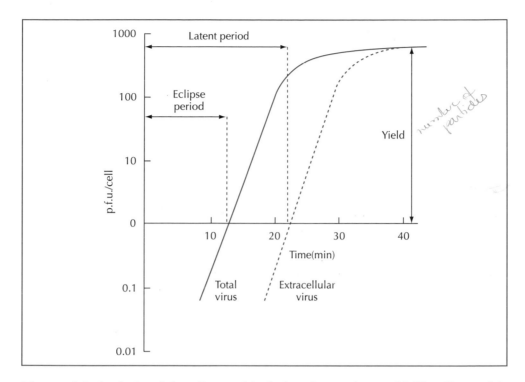

Figure 4.2 Analysis of data from a 'single-burst' experiment. Unlike Figure 4.1, which shows the total number of plaque-forming units (p.f.u.) produced, here the data is plotted as p.f.u./bacterial cell, which reflects the events occurring in a 'typical' infected cell in the population. The phases of replication named on the graph are defined in the text.

experiments. Examples of the use of such drugs will be given during the detailed consideration of the stages of virus replication later in this chapter.

The second key experiment on virus replication using **bacteriophages** was performed by Alfred Hershey and Martha Chase in 1952. Bacteriophage T2 was propagated in *Escherichia coli* cells which had been 'labelled' with one of two radioisotopes, either ^{35}S, which is incorporated into sulphur-containing amino acids in proteins, or ^{32}P, which is incorporated into nucleic acids (which do not contain any sulphur) (Figure 4.5). Particles labelled in each of these ways were used to infect bacteria. After a short period to allow attachment to the cells, the mixture was homogenized briefly in a blender which did not destroy the bacterial cells but was sufficiently vigorous to knock the phage coats off the outside of the cells. Analysis of the radioactive content in the cell pellets and culture supernatant (containing the empty phage coats) showed that most of the radioactivity in the ^{35}S-labelled particles remained in the supernatant, while in the ^{32}P-labelled particles, most of the radiolabel had entered the cells. This experiment indicated that it was the DNA **genome** of the bacteriophage that entered the cells and initiated the infection.

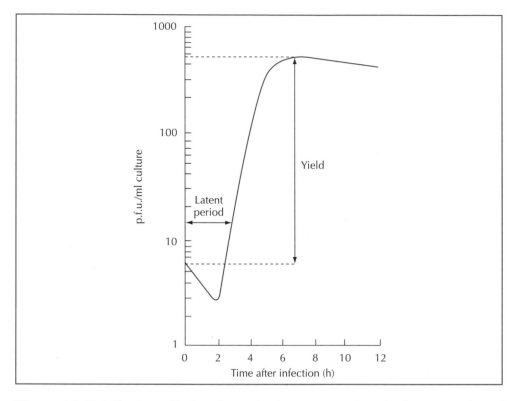

Figure 4.3 Replication of lytic eukaryotic viruses occurs in a similar way to that of bacteriophages. This figure shows a 'single-burst' type of experiment for a picornavirus (e.g. poliovirus). This type of data can only be produced from synchronous infections where a high **multiplicity of infection** is used.

Although this might seem obvious now, at the time this experiment settled a great controversy over whether a structurally simple polymer such as a nucleic acid, which was known to contain only four monomers, was complex enough to carry genetic information. (At the time, it was generally believed that proteins, which consist of a much more complex mixture of more than 20 different amino acids, were the carriers of the genes and that DNA was probably a structural component of cells and viruses.) Together, these two experiments illustrate the process of virus replication. Virus particles enter susceptible cells and release their genomic nucleic acids. These are replicated and packaged into virus particles consisting of newly synthesized virus proteins, which are then released from the cell.

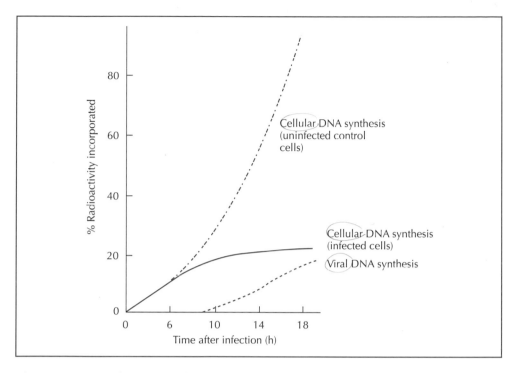

Figure 4.4 Biochemistry of virus infection. This graph shows the rate of cellular and virus DNA synthesis (based on the incorporation of radiolabelled nucleotides into high molecular weight material) in uninfected and herpesvirus–infected cells.

THE REPLICATION CYCLE

Virus replication can be divided into eight stages, as shown in Figure 4.6. It should be emphasized that these are purely arbitrary divisions, used here for convenience in explaining the replication cycle of a non-existent 'typical' virus. For the sake of clarity, this chapter concentrates on viruses which infect vertebrates. Viruses of bacteria, invertebrates and plants will be mentioned briefly, but the overall objective of this chapter is to illustrate similarities in the pattern of replication of different viruses. Regardless of their hosts, all viruses must undergo each of these stages in some form to successfully complete their replication cycles. Not all the steps described here are detectable as distinct stages for all viruses; often they blur together and appear to occur almost simultaneously. Some of the individual stages have been studied in great detail and a tremendous amount of information is known about them. Other stages have been much harder to study, and considerably less information is available.

Figure 4.5 The Hershey–Chase experiment, first performed in 1952, demonstrated that virus genetic information was encoded by nucleic acids and not proteins. Details of the experiment are given in the text.

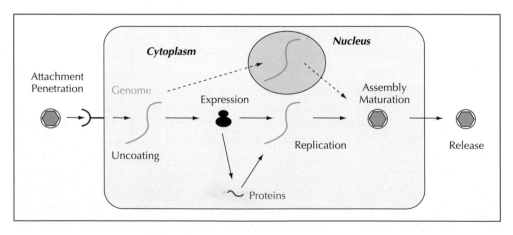

Figure 4.6 Generalized scheme for virus replication. See text for details.

Attachment

Because the stages of virus replication described here are purely arbitrary, and because complete replication necessarily involves a cycle, it is possible to begin discussion of virus replication at any point. Arguably, it is most logical to consider the first interaction of a virus with a new host cell as the starting point of the cycle. Technically, virus **attachment** consists of specific binding of a **virus-attachment protein** (or 'antireceptor') to a cellular **receptor** molecule. Many examples of virus receptors are now known, and a complete list is too long to be included here (see Figure 4.7 and references at end of this chapter).

Target receptor molecules on cell surfaces may be proteins (usually glycoproteins), or the carbohydrate residues present on glycoproteins or glycolipids. The former are usually specific receptors, in that a virus may use a particular protein as a receptor. Carbohydrate groups are usually less specific receptors because the same configuration of side-chains may occur on many different glycosylated membrane-bound molecules. Some complex viruses (e.g. poxviruses, herpesviruses) use more than one receptor and therefore have alternative routes of uptake into cells. Virus receptors fall into many different classes, e.g. immunoglobulin-like superfamily molecules, membrane-associated receptors and transmembrane transporters and channels. The one factor which unifies all virus receptors is that they did not evolve and are not manufactured by cells to allow viruses to enter cells. Rather, viruses have subverted molecules required for normal cellular functions.

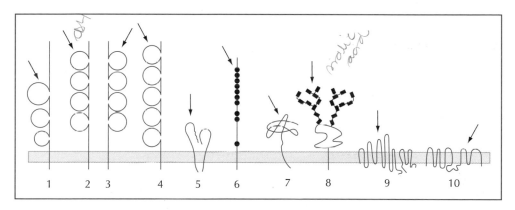

Figure 4.7 Schematic representation of some virus receptors. Arrows indicate virus attachment sites. (1) Poliovirus receptor (PVR); (2) CD4: HIV; (3) carcinoembryonic antigen(s): MHV (coronavirus); (4) ICAM-1: most rhinoviruses (1–4 are all immunoglobulin superfamily molecules). (5) VLA-2 integrin: echoviruses; (6) LDL receptor: some rhinoviruses; (7) aminopeptidase N: coronaviruses; (8) sialic acid (on glycoprotein): influenza, reoviruses, rotaviruses; (9) cationic amino acid transporter: murine leukaemia virus; (10) sodium–dependent phosphate transporter: gibbon ape leukaemia virus.

Plant viruses face special problems initiating an infection. The outer surfaces of plants are composed of protective layers of waxes and pectin, but more significantly, each cell is surrounded by a thick wall of cellulose overlying the cytoplasmic membrane. To date, no plant virus is known to use a specific cellular receptor of the type that animal and bacterial viruses use to attach to cells. Rather, plant viruses rely on a breach of the integrity of a cell wall to directly introduce a virus particle into a cell. This is achieved either by the vector associated with transmission of the virus or simply by mechanical damage to cells. After replication in an initial cell, the lack of receptors poses special problems for plant viruses in recruiting new cells to the infection. These are discussed in Chapter 6.

Some of the best understood examples of virus–receptor interactions are from the *Picornaviridae*. Picornaviruses are unusual in that the virus–receptor interaction has been studied intensively from the viewpoints of both the structural features of the virus responsible for receptor binding and those of the receptor molecule itself. The major *Human rhinovirus* (HRV) receptor molecule ICAM-1 (intercellular adhesion molecule 1), is an adhesion molecule whose normal function is to bind cells to adjacent substrates. Structurally, ICAM-1 is similar to an immunoglobulin molecule, with constant (C) and variable (V) domains homologous to those of antibodies and is regarded as a member of the immunoglobulin superfamily of proteins (Figure 4.7). Similarly, the poliovirus receptor is an integral membrane protein which is also a member of this family, with one variable and two constant domains. Unlike ICAM-1, the normal function of the poliovirus receptor is not known, but a murine homologue has been identified which is structurally similar to the human molecule but does not function as a receptor for poliovirus. However, the existence of two conserved molecules offers an opportunity for studying the molecular interaction of poliovirus with its receptor.

Since the structure of a number of picornavirus **capsids** is known at a resolution of a few angstroms (Chapter 2), it has been possible to determine the features of the virus responsible for **receptor** binding. In human rhinoviruses (HRVs), there is a deep cleft known as the 'canyon' in the surface of each triangular face of the **icosahedral** capsid, which is formed by the flanking monomers, VP1, VP2 and VP3 (Figure 4.8). There is biochemical evidence from a class of inhibitory drugs which block attachment of HRV particles to cells that the interaction between ICAM-1 and the virus particle occurs on the floor of this canyon. Unlike other areas of the virus surface, the amino acid residues forming the internal surfaces of the canyon are relatively invariant. It was suggested that these regions are protected from antigenic pressure because the antibody molecules are too large to fit into the cleft. This is important because radical changes here, although allowing the virus to escape an immune response, would disrupt receptor binding. Subsequently, it has been found that the binding site of the receptor extends well over the edges of the canyon, and the binding sites of neutralizing antibodies extend over the rims of the canyon. Nevertheless, the residues most significant for the binding site of the receptor and for

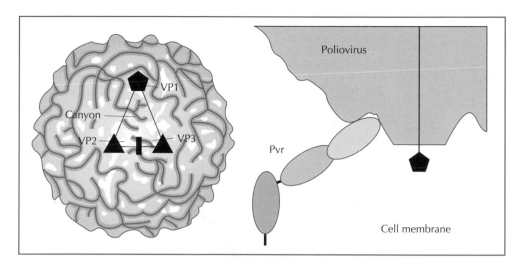

Figure 4.8 Rhinovirus particles have a deep surface cleft known as the 'canyon' between the three monomers (VP1, VP2 and VP3) making up each face of the particle. The poliovirus receptor (Pvr) binds to the base of the 'canyon'.

neutralizing antibodies are separated from each other. In polioviruses, there is a similar canyon which runs around each fivefold vertex of the capsid. The highly variant regions of the capsid to which antibodies bind are located on the 'peaks' on either side of this trough, which is again too narrow to allow antibody binding to the residues at its base. The invariant residues at the sides of the trough interact with the receptor.

Even within the *Picornaviridae* there is variation. Although 90 serotypes of HRV use ICAM-1 as their receptor, some 10 serotypes use proteins related to the low density lipoprotein (LDL) receptor. *Encephalomyocarditis virus* (EMCV) has been reported to use the immunoglobulin molecule vascular cell adhesion factor (VCAM-1) or glycophorin A. Several picornaviruses use integrins as receptors: some echoviruses use VLA-2 or fibronectin; foot-and-mouth disease viruses (FMDV) have been reported to use an unidentified integrin-like molecule. Other echoviruses use decay-accelerating factor (DAF, CD55), a molecule involved in complement function. This list is given to illustrate that even within one structurally related family of viruses, there is considerable variation in the receptor structures used.

Another well-studied example of virus–receptor interaction is that of influenza virus. The haemagglutinin protein forms one of the two types of glycoprotein spikes on the surface of influenza virus particles (see Chapter 2), the other type being formed by the neuraminidase protein. Each haemagglutinin spike is composed of a trimer of three molecules, while the neuraminidase spike consists of a tetramer (Figure 4.9). The haemagglutinin spikes are responsible for binding the influenza virus receptor, which is sialic acid (*N*-acetyl neuraminic acid), a sugar group commonly found on a variety of glycosylated molecules. As a result, there is little cell-type specificity imposed by this

Figure 4.9 Influenza virus glycoprotein spikes.

receptor interaction and therefore influenza viruses bind to a wide variety of different cell types (e.g. causing **haemagglutination** of red blood cells) in addition to the cells in which **productive infection** occurs.

The neuraminidase molecule of influenza virus and paramyxoviruses illustrates another feature of this stage of virus replication. Attachment to cellular receptors is in most cases a reversible process − if **penetration** of the cells does not ensue, the virus can elute from the cell surface. Some viruses have specific mechanisms for detachment and the neuraminidase protein is one of these. Neuraminidase is an esterase which cleaves sialic acid from sugar side-chains. This is particularly important for influenza. Because the receptor molecule is so widely distributed, the virus tends to bind inappropriately to a variety of cells and even cell debris. However, elution from the cell surface after receptor binding has occurred often leads to changes in the virus (e.g. loss or structural alteration of **virus–attachment protein**) which decrease or eliminate the possibility of subsequent attachment to other cells. Thus in the case of influenza, cleavage of sialic acid residues by neuraminidase leaves these groups bound to the active site of the haemagglutinin, preventing that particular molecule from binding to another receptor.

In many if not most cases, the expression (or absence) of receptors on the surface of cells largely determines the **tropism** of a virus, i.e. the type of host cell in which it is able to replicate. In some cases, intracellular blocks at later stages of replication are responsible for determining the range of cell types in which a virus can carry out a productive infection, but this is not common. Therefore, this initial stage of replication and the very first interaction between the virus and the host cell has a major influence on virus pathogenesis and in determining the course of a virus infection.

In some cases, interactions with more than one protein are required for virus entry. These are not examples of alternative **receptor** use since neither protein alone is a functional receptor – both are required to act in concert. An example is the process by which adenoviruses enter cells. This requires a two-stage process involving an initial interaction of the virion fibre protein with a range of cellular receptors, including the MHC (major histocompatibility complex) class I molecule and the coxsackievirus–adenovirus receptor (CAR). Another virion protein, the penton base, then binds to the integrin family of cell surface heterodimers, allowing internalization of the particle via receptor-mediated endocytosis. Most cells express primary receptors for the adenovirus fibre coat protein; however, the internalization step is more selective, giving rise to a degree of cell selection.

A similar observation has been made with HIV, although here the effects of receptors on determining cell tropism are more profound. The primary receptor for HIV is the helper T cell differentiation antigen, CD4. Transfection of human cells which do not normally express CD4 (such as epithelial cells) with recombinant CD4 expression constructs renders them permissive for HIV infection. However, transfection of rodent cells with human CD4 expression vectors does not permit productive HIV infection. If HIV **provirus** DNA is inserted into rodent cells by transfection, virus is produced, indicating that there is no intracellular block to infection. Therefore, there must be one or more accessory factors in addition to CD4 which are required to form a functional HIV receptor. These are a family of proteins known as β-chemokine receptors. Several members of this family have been shown to play a role in the entry of HIV into cells, and their distribution may be the primary control for the **tropism** of HIV for different cell types (lymphocytes, macrophages, etc.). Furthermore, there is evidence that in at least some cell types, HIV infection is not blocked by competing soluble CD4, indicating that in these cells a completely different receptor strategy may be being used. Several candidate molecules have been put forward to fill this role, e.g. galactosylceramide and various other candidate proteins. However, if any or all of these do allow HIV to infect a range of CD4-negative cells, this process is much less efficient than the interaction of the virus with its major receptor complex.

In some cases, specific receptor binding can be side-stepped by non-specific or inappropriate interactions between virus particles and cells. It is possible that virus particles can be 'accidentally' taken up by cells via processes such as pinocytosis or phagocytosis (see below). However, in the absence of some form of physical interaction which holds the virus particle in close association with the cell surface, the frequency with which these accidental events happen is very low. On occasions, antibody-coated virus particles binding to Fc receptor molecules on the surface of monocytes and other blood cells can result in virus uptake. This phenomenon has been shown to occur in a number of cases where antibody–dependent enhancement of virus uptake results in unexpected findings. For example, the presence of antivirus antibodies can occasionally result in increased virus uptake by cells and increased pathogenicity rather than virus neutralization, as would normally be expected. It has been suggested that this mechanism may also be important in the uptake of HIV by macrophages and monocytes and that this might be a factor in the pathogenesis of AIDS, although this is not yet certain.

Penetration

Penetration of the target cell normally occurs a very short time after attachment of the virus to its **receptor** in the cell membrane. Unlike attachment, cell penetration is generally an energy–dependent process, i.e. the cell must be metabolically active for this to occur. Three main mechanisms are involved:

1 Translocation of the entire virus particle across the cytoplasmic membrane of the cell (Figure 4.10). This process is relatively rare among viruses and is poorly understood. It must be mediated by proteins in the virus **capsid** and specific membrane receptors.

2 Endocytosis of the virus into intracellular vacuoles (Figure 4.11). This is probably the most common mechanism of virus entry into cells. It does not require any specific virus proteins (other than those already utilized for receptor binding) but relies on the normal formation and internalization of coated pits at the cell membrane. Receptor-mediated endocytosis is an efficient process for taking up and concentrating extracellular macromolecules.

3 **Fusion** of the virus **envelope** (only applicable to enveloped viruses) with the cell membrane, either directly at the cell surface or following endocytosis in a cytoplasmic vesicle (Figure 4.12). Fusion requires the presence of a specific fusion protein in the virus envelope, e.g. influenza haemagglutinin or retrovirus transmembrane (TM) glycoproteins. These proteins promote the joining of the cellular and virus membranes which results in the **nucleocapsid** being deposited directly in the cytoplasm. There are two types of virus-driven membrane fusion: one is pH–dependent and the other is pH–independent.

The process, of endocytosis is almost universal in animal cells and requires further consideration (Figure 4.11). The formation of coated pits results in the engulfment of a membrane-bounded vesicle by the cytoplasm of the cell. The lifetime of these initial coated vesicles is very short. Within seconds, most fuse with endosomes, releasing their contents into these larger vesicles. At this point, any virus contained within these structures is still cut off from the cytoplasm by a lipid bilayer and therefore has not strictly entered the cell. Moreover, as endosomes fuse with lysosomes, the environment inside these vessels becomes progressively more hostile as they are acid-

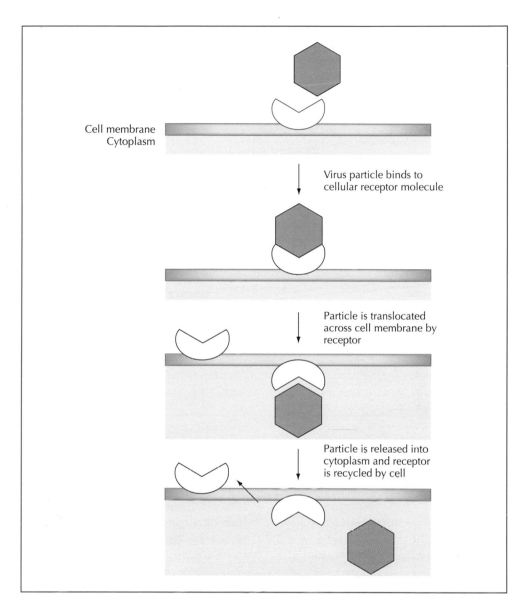

Cell membrane
Cytoplasm

Virus particle binds to
cellular receptor molecule

Particle is translocated
across cell membrane by
receptor

Particle is released into
cytoplasm and receptor
is recycled by cell

Figure 4.10 Translocation of entire virus particles across the cell membrane by cell
surface receptors.

ified and the pH falls, while the concentration of degradative enzymes rises. This
means that the virus must leave the vesicle and enter the cytoplasm before it is
degraded. There are a number of mechanisms by which this occurs, including membrane **fusion** and rescue by transcytosis. The release of virus particles from endosomes and their passage into the cytoplasm is intimately connected with (and often
impossible to separate from) the process of uncoating (see below).

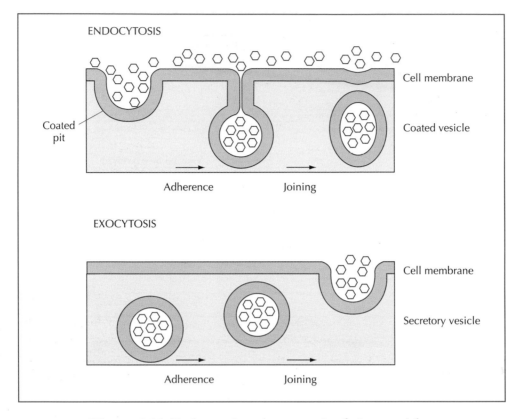

Figure 4.11 Endocytosis and exocytosis of virus particles.

Uncoating

Uncoating is a general term for the events which occur after **penetration**, in which the virus **capsid** is completely or partially removed and the virus **genome** exposed, usually in the form of a nucleoprotein complex. Unfortunately, uncoating is one of the stages of virus replication that has been least studied and is relatively poorly understood.

In one sense, the removal of a virus **envelope** which occurs during membrane fusion is part of the uncoating process. Fusion between virus envelopes and endosomal membranes is driven by virus fusion proteins. These are usually activated by the uncloaking of a previously hidden fusion domain as a result of conformational changes in the protein induced by the low pH inside the vesicle, although in some cases the fusion activity is triggered directly by **receptor** binding. The initial events in uncoating may occur inside endosomes, being triggered by the change in pH as the endosome is acidified, or directly in the cytoplasm. Ionophores such as monesin or nigericin or cations such as chloroquine and ammonium chloride can be used to block the acidification of these vesicles and to determine whether events are occur-

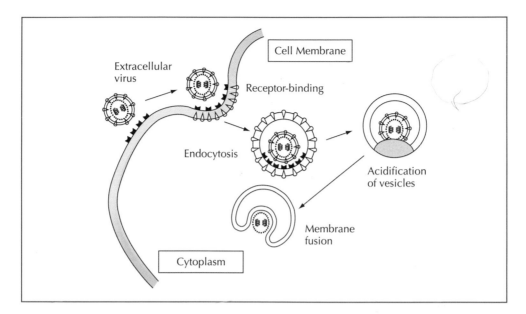

Figure 4.12 Virus–induced membrane fusion. This process is dependent on the presence of a specific fusion protein on the surface of the virus which, under particular circumstances (e.g. acidification of the virus-containing vesicle), becomes activated, inducing fusion of the vesicle membrane and the virus envelope.

ring following the acidification of endosomes (e.g. pH-dependent membrane fusion) or directly at the cell surface or in the cytoplasm (e.g. pH-independent membrane fusion). Endocytosis has some danger for viruses, since if they remain in the vesicle too long they will be irreversibly damaged by acidification or lysosomal enzymes. Some viruses can control this process, e.g. the influenza virus M2 protein is a membrane channel which allows entry of hydrogen ions into the **nucleocapsid**, facilitating uncoating. The M2 protein is multifunctional and also has a role in influenza virus **maturation** (below).

In picornaviruses, **penetration** of the cytoplasm by exit of virus from endosomes is tightly linked to uncoating (Figure 4.13). The acidic environment of the endosome causes a conformational change in the **capsid** which reveals hydrophobic domains not present on the surface of mature virus particles. The interaction of these hydrophobic patches with the endosomal membrane is believed to form pores through which the **genome** passes into the cytoplasm.

The product of uncoating depends on the structure of the virus nucleocapsid. In some cases, this might be relatively simple (e.g. picornaviruses have a small basic protein of approximately 23 amino acids (VPg) covalently attached to the 5′ end of the vRNA genome), or may be highly complex (e.g. retrovirus cores are highly ordered nucleoprotein complexes which contain, in addition to the diploid RNA genome, the reverse transcriptase enzyme responsible for converting the virus RNA genome

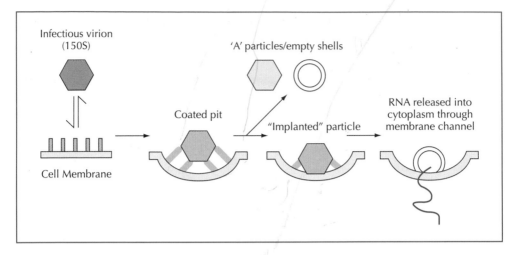

Figure 4.13 Cell penetration and uncoating of polioviruses.

into the DNA **provirus**). The structure and chemistry of the nucleocapsid determines the subsequent steps in replication. As discussed in Chapter 3, reverse transcription can only occur inside an ordered retrovirus core particle and cannot proceed with the components of the reaction free in solution. Herpesvirus, adenovirus and polyomavirus capsids undergo structural changes following **penetration**, but overall remain largely intact. These capsids contain sequences which are responsible for attachment to the cytoskeleton and this interaction allows the transport of the entire capsid to the nucleus. It is at the nuclear pores that uncoating occurs and the **nucleocapsid** passes into the nucleus. In reoviruses and poxviruses, complete uncoating does not occur, and many of the reactions of genome replication are catalysed by virus–encoded enzymes inside cytoplasmic particles which still resemble the mature **virions**.

Genome replication and gene expression

The replication strategy of any virus depends on the nature of its genetic material. In this respect, all viruses can be divided into seven groups. Such a scheme was first proposed by David Baltimore in 1971. Originally, this classification included only six groups, but it has since been extended to include the scheme of **genome** replication used by the hepadnaviruses and caulimoviruses. For viruses with RNA genomes in particular, genome replication and the expression of genetic information are inextricably linked. Therefore, both of these criteria are taken into account in the scheme below. The control of gene expression determines the overall course of a virus infection (acute, chronic, persistent or latent) and such is the emphasis placed on gene expression by molecular biologists that this subject is discussed in detail in Chapter 5. A schematic overview of the major events during replication of the different virus genomes is shown in Figure 4.14 and a complete list of all the families which constitute each class is given in Appendix 2 ⊘ .

- *Class I: Double-stranded DNA.* This class can be subdivided into two further groups:

  (a) Replication is exclusively nuclear (Figure 4.14). The replication of these viruses is relatively dependent on cellular factors.
  (b) Replication occurs in cytoplasm (*Poxviridae*). These viruses have evolved (or acquired) all the necessary factors for transcription and replication of their genomes and are therefore largely independent of the cellular machinery.

- *Class II: Single-stranded DNA* (Figure 4.15). Replication occurs in the nucleus, involving the formation of a double-stranded intermediate which serves as a template for the synthesis of single-stranded progeny DNA.
- *Class III: Double-stranded RNA* (Figure 4.16). These viruses have segmented genomes. Each segment is transcribed separately to produce individual **mono-cistronic** mRNAs.
- *Class IV: Single-stranded (+)sense RNA.* These can be subdivided into two groups:

  (a) Viruses with **polycistronic** mRNA (Figure 4.17). As with all the viruses in this class, the genome RNA forms the mRNA. This is translated to form a **polyprotein** product, which is subsequently cleaved to form the mature proteins.

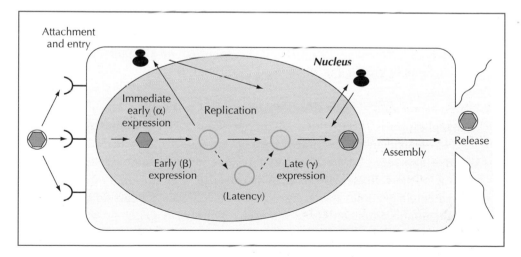

Figure 4.14 Schematic representation of the pattern of replication of Class I viruses. Details of the events which occur for genomes of each type are given in the text.

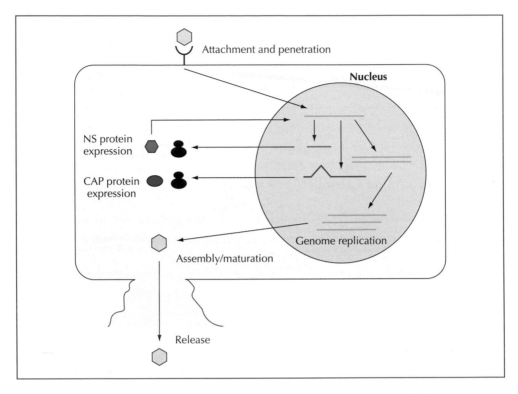

Figure 4.15 Schematic representation of the pattern of replication of Class II viruses.

(b) Viruses with complex transcription. Two rounds of translation (e.g. *Togavirus*) or subgenomic RNAs (e.g. *Tobamovirus*) are necessary to produce the genomic RNA.

■ *Class V: Single-stranded (−)sense RNA.* As discussed in Chapters 3 and 5, the genomes of these viruses can be divided into two types:

(a) Non-segmented genomes (order *Mononegvirales*) (Figure 4.18). The first step in replication is transcription of the (−)sense RNA genome by the virion RNA–dependent RNA polymerase to produce monocistronic mRNAs, which also serve as the template for subsequent genome replication. N.B. Some of these viruses also have an **ambisense** organization.

(b) Segmented genomes (*Orthomyxoviridae*). Replication occurs in the nucleus, with monocistronic mRNAs for each of the virus genes produced by the virus **transcriptase** from the full-length virus genome (see Chapter 5).

■ *Class VI: Single-stranded (+)sense RNA with DNA intermediate* (Figure 4.19). Retrovirus genomes are (+)sense RNA but unique in that they are diploid, and

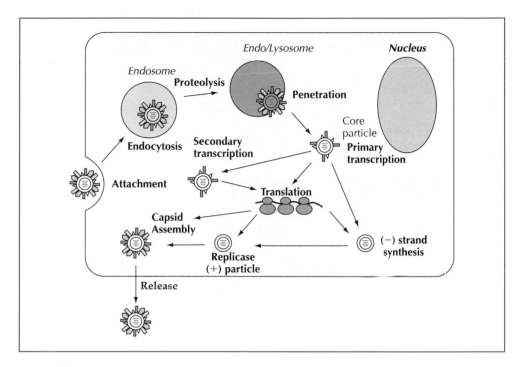

Figure 4.16 Schematic representation of the pattern of replication of Class III viruses.

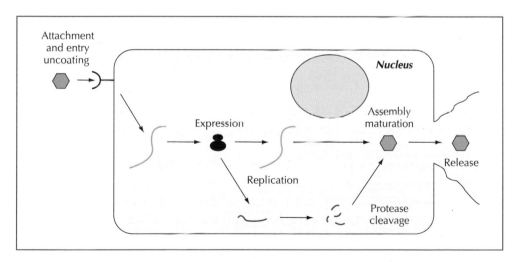

Figure 4.17 Schematic representation of the pattern of replication of Class IV viruses.

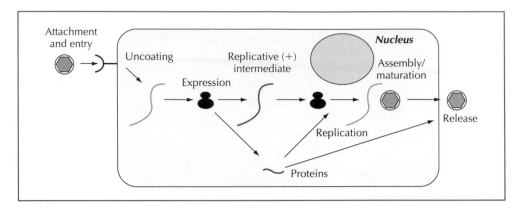

Figure 4.18 Schematic representation of the pattern of replication of Class V viruses.

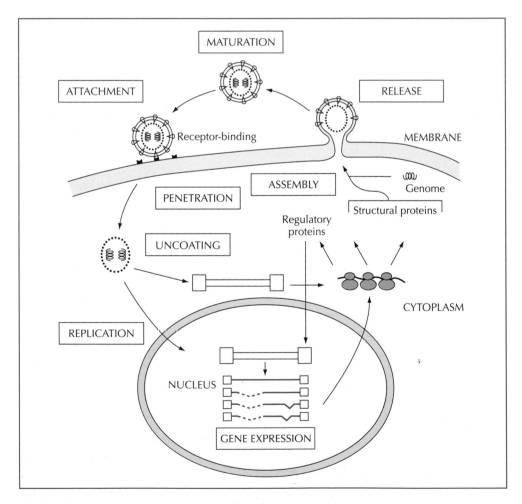

Figure 4.19 Schematic representation of the pattern of replication of Class VI viruses.

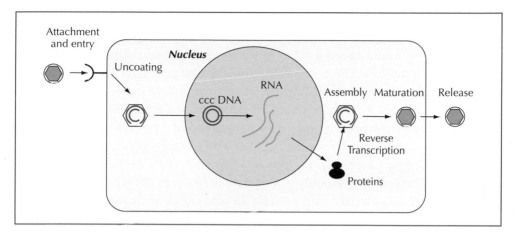

Figure 4.20 Schematic representation of the pattern of replication of Class VII viruses.

that they do not serve directly as mRNA, but as a template for reverse transcription into DNA (see Chapter 3).

- *Class VII: Double-stranded DNA with RNA intermediate* (Figure 4.20). This group of viruses also relies on reverse transcription, but unlike the retroviruses (class VI), this occurs inside the virus particle during maturation. On infection of a new cell, the first event to occur is repair of the gapped genome, followed by transcription (see Chapter 3).

Assembly

The **assembly** process involves the collection of all the components necessary for the formation of the mature **virion** at a particular site in the cell. During assembly, the basic structure of the virus particle is formed. The site of assembly depends on the site of replication within the cell and on the mechanism by which the virus is eventually released from the cell and varies for different viruses. For example in picornaviruses, poxviruses and reoviruses assembly occurs in the cytoplasm; in adenoviruses, polyomaviruses and parvoviruses it occurs in the nucleus.

As with the early stages of replication, it is not always possible to identify the assembly, **maturation** and **release** of virus particles as distinct and separate phases. The site of assembly has a profound influence on all these processes. In the majority of cases, cellular membranes are used to anchor virus proteins, and this initiates the process of assembly. In spite of considerable study, the control of virus assembly is generally not well understood. In general, it is thought that rising intracellular levels of virus proteins and **genome** molecules reach a critical concentration and this triggers the process. Many viruses achieve high levels of newly synthesized structural components by concentrating these into subcellular compartments, visible in light microscopes, which are known as **inclusion bodies**. These are a common feature of the late stages of infection of cells by many different viruses. The size and location of inclusion bodies in infected cells is often highly characteristic of particular viruses, e.g. rabies virus infection results in large perinuclear 'Negri bodies', first observed by Adelchi Negri in 1903. Alternatively, local concentrations of virus structural components can be boosted by lateral interactions between membrane-associated proteins. This mechanism is particularly important in **enveloped** viruses which are released from the cell by **budding** (see below).

As discussed in Chapter 2, the formation of virus particles may be a relatively simple process which is driven only by interactions between the subunits of the **capsid** and controlled by the rules of symmetry. In other cases, assembly is a highly complex, multi-step process involving not only virus structural proteins, but in addition virus-encoded and cellular scaffolding proteins which act as templates to guide the assembly of **virions**. The encapsidation of the virus genome may occur either early in the assembly of the particle (e.g. many viruses with **helical** symmetry are nucleated on the genome), or at a late stage, when the genome is stuffed into an almost completed protein shell.

Maturation

This is the stage of the life-cycle at which the virus becomes infectious. **Maturation** usually involves structural changes in the virus particle which may result from specific cleavages of **capsid** proteins to form the mature products or conformational changes in proteins during assembly. Such events frequently lead to substantial structural changes in the capsid which may be detectable by criteria such as differences in the antigenicity of incomplete and mature virus particles, which in some cases (e.g. picornaviruses) alters radically. Alternatively, internal structural alterations, for example the condensation of nucleoproteins with the virus **genome**, often results in such changes.

Virus proteases are frequently involved in maturation, although cellular enzymes or a mixture of virus and cellular enzymes are used in some cases. Clearly, there is a danger in relying on cellular proteolytic enzymes in that their relative lack of substrate specificity could easily completely degrade the capsid proteins. However, virus-encoded proteases are usually highly specific for particular amino acid sequences and structures, frequently only cutting one particular peptide bond in a large and complex virus capsid. Moreover, they are often further controlled by being packaged into virus particles during assembly and are only activated when brought into close contact with their target sequence by the conformation of the capsid, e.g. by being placed in a local hydrophobic environment or by changes of pH or metal ion concentration inside the **capsid**. Retrovirus proteases are good examples of enzymes involved in maturation which are under this tight control. The retrovirus core particle is composed of proteins from the gag gene and the protease is packaged into the core before its **release** from the cell on **budding**. At some stage of the budding process (the exact timing varies for different retroviruses) the protease cleaves the gag protein precursors into the mature products – the capsid, nucleocapsid and matrix proteins of the mature virus particle (Figure 4.21).

Not all protease cleavage events involved in maturation are this tightly regulated. Native influenza virus haemagglutinin undergoes post-translational modification (glycosylation in the Golgi apparatus) and at this stage exhibits receptor-binding activity. However, the protein must be cleaved into two fragments (HA1 and HA2) to be able to promote membrane **fusion** during infection. Cellular trypsin-like

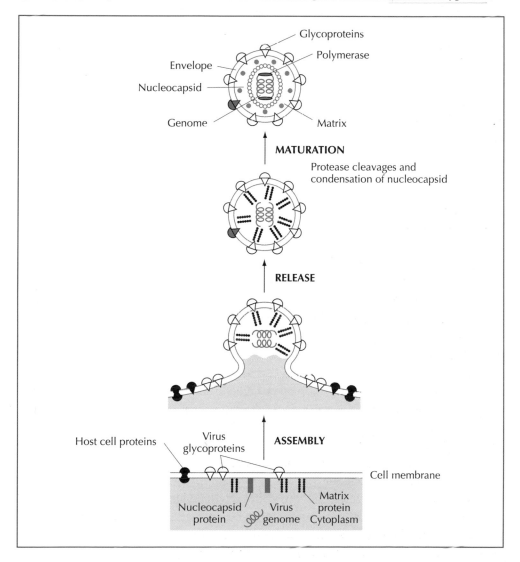

Figure 4.21 Virus release by budding. This is the process by which enveloped virus particles acquire their membranes and associated proteins.

enzymes are responsible for this process, which occurs in secretory vesicles as the virus buds into them prior to **release** at the cell surface. Amantadine and rimantadine are two drugs which are active against influenza A viruses (Chapter 6). The action of these closely related agents is complex and incompletely understood, but they are believed to block cellular membrane ion channels. The target for both drugs is the influenza matrix protein (M_2), but resistance to the drug may also map to the haemagglutinin gene. The replication of some strains of influenza virus is inhibited at the cell **penetration** stage and that of others at maturation. The biphasic action of these drugs results from the inability of drug-treated cells to lower the pH of the endosomal compartment (a function normally controlled by the M_2 gene product), and hence to cleave haemagglutinin during maturation. Similarly, retrovirus **envelope** glycoproteins require cleavage into the surface (SU) and transmembrane (TM) proteins for activity. This process is also carried out by cellular enzymes, but is in general poorly understood.

As already stated, for some viruses, assembly and maturation occur inside the cell and are inseparable, whereas for others, maturation events may occur only after release of the virus particle from the cell. In all cases, the process of maturation prepares the particle for the infection of subsequent cells.

Release

As described earlier, plant viruses face particular difficulties imposed by the structure of plant cell walls when it comes to leaving cells and infecting others. In response, they have evolved particular strategies to overcome this problem which are discussed in detail in Chapter 6. All other viruses escape the cell by one of two mechanisms. For **lytic** viruses (such as most non-enveloped viruses), **release** is a simple process – the infected cell breaks open and releases the virus. **Enveloped viruses** acquire their lipid membrane as the virus buds out of the cell through the cell membrane or into an intracellular vesicle prior to subsequent release. **Virion** envelope proteins are picked up during this process as the virus particle is extruded. This process is known as **budding**. Release of virus particles in this way may be highly damaging to the cell (e.g. paramyxoviruses, rhabdoviruses and togaviruses) or alternatively may not be (e.g. retroviruses), but in either case, the process is controlled by the virus - the physical interaction of the **capsid** proteins on the inner surface of the cell membrane forces the particle out through the membrane (Figure 4.15). As mentioned earlier, assembly, maturation and release are usually simultaneous processes for viruses which are released by budding. The type of membrane from which the virus buds depends on the virus concerned. In most cases, budding involves cytoplasmic membranes (retroviruses; togaviruses, orthomyxoviruses; paramyxoviruses; bunyaviruses; coronaviruses; rhabdoviruses; hepadnaviruses), but in some cases can involve the nuclear membrane (herpesviruses).

The release of mature virus particles from susceptible host cells by budding presents a problem in that these particles are designed to enter, rather than leave, cells.

How do these particles manage to leave the cell surface? The details are not known but there are clues as to how the process is achieved. Certain virus **envelope** proteins are involved in the **release** phase of replication as well as in the initiating steps. A good example of this is the neuraminidase protein of influenza virus. In addition to being able to reverse the attachment of virus particles to cells via haemagglutinin, neuraminidase is also believed to be important in preventing the aggregation of influenza virus particles and may well have a role in virus release. This process is targeted by the drug Relenza (Chapter 6).

In addition to using specific proteins, viruses which bud have also solved the problem of release by the careful timing of the assembly–maturation–release pathway. Although it may not be possible to separate these stages by means of biochemical analysis, this does not mean that careful spatial separation of these processes has not evolved as a means to solve this problem. Similarly, although we may not understand all the subtleties of the many conformation changes which occur in virus **capsids** and envelopes during these late stages of replication, virus replication clearly works, despite our deficiencies!

SUMMARY

In general terms, virus replication involves three broad stages which are carried out by all types of virus: the initiation of infection, replication and expression of the **genome**, and finally, the **release** of mature **virions** from the infected cell. At a detailed level, there are many differences between the replication processes of different viruses. These are imposed by the biology of the host cell and the nature of the virus genome. Nevertheless, it is possible to derive an overview of virus replication with common stages which, in one form or another, are followed by all viruses.

FURTHER READING

Berger, E.A., Murphy, P. M., Farber, J.M. (1999). Chemokine receptors as HIV-1 coreceptors: roles in viral entry, tropism, and disease. *Annual Review of Immunology* 17: 657–700.

Cann, A.J. (2000). *DNA Virus Replication: Frontiers in Molecular Biology*. Oxford University Press, Oxford. ISBN 019963713X.

Ellis, E.L. and Delbruck, M. (1939). The growth of bacteriophage. *Journal of General Physiology* 22: 365–384.

Guo, P. (Ed.) (1994). Virus assembly. *Seminars in Virology* 5: No.1.

Hershey, A.D. and Chase, M. (1952). Independent functions of viral protein and nucleic acid in growth of bacteriophage. *Journal of General Physiology* 26: 36–56.

Kasamatsu, H. and Nakanishi, A. (1998). How do animal DNA viruses get to the nucleus? *Annual Review of Microbiology* 52: 627–686.

Rossmann, M.G., Bella, J., Kolatkar, P. R., He, Y., Wimmer, E., Kuhn, R.J. and Baker, T.S.[HSJ1] (2000). Cell recognition and entry by rhino- and enteroviruses. *Virology* 269: 239–247.

Schneider-Schaulies, J. (2000). Cellular receptors for viruses: links to tropism and pathogenesis. *Journal of General Virology* 81: 1413–1429.

Sommerfelt, M.A. (1999). Retrovirus receptors. *Journal of General Virology* 80: 3049–3064.

Tang, H., Kuhen, K.L. and Wong-Staal, F. (1999). Lentivirus replication and regulation. *Annual Review of Genetics* 33: 133–170.

Self-Assessment Questions

(4.1) Virus replication involves the following distinct phases (true or false?):

T (a)   Initiation of infection.
T (b)   Replication of the virus genome.
T (c)   Expression of the virus genome.
F (d)   Cleavage of the virus genome.
T (e)   Release of mature virions from the infected cell.

(4.2) Are the following statements true or false?

F (a)   The 'single-burst' experiment was performed by Ellis and Delbruck in 1989.
T (b)   The 'single-burst' experiment demonstrates that new virus particles result from the intracellular assembly of preformed components and are released in a batch-like process.
T (c)   The 'single-burst' experiment demonstrates the essential phases of virus replication. "single-burst"
F (d)   The 'Hershey-Chase' experiment demonstrates the essential phases of virus replication.
T (e)   The 'Hershey-Chase' experiment demonstrates that nucleic acid is the genetic material.

(4.3) Are the following statements true or false?

F (a)   Viruses use proteins exclusively as their receptors. + sugars
F (b)   Viruses only have one type of receptor molecule.
F (c)   Plant viruses all use proteins as receptors. No known use receptors
F (d)   Sialic acid is the human rhinovirus receptor. influenza ICAM / LDL
T (e)   The expression of receptors on the surface of cells is the major factor which determines the tropism of a virus.

(4.4) The following are mechanisms by which virus particles penetrate cells (true or false?):

T (a)   Translocation
F (b)   Transfection
F (c)   Exocytosis
T (d)   Endocytosis
T (e)   Fusion.

(4.5) Are the following statements true or false?

T (a)   Virus penetration of cells is an energy-dependent process.
T (b)   Influenza haemagglutinin is a virus fusion protein.
F (c)   Uncoating can occur before or after penetration of the host cell.
F (d)   During uncoating, all proteins are removed from the virus genome.
F (e)   Fusion proteins are responsible for nuclear localization of virus
         genomes.

(4.6) Are the following statements true or false?

F (a)   There are six classes of virus genomes.
F (b)   Class I viruses have circular double-stranded DNA genomes.
T (c)   Class II viruses have (−)sense single-stranded DNA genomes.
F (d)   Class VI viruses (retroviruses) have (×)sense single-stranded RNA
         genomes.
F (e)   Class VII viruses have (+)sense single-stranded RNA genomes.

(4.7) Are the following statements true or false?

T (a)   Adenoviruses encode their own DNA polymerase but are dependent
         on cellular factors for genome replication.
F (b)   Poxviruses encode their own DNA polymerase but are dependent on
         cellular factors for genome replication.
F (c)   Reovirus genomes are transcribed by cellular RNA polymerase.
F (d)   RNA virus genomes always replicate in the cytoplasm of the host
         cell.
T (e)   Retrovirus genomes are transcribed by cellular RNA polymerase.

(4.8) The following viruses replicate their genomes in the <u>cytoplasm</u> of infected cells (true or false?):

T (a)   Picornaviruses, e.g. *Poliovirus.*
T (b)   Poxviruses, e.g. *Vaccinia virus.*
T (c)   Rhabdoviruses, e.g. *Rabies virus.*
T (d)   Paramyxoviruses, e.g. *Respiratory syncytial virus.*
F (e)   Hepadnaviruses, e.g. *Hepatitis B virus.*

(4.9)   The following viruses replicate their genomes in the nucleus of infected cells (true or false?):

T (a)   Herpesviruses, e.g. *Epstein–Barr virus*. ds DNA
T (b)   Parvoviruses, e.g. B19. ss DNA
T (c)   Orthomyxoviruses, e.g. influenza virus. (-) RNA
F (d)   Rotaviruses, e.g. group A rotaviruses. REOVIRIDAE; ds (RNA)
F (e)   Coronaviruses, e.g. OC43. (+) RNA CORONAVIRIDAE

(4.10)   Are the following statements true or false?

T (a)   Maturation usually involves structural changes in the virus particle.
T (b)   Maturation frequently involves protease cleavage of virus proteins.
T (c)   Enveloped viruses acquire their lipid membranes by budding
             through cellular membranes.
T (d)   Virus envelope proteins are acquired during the process of budding.
T (e)   Virus envelope proteins are involved in release from as well as
             attachment to host cells.

Answers to Self-Assessment Questions are given in Appendix 4.

CHAPTER 5

EXPRESSION

Learning Objectives

On completing this chapter, you should be able to:
- Describe a generalized replication cycle for each of the seven virus genome types
- Explain how the pattern of gene expression of a virus is determined by the structure of the virus genome and how it is replicated
- Understand the role of post-transcriptional events in controlling virus gene expression.

EXPRESSION OF GENETIC INFORMATION

The most critical interaction between a virus and its host cell is the requirement by the virus for the cellular apparatus of nucleic acid and protein synthesis. The course of virus replication is determined by tight control of gene expression. There are fundamental differences in the control of these processes in **prokaryotic** and **eukaryotic** cells. These differences inevitably affect the viruses that utilize them as hosts. In addition, the relative simplicity and compact size of virus **genomes** (compared with those of even the simplest cell) imposes further constraints. Cells have evolved varied and complex mechanisms for controlling gene expression by utilizing their extensive genetic capacity. Conversely, viruses have had to achieve highly specific quantitative, temporal, and spatial control of expression with much more limited genetic resources. Aspects of this problem have already been discussed in Chapters 3 and 4.

Viruses have counteracted their genetic limitations by the evolution of a range of solutions to these problems. These mechanisms include:

- Powerful positive and negative signals which promote or repress gene expression
- Highly compressed genomes in which overlapping reading frames are commonplace
- Control signals which are frequently nested within other genes
- Several strategies designed to create multiple polypeptides from a single messenger RNA.

Gene expression involves regulatory loops mediated by signals which act either in *cis* (affecting the activity of contiguous genetic regions) or in *trans* (giving rise to diffusible products which act on regulatory sites whether or not these are contiguous with the site from which they are produced). For example, transcription **promoters** are *cis*-acting sequences that are located adjacent to the genes whose transcription they control, while proteins such as 'transcription factors', which bind to specific sequences present on any stretch of nucleic acid present in the cell, are examples of *trans*-acting factors. The relative simplicity of virus **genomes** and the elegance of their control mechanisms are models that form the basis of our current understanding of genetic regulation.

This chapter assumes familiarity with the mechanisms involved in cellular control of gene expression. However, to illustrate the details of virus gene expression, a very brief summary of some pertinent aspects is given below.

CONTROL OF PROKARYOTE GENE EXPRESSION

Bacterial cells are second only to viruses in the specificity and economy of their genetic control mechanisms and possibly foremost in terms of the intensity with which these mechanisms have been studied. Genetic control is exercised both at the level of transcription and at subsequent (post-transcriptional) stages of gene expression.

The initiation of transcription is regulated primarily in a negative fashion by the synthesis of *trans*-acting repressor proteins, which bind to operator sequences upstream of protein-coding sequences. Collections of metabolically related genes are grouped together and co-ordinately controlled as 'operons'. Transcription of these operons typically produces a polycistronic **mRNA** that encodes several different proteins. During subsequent stages of expression, transcription is also regulated by a number of mechanisms which act, in Mark Ptashne's famous phrase, as 'genetic switches', turning on or off the transcription of different genes. Such mechanisms include antitermination, which is controlled by *trans*-acting factors that promote the synthesis of longer transcripts encoding additional genetic information, and by various modifications of RNA polymerase. Bacterial σ (sigma) factors are apoproteins which affect the specificity of the RNA polymerase holoenzyme for different **promoters**. Several **bacteriophages** (e.g. **phage** SP01 of *Bacillus subtilis*) encode proteins which function as alternative σ factors, sequestering RNA polymerase and altering the rate at which phage genes are transcribed. Phage T4 of *Escherichia coli* encodes an enzyme which carries out a covalent modification (ADP-ribosylation) of the host cell RNA polymerase. This is believed to eliminate the requirement of the polymerase holoenzyme for σ factor and to achieve an effect similar to the production of modified σ factors by other bacteriophages.

At a post-transcriptional level, gene expression in bacteria is also regulated by control of translation. The best known virus examples of this phenomenon come from study of bacteriophages of the family *Leviviridae*, such as R17, MS2 and Qβ. In these phages, the secondary structure of the single-stranded RNA phage **genome** not only regulates the quantities of different phage proteins that are translated, but also operates temporal control of a switch in the ratios between the different proteins produced in infected cells.

CONTROL OF EXPRESSION IN BACTERIOPHAGE λ

The **genome** of **phage** λ has probably been studied in more detail than any other and illustrates several of the mechanisms described above, including the action of repressor proteins in regulating **lysogeny** versus **lytic** replication and antitermination of transcription by phage-encoded *trans*-acting factors. Such has been the impact of these discoveries that no discussion of the control of virus gene expression could be considered complete without detailed examination of this phage.

Phage λ was discovered by Esther Lederberg in 1949. Experiments at the Pasteur Institute by André Lwoff in 1950 showed that some strains of *Bacillus megaterium*, when irradiated with ultraviolet light, stopped growing and subsequently lysed, releasing a crop of bacteriophage particles. Together with Francois Jacob and Jaques Monod, Lwoff subsequently showed that the cells of some bacterial strains carried a bacteriophage in a dormant form, known as a **prophage**, and that the phage could be made to alternate between the lysogenic (non-productive) and lytic (productive) growth cycles.

After many years of study, our understanding of λ has been refined into a picture that represents one of the best understood and most elegant genetic control systems yet to be investigated. A simplified genetic map of λ is shown in Figure 5.1. For regulation of the growth cycle of the phage, the structural genes encoding the head and tail components of the virus **capsid** can be ignored. The pertinent components involved in genetic control are as follows:

1 P_L is the promoter responsible for transcription of the left-hand side of the λ genome, including *N* and *cIII*.

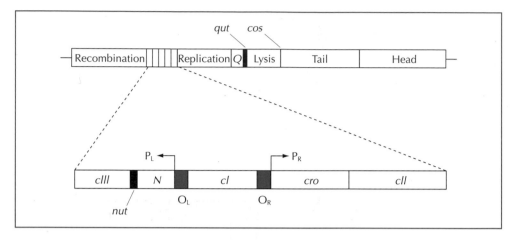

Figure 5.1 Simplified genetic map of bacteriophage λ.

2 O_L is a short, non-coding region of the phage genome (approximately 50 bp) which lies between the *cI* and *N* genes next to P_L.

3 P_R is the promoter responsible for transcription of the right-hand side of the λ genome, including *cro*, *cII*, and the genes encoding the structural proteins.

4 O_R is a short, non-coding region of the phage genome (approximately 50 bp) which lies between the *cI* and *cro* genes next to P_R.

5 *cI* is transcribed from its own promoter and encodes a repressor protein of 236 amino acids which binds to O_R preventing transcription of *cro* but allowing transcription of *cI*, and to O_L, preventing transcription of *N* and the other genes in the left-hand end of the genome.

6 *cII* and *cIII* encode activator proteins which bind to the genome, enhancing the transcription of the *cI* gene.

7 *cro* encodes a 66 amino acid protein which binds to O_R, blocking binding of the repressor to this site.

8 *N* encodes an antiterminator protein which acts as an alternative ρ (rho) factor for host cell RNA polymerase, modifying its activity and permitting extensive transcription from P_L and P_R.

9 *Q* is an antiterminator similar to *N*, but only permits extended transcription from P_R.

In a newly infected cell, *N* and *cro* are transcribed from P_L and P_R, respectively (Figure 5.2). The N protein allows RNA polymerase to transcribe a number of phage genes, including those responsible for DNA **recombination** and integration of the prophage, as well as *cII* and *cIII*. The N protein acts as a positive transcription regulator. In the absence of the N protein, the RNA polymerase holoenzyme stops at certain sequences located at the end of the *N* and *Q* genes, known as the *nut* and *qut* sites, respectively. However, RNA polymerase–N protein complexes are able to over-

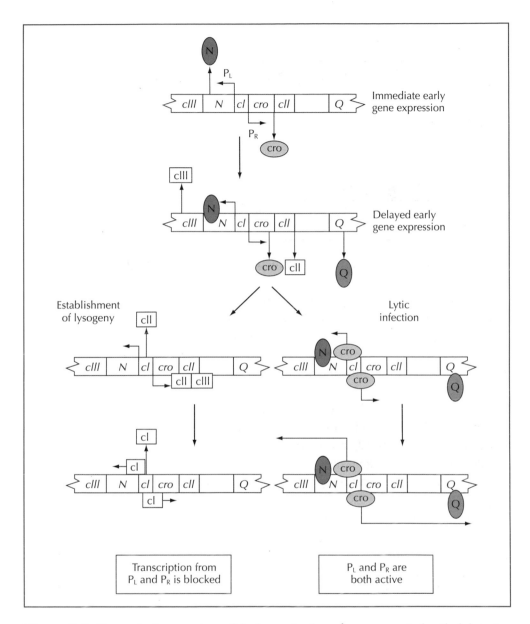

Figure 5.2 Control of expression of the bacteriophage λ genome. A detailed description of the events which occur in a newly infected cell and during lytic infection or lysogeny is given in the text.

come this restriction and permit full transcription from P_L and P_R. The RNA polymerase–Q protein complex results in extended transcription from P_R only. As levels of the cII and cIII proteins in the cell build up, transcription of the *cI* repressor gene from its own promoter is turned on.

It is at this point that the critical event occurs which determines the outcome of the infection. The cII protein is constantly degraded by proteases present in the cell. If levels of cII remain below a critical level, transcription from P_R and P_L continues and the phage undergoes a productive replication cycle which culminates in lysis of the cell and the **release** of phage particles. This is the sequence of events that occurs in the vast majority of infected cells. However, in a few rare instances, the concentration of cII protein builds up, transcription of *cI* is enhanced and intracellular levels of the cI repressor protein rise. The repressor binds to O_R and O_L, which prevents transcription of all phage genes (and in particular *cro*: see below) except itself. The level of cI protein is maintained automatically by a negative feedback mechanism, since at high concentrations the repressor also binds to the left-hand end of O_R and prevents transcription of *cI* (Figure 5.3). This autoregulation of cI synthesis keeps the cell in a stable state of **lysogeny**.

If this is the case, how do such cells ever leave this state and enter a productive, **lytic** replication cycle? Physiological stress and particularly ultraviolet irradiation of

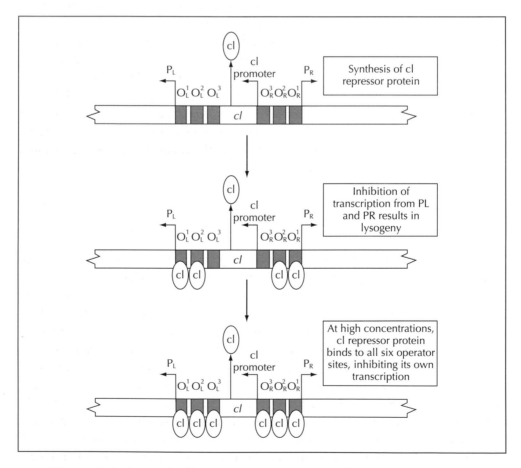

Figure 5.3 Control of lysogeny in bacteriophage λ. See text for details.

cells results in the induction of a host cell protein, RecA. This protein, whose normal function is to induce the expression of cellular genes which permit the cell to adapt to and survive in altered environmental conditions, cleaves the cI repressor protein. In itself, this would not be sufficient to prevent the cell re-entering the lysogenic state. However, when repressor protein is not bound to O_R, *cro* is transcribed from P_R. Cro also binds to O_R but unlike cI, which preferentially binds the right-hand end of O_R, the Cro protein binds preferentially to the left-hand end of O_R, preventing the transcription of *cI* and enhancing its own transcription in a positive feedback loop. Thus, the phage is locked into a lytic cycle and cannot return to the lysogenic state.

This description is a highly simplified version of the genetic control of expression in phage λ. A great deal of detail is known about the molecular mechanisms by which the above systems work, but since this could easily fill a whole book on its own there is insufficient space to recount all of it here. The molecular details of the λ system are not only of isolated interest, but have shaped our understanding of genetic regulation in **prokaryotic** and also in **eukaryotic** cells. Determination of the structures of the proteins involved in the above scheme has identified the fundamental principles by which many proteins from unrelated organisms can recognize and bind to specific sequences in DNA molecules. The concepts of proteins with independent DNA-binding and dimerization domains, protein cooperativity in DNA binding and DNA looping allowing proteins bound at distant sites to interact with one another have all arisen from the study of λ. It is important to read the references given at the end of this chapter to understand fully the nuances of gene expression in this complex bacteriophage, but also to remember the design and operation of this system when reading the examples of the regulation of gene expression described in the rest of this chapter.

CONTROL OF EUKARYOTE GENE EXPRESSION

Control of gene expression in **eukaryotic** cells is much more complex than in prokaryotic cells, and involves a 'multilayered' approach in which diverse control mechanisms exert their effects at multiple levels. The first level of control occurs prior to transcription and depends on the local configuration of the DNA. DNA in eukaryotic cells has an elaborate structure, forming complicated and dynamic but far from random complexes with numerous proteins to form **chromatin**. Although the contents of eukaryotic cell nuclei appear amorphous in electron micrographs (at least in interphase), they are actually highly ordered. Chromatin interacts with the structural backbone of the nucleus, the nuclear matrix, and these interactions are thought to be important in controlling gene expression. Locally, nucleosome configuration and DNA conformation, particularly the formation of left-handed helical 'Z–DNA', are also important. DNAse I digestion of chromatin does not give an even, uniform digestion pattern, but reveals particular 'DNAse hypersensitive' sites believed to indicate differences in the function of various regions of the chromatin. It is possible, for example, that retroviruses are more likely to integrate into the host cell genome at these sites than elsewhere. Transcriptionally active DNA is also hypomethylated, i.e. there is a relative paucity of nucleotides modified by the covalent attachment of methyl groups in these regions compared with the frequency of methylation in transcriptionally quiescent regions of the genome. The methylation of Moloney murine leukaemia virus sequences in pre-implantation mouse embryos has been shown to suppress the transcription of the **provirus** genome.

The second level of control rests in the process of transcription itself, which again is much more complex than in prokaryotes. There are three forms of RNA polymerase in eukaryotic cells which can be distinguished by their relative sensitivities to the drug α-amanitin and which show specificities for different classes of genes (Table 5.1). The rate at which transcription is initiated is a key control point in eukaryotic gene expression. Initiation is influenced dramatically by sequences upstream of the transcription start site, which function by acting as recognition sites for families of highly specific DNA-binding proteins, known colloquially as 'transcription factors'. Immediately upstream of the transcription start site is a relatively short region known as the **promoter**. It is at this site that transcription complexes, consisting of RNA polymerase plus accessory proteins, bind to the DNA and transcription begins. However, the sequences further upstream from the promoter influence the efficiency with which transcription complexes form. The rate of initiation depends on the combination of transcription factors bound to these transcription enhancers. The properties of these **enhancer sequences** are remarkable in that they can be inverted and/or moved around relative to the position of the transcription start site without losing their activity and can exert their influence even from a distance of several kilobases away. This emphasizes the flexibility of DNA, which allows proteins bound at distant sites to interact with one another, as also shown by the protein–protein interactions seen in regulation of phage λ gene expression (above). Transcription of eukaryotic genes results in the production of **monocistronic** mRNAs, each of which is transcribed from its own individual promoter.

Table 5.1 Forms of RNA polymerase in eukaryotic cells

RNA polymerase	sensitivity to α-amanatin	Cellular genes transcribed	Virus genes transcribed
I	Unaffected	Ribosomal RNAs	---
II	Highly sensitive	Most single-copy genes	Most DNA virus genomes
III	Moderately sensitive	5S rRNA, tRNAs	Adenovirus VA RNAs

At the next stage, gene expression is influenced by the structure of the mRNA produced. The stability of eukaryotic mRNAs varies considerably, some having comparatively long half-lives in the cell (e.g. many hours). The half-lives of others, typically those which encode regulatory proteins, may be very short (e.g. a few minutes). The stability of eukaryotic mRNAs depends on the speed with which they are degraded. This is determined by factors such as its terminal sequences, which consist of a methylated cap structure at the 5′ end and polyadenylic acid at the 3′ end, as well as on the overall secondary structure of the message. However, gene expression is also regulated by differential **splicing** of heterogeneous (heavy) nuclear RNA (**hnRNA**) precursors in the nucleus, which can alter the genetic 'meaning' of different mRNAs transcribed from the same gene. In eukaryotic cells, control is also exercised during export of RNA from the nucleus to the cytoplasm.

Finally, the process of translation offers further opportunities for control of expression. The efficiency with which different mRNAs are translated varies greatly. These differences result largely from the efficiency with which ribosomes bind to different mRNAs, recognize AUG translation initiation codons in different sequence contexts and the speed at which different sequences are converted into protein. Certain sequences act as translation **enhancers**, performing a function analogous to that of transcription enhancers.

The point of giving this extensive list of eukaryotic gene expression mechanisms is that they are all utilized by viruses to control gene expression. Examples of each type are given in the sections below. If this seems remarkable, it must be remembered that the control of gene expression in eukaryotic cells was unravelled largely by utilizing viruses as model systems. Therefore, finding examples of these mechanisms in viruses is really only a self-fulfilling prophecy.

GENOME CODING STRATEGIES

In Chapter 4, **genome** structure was one element of an arbitrary classification used to divide virus genomes into seven groups. The other part of such a scheme is the way in which the genetic information of each class of virus genomes is expressed. The replication and expression of virus genomes are inseparably linked, and this is particularly true in the case of RNA viruses. Here, the seven classes of virus genome described in Chapter 4 and Appendix 2 will be reviewed again, this time examining the way in which the genetic information of each class is expressed.

Class I: Double-stranded DNA

It was stated in Chapter 4 that this class of virus genomes can be subdivided into two further groups: those in which genome replication is exclusively nuclear (e.g. *Adenoviridae, Polyomaviridae, Herpesviridae*) and those in which replication occurs in the cytoplasm (*Poxviridae*). In one sense, all of these viruses can be considered as similar, since their genomes all resemble double-stranded cellular DNA, they are essentially transcribed by the same mechanisms as cellular genes. However, there are profound differences between them relating to the degree to which each family is reliant on the host cell machinery.

Polyomaviruses and papillomaviruses

Polyomaviruses are heavily dependent on cellular machinery both for replication and gene expression. They encode *trans*-acting factors (T-antigens) which stimulate transcription (and genome replication). Papillomaviruses in particular are dependent on the cell for replication, which only occurs in terminally differentiated keratinocytes and not in other cell types, although they do encode several *trans*-regulatory proteins (Chapter 7).

Adenoviruses

Adenoviruses are also heavily dependent on the cellular apparatus for transcription, but they possess various mechanisms that specifically regulate virus gene expression. These include *trans*-acting transcriptional activators such as the E1A protein, and post-transcriptional regulation of expression, which is achieved by alternative **splicing** of mRNAs and the virus-encoded VA (virus-associated) RNAs (Chapter 7). Adenovirus infection of cells is divided into two stages, early and late, the latter phase commencing at the time when genome replication occurs. However, in adenoviruses, these phases are less distinct than in herpesviruses (below).

Herpesviruses

These viruses are less reliant on cellular enzymes than the above groups. They encode many enzymes involved in DNA metabolism (e.g. thymidine kinase) and several *trans*-acting factors that regulate the temporal expression of virus genes, controlling the phases of infection. Transcription of the large, complex genome is sequentially regulated in a cascade fashion (Figure 5.4). At least 50 virus-encoded proteins are produced after transcription of the genome by host cell RNA polymerase II. Three distinct classes of mRNAs are made:

- α: Immediate-early (IE) mRNAs encode five *trans*-acting regulators of virus transcription
- β: (Delayed) early mRNAs encode further non-structural regulatory proteins and some minor structural proteins
- γ: Late mRNAs encode the major structural proteins.

Gene expression in herpesviruses is tightly and co-ordinately regulated, as indicated by the following observations (see Figure 5.4):

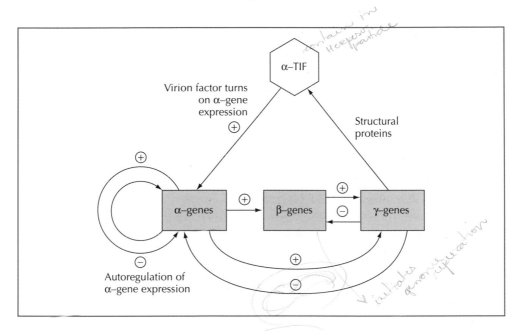

Figure 5.4 Control of expression of the herpesvirus genome. Herpesvirus particles contain a protein called α-TIF (α-gene transcription initiation factor), which turns on α-gene expression in newly infected cells, beginning a cascade of closely regulated events which control the expression of the entire complement of the 70-odd genes in the virus genome.

- If translation is blocked shortly after infection (e.g. by treating cells with cycloheximide), early mRNAs immediately accumulate in the nucleus but no further virus mRNAs are transcribed.
- Synthesis of the early gene product turns off the immediate-early products and initiates genome replication.
- Some of the late structural proteins (γ1) are produced independently of genome replication; others (γ2) are only produced after replication.

Both the immediate-early and early proteins are required to initiate genome replication. A virus-encoded DNA-dependent DNA polymerase and a DNA-binding protein are involved in genome replication, together with a number of enzymes (e.g. thymidine kinase) which alter cellular biochemistry. The production of all of these proteins is closely controlled.

Poxviruses

Genome replication and gene expression in poxviruses are almost independent of cellular mechanisms (except for the requirement for host cell ribosomes). Poxvirus genomes encode numerous enzymes involved in DNA metabolism, virus gene transcription, and post transcriptional modification of mRNAs. Many of these enzymes are packaged within the virus particle (which contains >100 proteins), enabling transcription and replication of the genome to occur in the cytoplasm (rather than in the nucleus, like all the families described above) almost totally under the control of the virus. Gene expression is carried out by virus enzymes associated with the core of the particle and is divided into two rather indistinct phases:

- *Early genes*: These comprise about 50% of the poxvirus genome and are expressed before genome replication inside a partially uncoated core particle (Chapter 2), resulting in the production of 5′ capped, 3′ polyadenylated but unspliced mRNAs.
- *Late genes*: These are expressed after genome replication in the cytoplasm, but their expression is also dependent on virus-encoded rather than on cellular transcription proteins (which are located in the nucleus). Like herpesviruses, late gene **promoters** are dependent on prior DNA replication for activity.

More detailed consideration of some of the mechanisms mentioned above is given later in this chapter (see Transcriptional Control of Expression and Post-Transcriptional Control of Expression below).

Class II: Single-stranded DNA

Both the autonomous and the helper virus-dependent parvoviruses are highly reliant on external assistance for gene expression and genome replication. This is presumably because the very small size of their genomes does not permit them to encode the necessary biochemical apparatus. Thus, they appear to have evolved an extreme form of parasitism, utilizing the normal functions present in the nucleus of their host cells for both expression and replication (Figure 5.5). The members of the replication-defective *Dependovirus* genus of the *Parvoviridae* are entirely dependent on adenovirus or herpesvirus **superinfection** for the provision of further helper functions essential for their replication. The adenovirus genes required as helpers are the early, transcriptional regulatory genes such as E1A rather than late structural genes, but it has been shown that treatment of cells with UV, cycloheximide, or some carcinogens can replace the requirement for helper viruses. Therefore, the help required appears to be for a modification of the cellular environment (probably affecting transcription of the defective parvovirus genome) rather than for a specific virus protein.

The *Geminiviridae* also fall into this class of genome structures (Figure 3.15). The expression of their genomes is quite different from that of parvoviruses, but nevertheless still relies heavily on host cell functions. There are open reading frames in both orientations in the virus DNA, which means that both (+) and (−)sense strands are transcribed during infection. The mechanisms involved in control of gene expression have not been fully investigated, but at least some geminiviruses (subgroup I) may use **splicing**

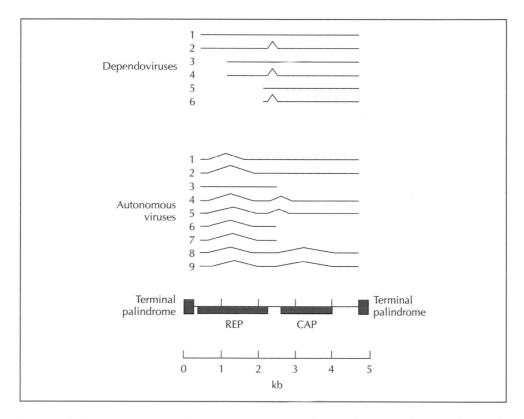

Figure 5.5 Transcription of parvovirus genomes is heavily dependent on host cell factors and results in the synthesis of a series of spliced, subgenomic mRNAs which encode two proteins: rep, which is involved in genome replication and cap, the capsid protein (see text).

Class III: Double-stranded RNA

All viruses with RNA genomes differ fundamentally from their host cells, which of course possess double-stranded DNA genomes. Therefore, although each virus must be biochemically 'compatible' with its host cell, there are fundamental differences in the mechanisms of virus gene expression from those of the host cell. Reoviruses have multipartite genomes (see Chapter 3) and replicate in the cytoplasm of the host cell. Characteristically for viruses with segmented RNA genomes, a separate **mono-cistronic** mRNA is produced from each segment (Figure 5.6).

Early in infection, transcription of the **ds** RNA genome segments by virus-specific **transcriptase** activity occurs inside partially uncoated subvirus particles. At least five enzymatic activities are present in reovirus particles to carry out this process, although these are not necessarily all separate peptides (Table 5.2, Figure 2.14). This primary transcription results in capped transcripts that are not polyadenylated and

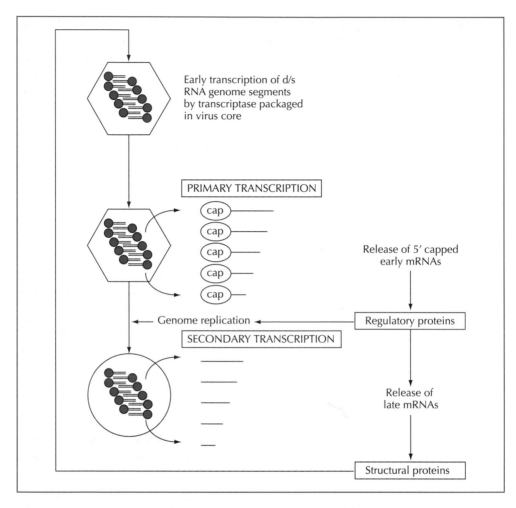

Figure 5.6 Expression of reovirus genomes is initiated by a transcriptase enzyme packaged inside every virus particle. Subsequent events occur in a tightly regulated pattern, the expression of late mRNAs encoding the structural proteins being dependent on prior genome replication.

Table 5.2 Enzymes in Reovirus Particles		
Activity	**Virus protein**	**Encoded by genome segment**
d/s RNA-dependent RNA polymerase (*pol*)	λ3	L3
RNA triphosphatase	μ2	M1
Guanyltransferase (*cap*)	λ2	L2
Methyltransferase	λ2	L2
Helicase (*hel*)	λ1	L1

which leave the virus core to be translated in the cytoplasm. The various genome segments are transcribed/translated at different frequencies, which is perhaps the main advantage of a segmented genome. RNA is transcribed conservatively, i.e. only (−)sense strands are used, resulting in synthesis of (+)sense mRNAs, which are capped inside the core (all this occurs without *de novo* protein synthesis). Secondary transcription occurs later in infection inside new particles produced in infected cells and results in uncapped, non-polyadenylated transcripts. The genome is replicated in a conservative fashion (cf. semi-conservative DNA replication). An excess of (+)sense strands are produced which serve as late mRNAs and as template for (−)sense strand synthesis (i.e. each (−) strand leads to many (+) strands, not one-for-one as in semi-conservative replication).

Class IV: Single-stranded (+)sense RNA

This type of genome occurs in many animal viruses and plant viruses (Appendix 2). In terms of both the number of different families and the number of individual viruses, this is the largest single class of virus genome. Fundamentally, these virus genomes act as messenger RNAs and are themselves translated immediately after infection of the host cell (Chapter 3). Not surprisingly with so many representatives, this class of genomes displays a very diverse range of strategies for controlling gene expression and genome replication. However, in very broad terms, the viruses in this class can be subdivided into two groups as follows:

1 Production of a **polyprotein** encompassing the whole of the virus genetic information, which is subsequently cleaved by proteases to produce precursor and mature polypeptides. These cleavages can be a subtle way of regulating the expression of genetic information. Alternative cleavages result in the production of various proteins with distinct properties from a single precursor, e.g. in picornaviruses and potyviruses (Figure 5.7). Certain plant viruses with multipartite genomes utilize a very similar strategy for controlling gene expression, although a separate polyprotein is produced from each of the genome segments. The best-studied example of this is the comoviruses, whose genome organization is very similar to that of the picornaviruses and may represent another member of this 'superfamily' (Figure 5.7).

2 Production of subgenomic mRNAs, resulting from two or more rounds of translation of the genome. This strategy is used to achieve temporal separation of what are essentially 'early' and 'late' phases of replication, in which non-structural proteins, including a virus **replicase**, are produced during the 'early' phase followed by structural proteins in the 'late' phase (Figure 5.8). The proteins produced in each of these phases may result from proteolytic processing of a polyprotein precursor, although this encompasses only part of the virus genome rather than the entire genome, as above. Proteolytic processing offers further opportunities for

Figure 5.7 Positive-sense RNA virus genomes are frequently translated to form a long polyprotein, which is subsequently cleaved by a highly specific virus-encoded protease to form the mature polypeptides.

regulation of the ratio of different polypeptides produced in each phase of replication (e.g. in togaviruses and tymoviruses). In addition to proteolysis, some viruses employ another strategy to produce alternative polypeptides from a subgenomic mRNA, either by read-through of a 'leaky' translation stop codon, e.g. tobamoviruses such as TMV (Figure 3.12), or by deliberate ribosomal frameshifting at a particular site (see Post-Transcriptional Control of Expression below).

All the viruses in this class have evolved mechanisms that allow them to regulate their gene expression both in terms of the ratios of different virus-encoded proteins and the stage of the replication cycle when they are produced. Compared with the two classes of DNA virus genomes described above, these mechanisms operate largely independently of those of the host cell. The power and flexibility of these strategies is reflected very clearly in the overall success of the viruses in this class, as determined

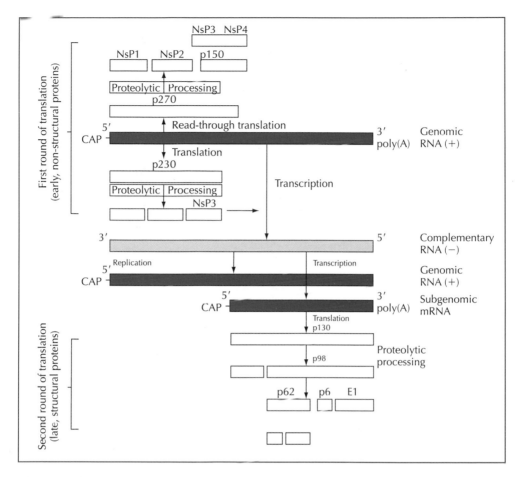

Figure 5.8 Some positive-sense RNA virus genomes (e.g. togaviruses) are expressed by two separate rounds of translation, involving the production of a subgenomic mRNA at a later stage of replication.

by the number of different representatives known and the number of different hosts they infect.

Class V: Single-stranded (−)sense RNA

As discussed in Chapter 3, the genomes of these viruses may be either segmented or non-segmented. The first step in the replication of segmented orthomyxovirus genomes is transcription of the (−)sense vRNA by the virion-associated RNA-dependent RNA polymerase to produce (predominantly) **monocistronic** mRNAs, which also serve as the template for subsequent genome replication (Figure 5.9). As with all (−)sense RNA viruses, packaging of this virus-specific **transcriptase/replicase** within the virus **nucleocapsid** is essential because no host cell contains any enzyme capable of decoding and copying the RNA genome.

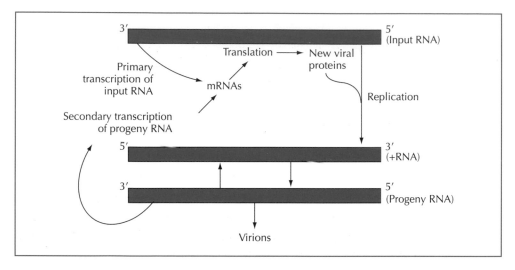

Figure 5.9 Generalized scheme for the expression of negative-sense RNA virus genomes.

In the other families that have non-segmented genomes, monocistronic mRNAs are also produced. Here, however, these messages must be produced from a single, long (−)sense RNA molecule. Exactly how this is achieved is not clear. It is possible that a single, genome-length transcript is cleaved after transcription to form the separate mRNAs, but it is more likely that these are produced individually by a stop and start mechanism of transcription regulated by the conserved intergenic sequences present between each of the virus genes (Chapter 3). **Splicing** mechanisms cannot be used because these viruses replicate in the cytoplasm.

On the surface, such a scheme of gene expression might appear to offer few opportunities for regulation of the relative amounts of different virus proteins. If this were true, it would be a major disadvantage, since all viruses require far more copies of the structural proteins (e.g. **nucleocapsid** protein) than of the non-structural proteins (e.g. polymerase) for each **virion** produced. In practice, the ratio of different proteins is regulated both during transcription and afterwards. In paramyxoviruses for example, there is a clear polarity of transcription from the 3′ end of the virus genome to the 5′ end, which results in the synthesis of far more mRNAs for the structural proteins encoded in the 3′ end of the genome than for the non-structural proteins located at the 5′ end (Figure 5.10). Similarly, the advantage of producing **monocistronic** mRNAs is that the translational efficiency of each message can be varied with respect to the others (see Post-Transcriptional Control of Expression below).

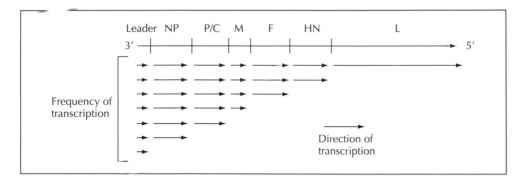

Figure 5.10 Paramyxovirus genomes exhibit 'transcriptional polarity'. Transcripts of genes at the 3′ end of the virus genome are more abundant than those of genes at the 5′ end of the genome, permitting regulation of the relative amounts of structural (3′ genes) and nonstructural (5′ genes) proteins produced.

Class VI: Single-stranded (+)sense RNA with DNA intermediate

The retroviruses are perhaps the ultimate case of reliance on host cell transcription machinery. The RNA genome forms a template for reverse transcription to DNA – these are the only (+)sense RNA viruses whose genome does not serve as mRNA on entering the host cell (Chapter 3). Once integrated into the host cell genome, the DNA **provirus** is under the control of the host cell and is transcribed exactly as are other cellular genes. Some retroviruses, however, have evolved a number of transcriptional and post-transcriptional mechanisms that allow them to control the expression of their genetic information and these are discussed in detail in the relevant sections later in this chapter.

Class VII: Double-stranded DNA with RNA intermediate

Expression of the genomes of these viruses is complex and relatively poorly understood. The hepadnaviruses contain a number of overlapping reading frames clearly designed to squeeze as much coding information as possible into a compact genome. The X gene encodes a transcriptional *trans*-activator believed to be analogous to the HTLV tax protein (below). At least two mRNAs are produced from independent **promoters**, each of which encodes several proteins and the larger of which is also the template for reverse transcription during the formation of the virus particle (Chapter 3).

Expression of *Caulimovirus* genomes is similarly complex, although there are similarities with hepadnaviruses in that two major transcripts are produced, 35S and 19S. Each of these encodes several polypeptides and the 35S transcript is the template for reverse transcription during the formation of the virus genome.

TRANSCRIPTIONAL CONTROL OF EXPRESSION

Having reviewed the general strategies used by different groups of viruses to regulate gene expression, the rest of this chapter will concentrate on more detailed explanations of specific examples from some of the viruses mentioned above, beginning with control of transcription in SV40, a member of the *Polyomaviridae*.

Few other **genomes**, virus or cellular, have been studied in such detail as that of SV40, which has been a paradigm for the study of **eukaryotic** transcription mechanisms (and particularly, DNA replication: see Chapter 6) for many years. In this sense, SV40 provides a eukaryotic parallel with the bacteriophage λ genome. *In vitro* systems exist for both transcription and replication of the SV40 genome and it is believed that all the virus and cellular DNA-binding proteins involved in both of these processes are known. The SV40 genome encodes two T-antigens ('tumour antigens') known as large T-antigen and small T-antigen after the sizes of the proteins (Figure 5.11). Replication of the double-stranded DNA genome of SV40 occurs in the nucleus of the host cell. Transcription of the genome is carried out by host cell RNA polymerase II and large T-antigen plays a vital role in regulating transcription of the virus genome. Small T-antigen is not essential for virus replication, but allows virus DNA to accumulate in the nucleus. Both proteins contain 'nuclear localization signals' which results in their accumulation in the nucleus, where they migrate after being synthesized in the cytoplasm.

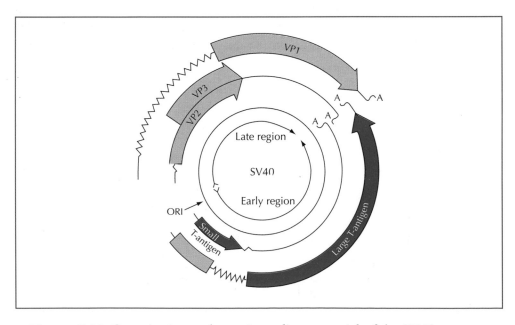

Figure 5.11 Organization and protein-coding potential of the SV40 genome.

Soon after infection of permissive cells, early mRNAs are expressed from the early **promoter**, which contains a strong transcription **enhancer element** (the 72 bp sequence repeats), allowing it to be active in newly infected cells (Figure 5.12). The early proteins synthesized are the two T-antigens. As the concentration of large T-antigen builds up in the nucleus, transcription of the early genes is repressed by direct binding of the protein to the origin region of the virus **genome**, preventing transcription from the early promoter and causing the switch to the late phase of infection. As already mentioned, large T-antigen is also required for replication of the genome, which is considered further in Chapter 7. After DNA replication has occurred, transcription of the late genes occurs from the late promoter and results in the synthesis of the structural proteins, VP1, VP2 and VP3. Therefore, the role of the SV40 T-antigen in controlling the transcription of the genome is comparable to that of a 'switch' and readers should compare the functioning of this system with the description of bacteriophage λ gene expression control given earlier.

Another area where control of virus transcription has received much attention is in the human retroviruses *Human T-cell leukaemia virus* (HTLV) and *Human immuno-deficiency virus* (HIV). Integrated DNA **proviruses** are formed by reverse transcription of the RNA retrovirus **genome**, as described in Chapter 3. The presence of numerous binding sites for cellular transcription factors in the long terminal repeats (LTRs) of these viruses have been analysed by 'DNAse I footprinting' and 'gel–shift' assays (Figure 5.13). Together, the 'distal' elements (such as NFκB and SP1 binding sites) and 'proximal' elements (such as the TATA box) make up a functional transcription **promoter** in the U3 region of the LTR (Chapter 3). However, the basal activity of these promoters on their own is relatively weak, and results in only limited transcription of the provirus genome by RNA polymerase II. Both HTLV and HIV encode proteins which are *trans*–acting positive regulators of transcription: the tax protein of HTLV and the HIV tat protein (Figure 5.14). These proteins act to

Figure 5.12 Control of transcription of the SV40 genome.

Figure 5.13 Cellular transcription factors which interact with retrovirus LTRs. These cellular DNA-binding proteins are involved in regulating both the basal and *trans*-activated levels of transcription from the promoter in the U3 region of the LTR.

increase transcription from the virus LTR by a factor of at least 50–100 times that of the basal rate from the 'unaided' promoter. Unlike T-antigen and the early promoter of SV40, neither the tax nor the tat protein (which have no structural similarity to one another) bind directly to their respective LTRs. Recent work has illustrated how these proteins act.

HTLV tax binds directly to three 21 bp GC-rich CRE (cyclic AMP-response element) sequences in the virus LTR. However, tax also forms protein–protein interactions with a considerable number of different cellular transcription factors, e.g. p105, an inactive precursor of transcription factor NFκB. NFκB plays a central role in controlling transcription and immune activation of lymphoid cells. Antisense inhibition of NFκB has been shown to ablate tax-transformed tumours transplanted into mice, indicating the importance of this protein for tax function. The promiscuous nature of tax *trans*-activation is also explained by a report that tax enhances dimerization of 'bZIP' proteins that bind to DNA via a basic domain–leucine zipper region. Such proteins include a number of factors known to be involved in transcription of the HTLV **genome**. Dimerization of these proteins is required for DNA binding and thus for transcriptional activation, and tax stimulates this process, even in the absence of DNA.

The HIV tat protein binds to a stem–loop structure at the 5′ end of mRNAs transcribed from the LTR, known as the TAR (*trans*-activation response) element. Several cellular proteins also bind to TAR, although the way in which they interact with tat has not been clearly defined. Tat is the first documented example of the regulation of virus gene expression through control of elongation by RNA polymerase

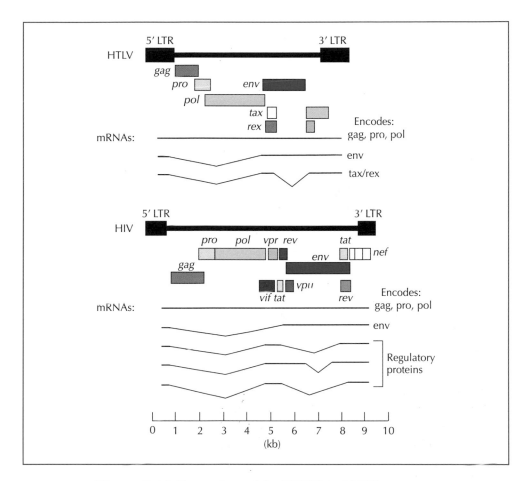

Figure 5.14 Expression of the HTLV and HIV genomes.

II. In the absence of tat, initiation from the LTR is efficient, but transcription is impaired because the promoter forms a poorly processive polymerase complex which falls off the DNA template prematurely. In the presence of tat bound to TAR, a different transcription initiation complex forms which is competent to complete transcription of the HIV genome.

The HTLV tax and HIV tat proteins are positive regulators of the basal promoter in the **provirus** LTR and are under the control of the virus, since synthesis of these proteins is dependent on the promoters which they themselves activate (Figure 5.15). On its own, this would be an unsustainable system because it would result in unregulated positive feedback, which might be acceptable in a **lytic** replication cycle, but would not be appropriate for a retrovirus integrated into the genome of the host cell. Therefore, these viruses each encode an additional protein, the rex and rev proteins in HTLV and HIV, respectively, which further regulate gene expression at a post-transcriptional level (see Post-Transcriptional Control of Expression).

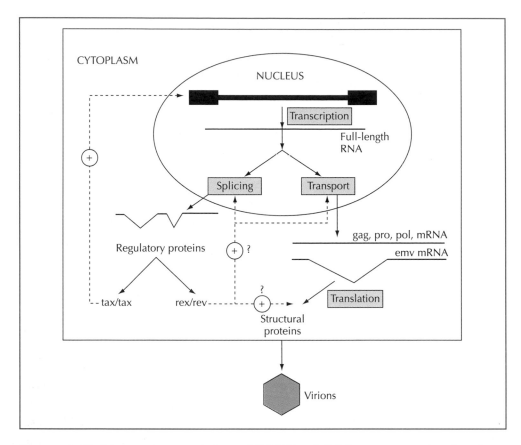

CYTOPLASM

NUCLEUS

Transcription

Full-length
RNA

Splicing   Transport

Regulatory proteins   + ?

gag, pro, pol, mRNA

emv mRNA

- - tax/tax   rex/rev - - - - -   ?
                                   + - - ▶   Translation

Structural
proteins

Virions

Figure 5.15 *Trans*-acting regulation of HTLV and HIV gene expression by virus-encoded proteins. The tax and tat proteins (from HTLV and HIV respectively) act at a transcriptional level and stimulate the expression of all virus genes. The rex (HTLV) and rev (HIV) proteins act post-transcriptionally and regulate the balance of expression between virion proteins and regulatory proteins.

Control of transcription is a critical step in virus replication and in all cases, is closely regulated. Even some of the simplest virus **genomes**, such as SV40, encode proteins that regulate their transcription. Many virus genomes encode *trans*-acting factors that modify and/or direct the cellular transcription apparatus. Examples of this include HTLV and HIV as described above, but also the X protein of hepadna-viruses, rep protein of parvoviruses, E1A protein of adenoviruses (see below) and the immediate-early proteins of herpesviruses. The expression of RNA virus genomes is similarly tightly controlled, but this process is carried out by virus-encoded **transcriptases** and has been less intensively studied and is generally much less well understood than transcription of DNA genomes.

POST-TRANSCRIPTIONAL CONTROL OF EXPRESSION

In addition to control of the process of transcription itself, the expression of virus genetic information is also governed at a number of additional stages between the formation of the primary RNA transcript and the completion of the finished polypeptide. There are many generalized, subtle controls, such as the differential stability of various mRNAs, which are undoubtedly employed by viruses to regulate the flow of genetic information from their **genomes** into proteins. This section, however, will describe only a few well-researched specific examples of post-transcriptional regulation.

Many DNA viruses that replicate in the nucleus encode mRNAs which must be spliced by cellular mechanisms to remove intervening sequences (**introns**) before being translated. This type of modification applies only to viruses which replicate in the nucleus (and not, for example, to poxviruses) since it requires the processing of mRNAs by nuclear apparatus before they are transported into the cytoplasm for translation. However, several virus families have taken advantage of this capacity of their host cells to compress more genetic information into their genomes. Some of the best examples of such a reliance on **splicing** are the parvoviruses, transcription of which results in multiple spliced, polyadenylated transcripts in the cytoplasm of infected cells, enabling them to produce multiple proteins from their 5 kb genomes (Figure 5.5), and similarly, polyomaviruses such as SV40 (Figure 5.11). In contrast, the large genetic capacity of herpesviruses makes it possible for these viruses to produce mostly unspliced **monocistronic** mRNAs, each of which is expressed from its own **promoter**, thereby rendering unnecessary extensive splicing to produce the required repertoire of proteins.

One of the best-studied examples of the **splicing** of virus mRNAs is the expression of the adenovirus **genome** (Figure 5.16). Several 'families' of adenovirus genes are expressed via differential splicing of precursor **hnRNA** transcripts. This is particularly true for the early genes that encode *trans-acting* regulatory proteins expressed immediately after infection. The first proteins to be expressed, E1A and E1B, are encoded by a transcriptional unit on the r-strand at the extreme left-hand end of the adenovirus genome (Figure 5.16). These proteins are primarily transcriptional *trans*-regulatory proteins comparable to the tax and tat proteins described above, but are also involved in **transformation** of adenovirus-infected cells (Chapter 6). Five polyadenylated, spliced mRNAs are produced (13S, 12S, 11S, 10S, 9S) which encode five related E1A polypeptides (containing 289, 243, 217, 171 and 55 amino acids respectively) (Figure 5.17).

All of these proteins are translated from the same reading frame and have the same amino- and carboxy-termini. The differences between them are a consequence of differential splicing of the E1A transcriptional unit and result in major differences in their functions. The 289 and 243 amino acid peptides are transcriptional activators. Although these proteins activate transcription from all the early

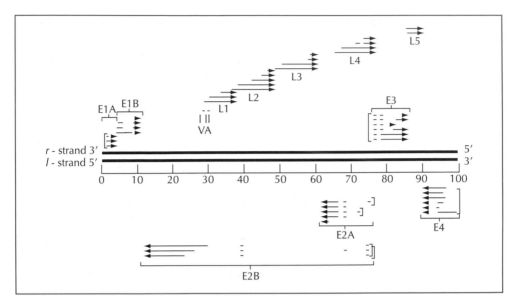

Figure 5.16 Transcription of the adenovirus genome. The arrows show the position of exons in the virus genome which are joined by splicing to produce families of virus proteins.

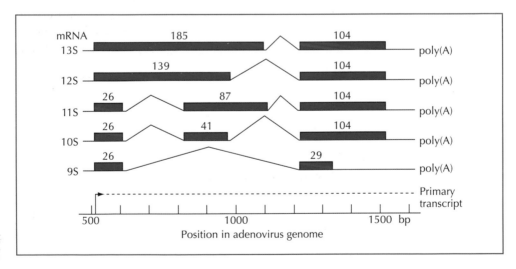

Figure 5.17 Expression of the adenovirus E1A proteins. Numbers shown above each box are the number of amino acids encoded by each exon.

adenovirus promoters, it has been discovered that they also seem to be 'promiscuous', activating most RNA polymerase II-responsive promoters that contain a TATA box. There are no obvious common sequences present in all of these promoters and there is no evidence that the E1A proteins bind directly to DNA. E1A proteins from different adenovirus serotypes contain three conserved domains: CR1, CR2 and CR3. The E1A proteins interact with many other cellular proteins, primarily through binding to the three conserved domains. By binding to components of the basal transcription machinery, activating proteins that bind to upstream promoter and enhancer sequences and regulatory proteins that control the activity of DNA-binding factors, E1A can both activate and repress transcription.

Synthesis of E1A starts a cascade of transcriptional activation by turning on transcription of the other adenovirus early genes, E1B, E2, E3 and E4 (Figure 5.16). After the virus **genome** has been replicated, this cascade eventually results in transcription of the late genes encoding the structural proteins. The transcription of the E1A itself is a balanced, self-regulating system. The immediate early genes of DNA viruses typically have strong **enhancer elements** upstream of their promoters. This is because in a newly infected cell, there are no virus proteins present and the enhancer is required to 'kick-start' expression of the virus genome. The immediate-early proteins synthesized are transcriptional activators that turn on expression of other virus genes, and E1A functions in exactly this way. However, although E1A *trans*-activates its own promoter, the protein represses the function of the upstream enhancer element and therefore at high concentrations, also downregulates its own expression (Figure 5.18).

The next stage at which expression can be regulated is during export of mRNA from the nucleus and preferential translation in the cytoplasm. Again, the best-studied example of this phenomenon comes from the *Adenoviridae*. The VA (virus-associated) genes encode two small (~160 nt) RNAs transcribed from the r-strand of the genome by RNA polymerase III (whose normal function is to transcribe similar small RNAs

Figure 5.18 Regulation of adenovirus gene expression.

such as 5S ribosomal RNA and tRNAs) during the late phase of virus replication (Figure 5.16). Both VA RNA I and VA RNA II have a high degree of secondary structure and neither molecule encodes any polypeptide – in these two respects they are similar to tRNAs – and accumulate to high levels in the cytoplasm of adenovirus–infected cells. The way in which these two RNAs act is not completely understood, but their net effect is to boost the synthesis of adenovirus late proteins. Virus infection of cells stimulates the production of interferons (Chapter 6). One of the actions of interferons is to activate a cellular protein kinase known as PKR that inhibits the initiation of translation. VA RNA I binds to this kinase, preventing its activity and therefore relieves the inhibition on translation. The effects of interferons on the cell are generalized (discussed in Chapter 6), and result in inhibition of the translation of both cellular and virus mRNAs. The VA RNAs may be able to promote selectively the translation of adenovirus mRNAs at the expense of cellular mRNAs whose translation remains inhibited.

The HTLV rex and HIV rev proteins mentioned earlier also act to promote the selective translation of specific virus mRNAs. These proteins regulate the differential expression of the virus **genome** but do not, as far as is known, substantially alter the expression of cellular mRNAs. Both of these proteins appear to function in a similar way, and although not related to one another in terms of their amino acid sequences, the HTLV rex protein has been shown to be able to substitute functionally for the HIV rev protein. Negative-regulatory sequences in the HIV and HTLV genomes cause the retention of virus mRNAs in the nucleus of the infected cell. These sequences are located in the **intron** regions that are removed from spliced mRNAs encoding the tax/tat and rex/rev proteins (Figure 5.14). Therefore, these proteins are expressed immediately after infection. Tax and tat stimulate enhanced transcription from the virus LTR (Figure 5.15). However, unspliced or singly spliced mRNAs encoding the gag, pol and env gene products are only expressed when sufficient rex/rev protein is present in the cell. Both proteins bind to a region of secondary structure formed by a particular sequence in the mRNA and shuttle between the nucleus and the cytoplasm since they contain both a nuclear localization signal and a nuclear export signal, increasing the export of unspliced virus mRNA to the cytoplasm where it is translated and acts as the virus genome during particle formation.

The efficiency with which different mRNAs are translated varies considerably. This is determined by a number of factors, including the stability and secondary structure of the RNA, but the main one appears to be the particular nucleotide sequence surrounding the AUG translation initiation codon which is recognized by ribosomes. The most favourable sequence for initiation is GCC(A/G)CCAUGGG, although there can be considerable variation within this sequence. A number of viruses use variations of this sequence to regulate the amounts of protein synthesized from a single mRNA. Examples of this are the tax and rex proteins of HTLV, which are encoded by overlapping reading frames in the same doubly spliced 2.1 kb mRNA (Figure 5.14). The AUG initiation codon for the rex protein is upstream of that for tax, but provides a less favourable context for initiation of translation than the sequence surrounding the tax AUG codon. This is known as the 'leaky scanning' mechanisms because it is believed that the ribosomes scan along the mRNA before initiating translation. Therefore, the relative abundance of rex protein in HTLV-infected cells is considerably less than that of the tax protein, even though both are encoded by the same mRNA.

Picornavirus **genomes** illustrate an alternative mechanism for controlling the initiation of translation. Although these genomes are genetically economical (i.e. have discarded most *cis*-**acting** control elements and express their entire coding capacity as a single **polyprotein**), they have retained very long non-coding regions at their 5′ ends (5′ NCR), comprising approximately 10% of the entire genome. These sequences are involved in the replication and possibly packaging of the virus genome. Translation of most cellular mRNAs is initiated when ribosomes recognize the 5′ end of the mRNA and scan along the nucleotide sequence until they reach an AUG initiation codon. Picornavirus genomes are not translated in this way. The 5′ end of the RNA is not capped and thus is not recognized by ribosomes in the same way as other mRNAs, but is modified by the addition of the VPg protein (see Chapters 3 and 6). There are also multiple AUG codons in the 5′ NCR upstream of the start of the polyprotein coding sequences which are not recognized by ribosomes. In picornavirus-infected cells, a virus protease cleaves the 220 kDa 'cap-binding complex' (CBC) involved in binding the m7G cap structure at the 5′ end of the mRNA during initiation of translation. Translation of artificially mutated picornavirus mRNAs *in vitro* and the construction of bicistronic picornavirus genomes bearing additional 5′ NCR signals in the middle of the polyprotein have resulted in the concept of the ribosome 'landing pad', or internal ribosomal entry site (**IRES**). Rather than scanning along the RNA from the 5′ end, ribosomes bind to the RNA via the IRES and begin translation internally. This is a precise method for controlling the translation of virus proteins. Very few cellular mRNAs utilize this mechanism but it has been shown to be used by a variety of viruses, including picornaviruses, hepatitis C virus, coronaviruses and flaviviruses.

Many viruses belonging to different families compress their genetic information by encoding different polypeptides in overlapping reading frames. The problem with this strategy lies in decoding the information. If each polypeptide is expressed from a **monocistronic** mRNA transcribed from its own **promoter**, the additional *cis*-acting sequences required to control and co-ordinate expression might cancel out any genetic advantage gained. More importantly, there is the problem of co-ordinately regulating the transcription and translation of multiple different messages. Therefore, it is highly desirable to express several polypeptides from a single RNA transcript, and the examples described above illustrate several mechanisms by which this can be achieved, namely, differential **splicing** and control of RNA export from the nucleus or initiation of translation.

There is, however, an additional mechanism, known as ribosomal frameshifting, used by several groups of viruses to achieve the same end. The best-studied examples of this phenomenon come from retrovirus **genomes**, but many viruses use a similar mechanism. Such frameshifting was first discovered in viruses, but is now known to occur also in **prokaryotic** and **eukaryotic** cells. Retrovirus genomes are transcribed to produce at least two 5′ capped, 3′ polyadenylated mRNAs. Spliced mRNAs encode the **envelope** proteins and, in more complex retroviruses such as HTLV and HIV, additional proteins such as tax/tat and rex/rev proteins (Figure 5.14). A long, unspliced transcript encodes the *gag*, *pro* and *pol* genes and also forms the genomic RNA packaged into **virions**. The problem faced by retroviruses is how to express three different proteins from one long transcript. The arrangement of the three genes varies in different viruses. In some cases (e.g. HTLV), they occupy three different reading frames, while in others (e.g. HIV), the protease (*pro*) gene forms an extension at the 5′ end of the *pol* gene (Figure 5.19). In the latter case, the protease and polymerase (i.e. reverse transcriptase) are expressed as a **polyprotein** which is auto-catalytically cleaved into the mature proteins in a process that is similar to the cleavage of picornavirus polyproteins.

At the boundary between each of the three genes there is a particular sequence which usually consists of a tract of reiterated nucleotides, such as UUUAAAC (Figure

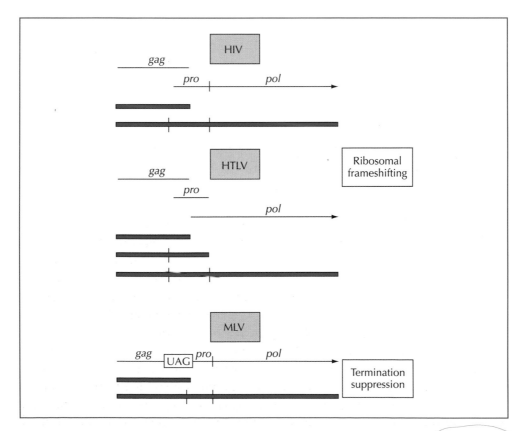

Figure 5.19 Ribosomal frameshifting and termination suppression in retroviruses.

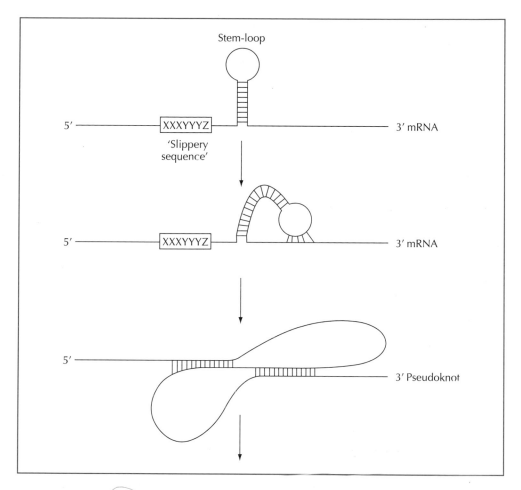

Figure 5.20 RNA pseudoknot formation – the mechanism by which ribosomal frameshifting occurs.

5.20). Remarkably, this sequence is rarely found in protein-coding sequences and therefore appears to be specifically used for this type of regulation. Most ribosomes encountering this sequence will translate it without difficulty and continue on along the transcript until a translation stop codon is reached. However, a proportion of the ribosomes which attempt to translate this sequence will slip back by one nucleotide before continuing to translate the message, but now in a different (i.e. −1) reading frame. Because of this, the UUUAAAC sequence has been termed the 'slippery sequence', and the result of this −1 frameshifting is the translation of a polyprotein containing alternative information from a different reading frame. This mechanism also allows the virus to control the ratios of the proteins produced. Because only a proportion of ribosomes undergo frameshifting at each slippery sequence, there is a gradient of translation from the reading frames at the 5′ end of the mRNA to those at the 3′ end.

However, the slippery sequence alone only results in a low frequency of frameshifting, which appears to be inadequate to produce the amount of protease and reverse transcriptase protein required by the virus. Therefore, there are additional sequences that further regulate this system and increase the frequency of frameshift events. A short distance downstream of the slippery sequence there is an inverted repeat which allows the formation of a stem–loop structure in the mRNA (Figure 5.20). A little further on there is an additional sequence complementary to the nucleotides in the loop which allows base-pairing between these two regions of the RNA. The net result of this combination of sequences is the formation of what is known as an RNA **pseudoknot**. This secondary structure in the mRNA causes ribosomes translating the message to pause at the position of the slippery sequence upstream, and this slowing or pausing of the ribosome during translation increases the frequency at which frameshifting occurs, thus boosting the relative amounts of the proteins encoded by the downstream reading frames. It is easy to imagine how this system can be fine-tuned by subtle mutations that alter the stability of the pseudoknot structure and thus the relative expression of the different genes.

The final method of translational control to be considered is termination **suppression**. This is a mechanism similar in many respects to frameshifting and permits multiple polypeptides to be expressed from individual reading frames in a single mRNA. In some retroviruses, such as *Murine leukaemia virus* (MLV), the *pro* gene is separated from the *gag* gene by a UAG termination codon rather than a 'slippery sequence' and pseudoknot (Figure 5.19). In the majority of cases, translation of MLV mRNA terminates at this sequence, giving rise to the gag proteins. However, in a few instances, the UAG stop codon is suppressed and translation continues, producing a gag–pro–pol **polyprotein**, which subsequently cleaves itself to produce the mature proteins. The overall effect of this system is much the same as ribosomal frameshifting, with the relative ratios of gag and pro/pol proteins being controlled by the frequency with which ribosomes traverse or terminate at the UAG stop codon.

SUMMARY

Control of gene expression is a vital element of virus replication. Co-ordinate expression of groups of virus genes results in successive phases of gene expression. Typically, immediate-early genes encode 'activator' proteins, early genes encode further regulatory proteins and late genes encode virus structural proteins. Viruses make use of the biochemical apparatus of their host cells to express their genetic information as proteins and, consequently, utilize the appropriate biochemical language recognized by the cell. Thus viruses of **prokaryotes** produce **polycistronic** mRNAs while viruses with **eukaryotic** hosts produce mainly **monocistronic** mRNAs. Some viruses of eukaryotes do produce polycistronic mRNA to assist with the co-ordinate regulation of multiple genes. In addition, viruses rely on specific *cis-* and *trans-*acting mechanisms to manipulate the biology of their host cells and to enhance and co-ordinate the expression of their own genetic information.

FURTHER READING

Alberts, B., Bray, D., Lewis, J., Raff, M,. Roberts, K. and Watson, J.D. (Eds) (1994). *Molecular Biology of the Cell* (3rd edn). Garland, New York. ISBN 0815316194.

Cann, A.J. and Chen, I.S.Y. (1996). Human T-cell leukemia virus types I and II. In Fields, B.N., Knipe D.M. and Howley, P. M. (Eds) *Virology* (3rd edn), pp. 1849-1880. Raven Press, New York.

Farabaugh, F.J. (1996). Programmed translational frameshifting. *Annual Review of Genetics* 30: 507–528.

Flint, J. and Shenk, T. (1997). Viral transactivating proteins. *Annual Review of Genetics* 31: 177–212.

Karn, J. (1999). Tackling tat. *Journal of Molecular Biology* 293: 235–254.

Latchman, D.S. (1999). *Eukaryotic Transcription Factors*. Academic Press, London. ISBN 0124371779.

Pollard, V.W. and Malim, M.H. (1998). The HIV-1 rev protein. *Annual Review of Microbiology* 52: 491–532.

Ptashne, M. (1992). *A Genetic Switch: Phage and Higher Organisms* (2nd edn). Cell Press/Blackwell Scientific, Oxford. ISBN 0865422095.

SELF-ASSESSMENT QUESTIONS

(5.1) Are the following statements true or false?

(a)   The course of virus replication is independent of virus gene expression.

(b)   Transcription promoters are *cis*-acting sequences located adjacent to the genes whose transcription they control.

(c)   Transcription factors are *trans*-acting proteins which bind to specific sequences present anywhere in the cell.

(d)   Transcription of bacterial operons typically produces polycistronic mRNAs.

(e)   Gene expression in bacteria is regulated exclusively at the level of transcription.

(5.2) Viruses have counteracted their genetic limitations by evolving of a range of solutions to these problems, including (true or false?):

(a)   Powerful positive *cis-* and *trans*-acting signals which promote gene

expression.
(b)   Powerful *cis*-acting negative signals which repress gene expression.
(c)   Highly compressed genomes with overlapping reading frames common.
(d)   Control signals which are frequently nested within other genes.
(e)   Several strategies designed to create multiple polypeptides from a single mRNA.

(5.3) Are the following statements true or false?
(a)   Bacteriophage λ can alternate between the lysogenic and lytic growth cycles.
(b)   The λ N protein acts as a negative transcription regulator.
(c)   In the absence of the N protein, RNA polymerase stops at the nut site.
(d)   The *cI* repressor protein binds to O_R but not O_L.
(e)   Lysogeny is maintained by autoregulation of *cI* transcription.

(5.4) Are the following statements true or false?
(a)   Transcription of eukaryotic cellular genes results in monocistronic mRNAs, each transcribed from its own promoter.
(b)   Post-transcriptional control of gene expression in eukaryotes is achieved by splicing of hnRNA and differential export of mRNA from the nucleus to the cytoplasm.
(c)   Eukaryotic mRNAs are translated with variable efficiency owing to the speed at which ribosomes are degraded.
(d)   The stability of eukaryotic mRNAs depends on the speed at which they are degraded.
(e)   Translation enhancers perform a function analogous to that of transcription enhancers.

(5.5) Are the following statements true or false?
(a)   Polyomaviruses are heavily dependent on cellular machinery for gene expression.
(b)   Herpesviruses make three classes of mRNA: early, late and structural.
(c)   Geminivirus genomes are replicated and expressed in the nucleus of infected cells because they are heavily reliant on host cell functions.
(d)   Reovirus transcription occurs inside virus core particles.
(e)   Segmented virus genomes are usually transcribed to produce monocistronic mRNAs.

(5.6) Viruses with (+)sense RNA genomes (true or false?):
(a)   are heavily dependent on cellular mechanisms for control of gene expression.
(b)   are all translated to produce a long polyprotein.

(c)   are all transcribed to produce subgenomic RNAs.
(d)   are all non-segmented.
(e)   can only produce an equal ratio of all the polypeptides they encode.

(5.7)   Are the following statements true or false?
(a)   Viruses with non-segmented (−)sense genomes produce mono-cistronic mRNAs.
(b)   Viruses with (−)sense genomes all contain a virus-specific transcriptase/replicase within the virus nucleocapsid.
(c)   Viruses with non-segmented (−)sense genomes can only produce an equal ratio of all the polypeptides they encode.
(d)   Retroviruses are the only RNA viruses whose genomes are transcribed by cellular RNA polymerase.
(e)   Hepadnavirus and caulimovirus genomes contain a number of overlapping reading frames.

(5.8)   Are the following statements true or false?
(a)   SV40 large T-antigen binds to the origin of replication in the virus genome.
(b)   SV40 large T-antigen represses transcription of the virus early genes.
(c)   SV40 large T-antigen promotes export of virus mRNAs from the nucleus to the cytoplasm.
(d)   The HTLV tax protein binds to the TAR sequence in the provirus genome.
(e)   The HIV tat protein binds to cellular transcription factors, not virus mRNAs.

(5.9)   Are the following statements true or false?
(a)   With the exception of retroviruses, no RNA virus genome undergoes splicing.
(b)   The HTLV rex protein promotes the export of virus structural protein mRNAs from the nucleus.
(c)   The abbreviation 'IRES' stands for initial replication exit site.
(d)   All (+)sense RNA viruses contain an IRES element.
(e)   All eukaryotic mRNAs contain an IRES element.

(5.10) Are the following statements true or false?
(a)   Ribosomal frameshifting allows viruses to produce several different proteins from a polycistronic mRNA.
(b)   Ribosomal frameshifting allows viruses to produce varying amounts of different proteins from a polycistronic mRNA.

(c)   RNA pseudoknots are produced by *trans*-acting proteins such as the HIV tat protein.

(d)   RNA pseudoknots increase the frequency of ribosomal frameshifting.

(e)   Suppression of termination codons allows some viruses to produce multiple proteins from a polycistronic mRNA.

Answers to Self-Assessment Questions are given in Appendix 4.

CHAPTER 6

INFECTION

Learning Objectives

On completing this chapter, you should be able to:
- Describe the course taken by different virus infections
- Explain the scientific basis for therapeutic interventions against virus diseases
- Summarize the major responses of plants and animals to virus infections.

Virus infection of higher organisms is the cumulative result of all the processes of replication and gene expression described in earlier chapters. Together, these determine the overall course (or 'natural history') of each infection. Virus infections range in complexity and duration from a very brief, superficial interaction between the virus and its host to infections which may encompass the entire life of the host organism, from before birth to its eventual death and in which many different tissues and organs are infected. One of the most common misconceptions is that virus infection inevitably results in disease. In reality, the converse is true – only a small minority of virus infections give rise to any disease symptoms.

This chapter provides an overview of the numerous patterns of virus infection and forms an introduction to the consideration of virus pathogenesis in Chapter 7. Most of this chapter is concerned with the infection of eukaryotes by viruses. Unlike previous and subsequent chapters, this chapter deals primarily with the interaction of viruses with intact organisms rather than with the molecular biologist's usual concern about the interaction between a virus and the cell.

Virus Infections of Plants

The overall course of virus replication is determined by a dynamic interaction between the virus and its host organism. Clearly, there are major differences between virus infections of plants and those of vertebrates. In economic terms, viruses are only of importance if it is likely that they will spread to crops during their commercial lifetime, which of course varies greatly between very short extremes in horticultural production and very long extremes in forestry. Some estimates put total worldwide damage due to plant viruses as high as US\$60 billion per year. The mechanism by which plant viruses are transmitted between hosts is therefore of great importance. There are a number of routes by which plant viruses may be transmitted:

- *Seeds*: These may transmit virus infection either by external contamination of the seed with virus particles, or by infection of the living tissues of the embryo. Transmission by this route leads to early outbreaks of disease in new crops which are usually initially focal in distribution, but may subsequently be transmitted to the remainder of the crop by other mechanisms (below).
- *Vegetative propagation/grafting*: These techniques are cheap and easy methods of plant propagation, but provide the ideal opportunity for viruses to spread to new plants.
- *Vectors*: Many different groups of living organisms can act as vectors and spread viruses from one plant to another:

  - Bacteria (e.g. *Agrobacterium tumefaciens* – the Ti plasmid of this organism has been used experimentally to transmit virus genomes between plants)
  - Fungi
  - Nematodes
  - Arthropods, including insects (aphids, leafhoppers, planthoppers, beetles, thrips, etc.) and arachnids (mites).

- *Mechanical*: Mechanical transmission of viruses is the most widely used method for experimental infection of plants and is usually achieved by rubbing virus-containing preparations into the leaves, which in most plant species are particularly susceptible to infection. However, this is also an important natural method of transmission. Virus particles may contaminate soil for long periods and may be transmitted to the leaves of new host plants as wind-blown dust or as rain-splashed mud.

The problems plant viruses face in initiating infections of host cells have already been described (Chapter 4), as has the fact that no known plant virus employs a specific cellular receptor of the types that animal and bacterial viruses use to attach to cells. Transmission of plant viruses by insects is therefore of particular agricultural importance. Extensive areas of monoculture and the inappropriate use of pesticides which kill natural predators can result in massive population booms of insects such as aphids. Plant viruses rely on a mechanical breach of the integrity of a cell wall to directly introduce a virus particle into a cell. This is achieved either by the vector associated with transmission of the virus or simply by mechanical damage to cells. Transfer by insect vectors is a particularly efficient means of virus transmission. In some instances, viruses are transmitted mechanically from one plant to the next by the vector and the insect is merely a means of distribution, through flying or being carried on the wind for long distances (sometimes hundreds of miles). Insects which bite or suck plant tissues are, of course, the ideal means of transmitting viruses to new hosts. This is known as non-propagative transmission. However, in other cases (e.g. many plant rhabdoviruses) the virus may also infect and multiply in the tissues of the insect (propagative transmission) as well as those of host plants. In these cases, the vector serves as a means not only of distributing the virus, but also of amplifying the infection.

Initially, most plant viruses multiply at the site of infection, giving rise to localized symptoms such as necrotic spots on the leaves. The virus may subsequently be distributed to all parts of the plant either by direct cell-to-cell spread or by the vascular system, resulting in a systemic infection involving the whole plant. However, the problem these viruses face in reinfection and recruitment of new cells is the same problem as they face initially – how to cross the barrier of the plant cell wall. Plant cell walls necessarily contain channels called plasmodesmata which allow plant cells to communicate with each other and to pass metabolites between them. However, these channels are too small to allow the passage of virus particles or genomic nucleic acids. Many (if not most) plant viruses have evolved specialized movement proteins which modify the plasmodesmata. One of the best-known examples of this is the 30k protein of *Tobacco mosaic virus* (TMV). This protein is expressed from a subgenomic mRNA (Figure 3.12) and its function is to modify plasmodesmata, causing genomic RNA coated with 30k protein to be transported from the infected cell to neighbouring cells (Figure 6.1). Other viruses, such as *Cowpea mosaic virus* (CPMV, *Comoviridae*) have a similar strategy but employ a different molecular mechanism. In CPMV, the 58/48k proteins form tubular structures allowing intact virus particles to pass from one cell to another (Figure 6.1).

Typically, virus infections of plants might result in effects such as growth retardation, distortion, mosaic patterning on the leaves, yellowing, wilting, etc. These macroscopic symptoms result from:

- Necrosis of cells, caused by direct damage due to virus replication
- Hypoplasia, i.e. localized retarded growth frequently leading to mosaicism (the appearance of thinner, yellow areas on the leaves)
- Hyperplasia, which is excessive cell division or the growth of abnormally large cells, resulting in the production of swollen or distorted areas of the plant.

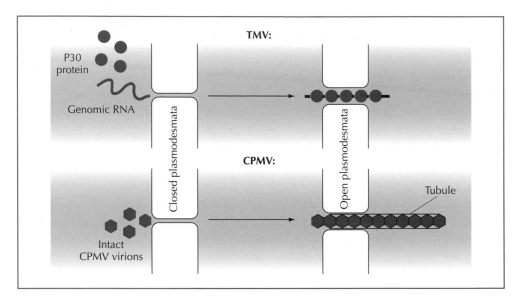

Figure 6.1 Plant movement proteins.

Plants might be seen as sitting targets for virus infection – unlike animals, they cannot run away. However, plants exhibit a range of responses to virus infections designed to minimize their effects. Initially, infection results in a 'hypersensitive response', manifested as:

- the synthesis of a range of new proteins, the 'PR' (pathogenesis-related) proteins;
- an increase in the production of cell wall phenolics;
- the release of active oxygen species;
- the production of phytoalexins; and
- the accumulation of salicylic acid. (Amazingly, plants can even warn each other that viruses are coming by airborne signalling with volatile compounds such as methylsalicylate.)

Although this system is poorly understood, at least some of the PR proteins have been characterized and have been shown to be proteases, which presumably destroy virus proteins, limiting the spread of the infection. There is some similarity here between this response and the production of interferons by animals (see below).

Systemic resistance to virus infection is a naturally occurring phenomenon in some strains of plant. This is clearly a highly desirable characteristic and is highly prized by plant breeders, who try to spread this attribute to economically valuable crop strains. There are probably many different mechanisms involved in systemic resistance, but in general terms there is a tendency towards increased local necrosis, as substances such as proteases and peroxidases are produced by the plant to destroy the virus and to prevent its spread and subsequent systemic disease. An example of this is the tobacco *N* gene, which encodes a cytoplasmic protein with a nucleotide-binding site which interferes with the TMV replicase. When present in plants, this gene causes TMV to produce a localized, necrotic infection rather than the systemic mosaic symptoms normally seen.

Virus-resistant plants have been created by the production of transgenic plants expressing recombinant virus proteins or nucleic acids which interfere with virus replication without producing the pathogenic consequences of infection. Some examples of these are:

- Virus coat proteins, which have a variety of complex effects, including inhibition of virus uncoating and interference of expression of the virus at the level of RNA ('gene silencing' by 'untranslatable' RNAs)
- Intact or partial virus replicases, which interfere with genome replication
- Antisense RNAs
- Defective virus genomes
- Satellite sequences (see Chapter 8)
- Catalytic RNA sequences (ribozymes)
- Modified movement proteins.

This is a very promising technology which offers the possibility of substantial increases in agricultural production without the use of expensive, toxic and ecologically damaging chemicals (fertilizers, herbicides or pesticides), but it is still in its infancy.

IMMUNE RESPONSES TO VIRUS INFECTIONS IN ANIMALS

The most significant response to virus infection in vertebrates is the activation of both the cellular and humoral arms of the immune system. A thorough description of all the events involved in the immune response to the presence of foreign antigens in the body is beyond the scope of this chapter. Readers should refer to the books cited under Further Reading to ensure that they are familiar with all the immune mechanisms (and jargon!) described below. However, a brief summary of some of the more pertinent aspects is well worth considering, beginning with the humoral immune response, which results in the production of antibodies.

The major impact of the humoral immune response is the eventual clearance of virus from the body, i.e. serum neutralization stops the spread of virus to uninfected cells and allows other defence mechanisms to mop up the infection. Figure 6.2 shows a grossly simplified version of the mammalian humoral response to infection. Virus infection induces at least three classes of antibody: immunoglobulin G (IgG), IgM and IgA. IgM is a large, multivalent molecule which is most effective at cross-linking large targets (e.g. bacterial cell walls or flagella), but is probably less important in combating

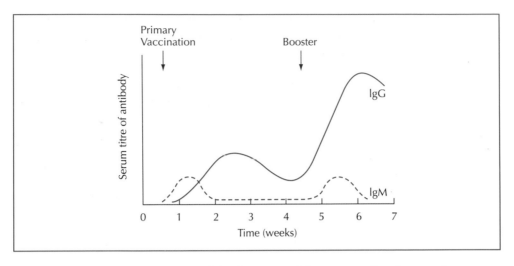

Figure 6.2 Simplified version of the kinetics of the mammalian humoral response to a 'typical' foreign virus (or other) antigen.

virus infections. In contrast, the production of IgA is very important for initial protection from virus infection. Secretory IgA is produced at mucosal surfaces and results in 'mucosal immunity', an important factor in preventing infection from occurring. Induction of mucosal immunity depends to a large extent on the way in which antigens are presented to and recognized by the immune system. Similar antigens incorporated into different vaccine delivery systems (see Prevention and Therapy of Virus Infection) can lead to very different results in this respect and mucosal immunity is such an important factor that similar vaccines may vary considerably in their efficacy. IgG is probably the most important class of antibody for direct neutralization of virus particles in serum and other body fluids (into which it diffuses).

Direct virus neutralization by antibodies results from a number of mechanisms, including conformational changes in the virus capsid caused by antibody binding, or blocking of the function of the virus target molecule (e.g. receptor binding) by steric hindrance. A secondary consequence of antibody binding is phagocytosis of antibody-coated ('opsonized') target molecules by mononuclear cells or polymorphonuclear leukocytes. This process is mediated by the presence of the Fc receptor on the surface of these cells, but as has already been noted in Chapter 4, in some cases opsonization of virus by the binding of non-neutralizing antibodies can result in enhanced virus uptake. This has been shown to occur with rabies virus and in the case of HIV may promote uptake of the virus by macrophages. Antibody binding also leads to the activation of the complement cascade, which assists in the neutralization of virus particles. The morphological alterations induced by the disruption of viruses by complement can sometimes be visualized directly by electron microscopy. Complement is particularly important early in virus infection when limited amounts of low–affinity antibody are made – complement potentiates the action of these.

   Despite all the above mechanisms, in overall terms, cell-mediated immunity is probably more important than humoral immunity in the control of virus infections. This is demonstrated by the following observations:

■ Congenital defects in cell-mediated immunity tend to result in predisposition to virus (and parasitic) infections, rather than to bacterial infections.
■ The functional defect in acquired immune deficiency syndrome (AIDS) is a reduction in the ratio of T helper ($CD4^+$):T suppressor ($CD8^+$) cells from the normal value of about 1.2 to 0.2. AIDS patients commonly suffer many opportunistic virus infections (e.g. various herpesviruses such as HSV, CMV and EBV), which may have been present before the onset of AIDS but were previously suppressed by the intact immune system.

Cell-mediated immunity is effected through three main systems (Figure 6.3):

1 Non-specific cell killing (mediated by 'natural killer' (NK) cells)
2 Specific cell killing (mediated by cytotoxic T lymphocytes, CTLs)
3 Antibody-dependent cellular cytotoxicity (ADCC)

by mechanisims which will be explained later (see Virus and Apoptosis).

Natural killer cells

NK cells mediate cell lysis independently of conventional immunological specificity, i.e. clonal antigen recognition. They are not MHC-restricted (i.e. only able to recognize a specific antigen in the context of MHC antigens plus the T-cell receptor

Figure 6.3 Diagram illustrating the three main mechanisms by which cell-mediated immunity is effected.

(TCR)/CD3 complex). The advantages of this are that they have broad specificity and are active without the requirement for sensitizing antibodies. They are therefore the first line of defence against virus infection. NK cells are most active in the early stages of infection (i.e. the first few days) and their activity is stimulated by interferon-α/β (IFN-α/β) (see below). NK cells are not directly induced by virus infection – they exist even in immunologically naive individuals and are 'revealed' in the presence of interferon-α/β. They are thus part of the 'innate' immune response. Their function is complementary to and is later taken over by CTLs (below), which are part of the 'adaptive' immune response. The target for NK cells on the surface of infected cells is not known, but their action is inhibited by MHC class I antigens (which are present on all nucleated cells), allowing recognition of 'self' and preventing total destruction of the body. It is known that some virus infections disturb normal cellular MHC class I expression and this is one possible mechanism of NK recognition of infected cells. NK cell cytotoxicity is activated by IFN-α/β, thus directly linking NK activity to virus infection (see below).

Cytotoxic T lymphocytes

Cytotoxic T lymphocytes (CTLs) are usually of CD8$^+$ (suppressor) phenotype. CTLs are the major cell-mediated immune response to virus infections and are MHC-restricted, i.e. clones of cells recognize a specific antigen only when presented by MHC class I antigen on the target cell to the TCR/CD3 complex on the surface of the CTL. (MHC class I antigens are expressed on all nucleated cells in the body; MHC class II antigens are expressed only on the surface of the antigen-presenting cells of the immune system – T cells, B cells and macrophages.) CTL activity requires 'help' (i.e. cytokine production) from T helper cells. The CTLs themselves recognize foreign antigens through the TCR/CD3 complex, which 'docks' with antigen presented by MHC class I on the surface of the target cell (Figure 6.4). However, the mechanism of cell killing by CTLs is similar to that of NK cells (see below). The induction of a CTL response also results in the release of many different cytokines from T helper cells, some of which result in clonal proliferation of antigen-specific CTLs and others which have direct antiviral effects, for example, interferons (see below). The kinetics of the CTL response (which peak at about 7 days after infection) are somewhat slower than those of the NK response (e.g. 3–7 days, cf. 0.5–3 days for NK cells) and therefore these are complementary systems.

The induction of a CTL response is dependent on recognition of specific T-cell epitopes by the immune system. These are distinct from the B-cell epitopes recognized by the humoral arm of the immune system. T-cell epitopes are frequently more highly conserved (less variable) than B-cell epitopes, which are frequently able to mutate quickly to escape immune pressure. These are important considerations in the design of antiviral vaccines. The specificity of killing by CTLs is not absolute. Although they are better 'behaved' than NK cells, diffusion of perforin and local

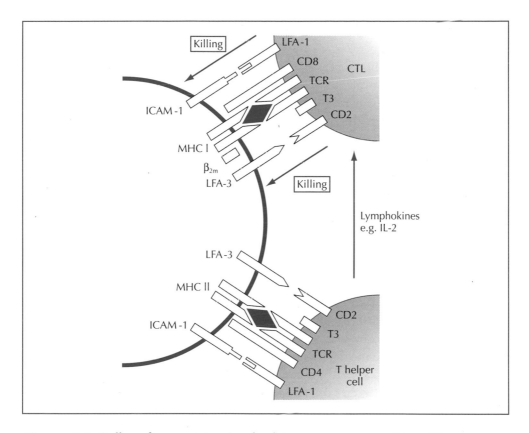

Figure 6.4 Cell surface proteins involved in immune recognition. Close contact between cells results in cell-to-cell signalling which regulates the immune response.

cytokine production frequently results in inflammation and bystander cell damage. This is a contributory cause of the pathology of many virus diseases (see Chapter 7), but the less attractive alternative is to allow virus replication to proceed unchecked.

Antibody-dependent cellular cytotoxicity

ADCC is less well understood than either of the above two mechanisms. It can be mediated either by NK cells or by CTLs. The mechanism of cell killing is the same, although complement may also be involved in ADCC. However, this mechanism is dependent on the recognition of antigen on the surface of the target cell by antibody on the surface of the effector cell. The antibody involved is usually IgG, which is bound to Fc receptors on the surface of the T cell. ADCC therefore requires a pre-existing antibody response and hence does not occur early during primary virus infections – it is part of the adaptive immune response. The overall contribution of ADCC to the control of virus infections is not clear, although it is now believed that it plays a significant part in their control.

VIRUSES AND APOPTOSIS

Apoptosis, or 'programmed cell death', is a critical mechanism in tissue remodelling during development and in cell killing by the immune system. There are two ways in which a cell can die: necrosis or apoptosis.

Necrosis is the normal response of cells to injury caused by toxins or environmental stress. It is marked by a non-specific changes such as disruption of the plasma membrane and nuclear envelope, rupture of membrane-bounded organelles such as mitochondria and lysosomes, cell swelling, random fragmentation of DNA/RNA, influx of calcium ions into the cell and loss of membrane electrical potential. The release of cellular components from the dying cell causes a localized inflammatory response by the cells of the immune system. This frequently leads to damage to adjacent cells/tissue – 'bystander' cell damage.

Apoptosis is, in contrast, a tightly regulated process which relies on complex molecular cascades for its control. It is marked by cell shrinkage, condensation and clumping of chromatin, a regular pattern of DNA fragmentation, 'bubbling off' of cellular contents into small, membrane-bounded vesicles ('blebbing'), which are subsequently phagocytosed by macrophages, preventing inflammation.

When triggered by the appropriate signals, immune effector cells such as CTLs and NK cells release previously manufactured lytic granules stored in their cytoplasm. These act on the target cell and induce apoptosis by two mechanisms:

1 *Release of cytotoxins*, such as perforin and granzymes: Perforin (also known as cytolysin), a peptide related to complement component C9, polymerizes on release to form polyperforin, which forms transmembrane channels, resulting in permeability of the target cell membrane. The membrane pores allow the entry into the cell of granzymes, which are serine proteases related to trypsin. Thus these two effectors act collaboratively. The membrane channels also allow the release of intracellular calcium from the target cell, which acts to trigger apoptotic pathways.
2 *Fas ligand expression*: CTLs (but not NK cells) express Fas ligand on their surface. This binds to Fas (CD95) on the surface of the target cell, triggering apoptosis. Binding of Fas ligand on the effector cell to Fas on the target cell results in activation of cellular proteases known as caspases, which in turn trigger a cascade of events leading to apoptosis.

Induction and repression of apoptosis during virus infection has received much attention during the last few years. It is now recognized that this is an important innate response to virus infection. The regulation of apoptosis is a complex issue which it is not possible to describe fully here (see Further Reading and Figure 6.5 for a summary), but it is important to be aware that virus infections perturb cellular biochemistry and frequently trigger an apoptotic response:

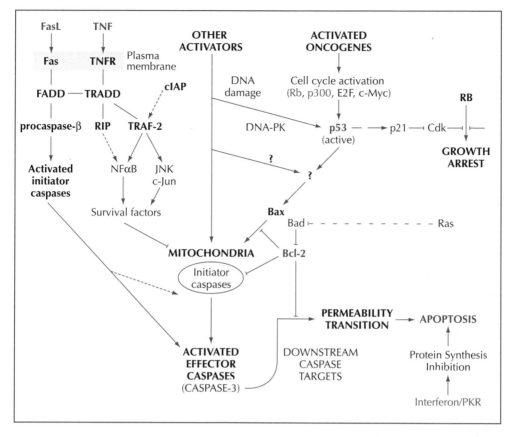

Figure 6.5 Overview of apoptosis. Items in blue type are of major significance in virus infection.

- *Receptor signalling*: Binding of virus particles to cellular receptors may trigger signalling mechanisms resulting in apoptosis (e.g. HIV (Chapter 7), reovirus).
- *PKR activation*: The interferon effector PKR (see below) may be activated by some viruses (e.g. HIV, reovirus).
- *p53 activation*: Viruses which interact with p53 (Chapter 7) may cause either growth arrest or apoptosis (e.g. adenoviruses, SV40, papillomaviruses).
- *Transcriptional disregulation*: Viruses which encode transcriptional regulatory proteins may trigger an apoptotic response (e.g. HTLV tax).
- *Foreign protein expression*: Overexpression of virus proteins at late stages of the replication cycle can also cause apotosis by a variety of mechanisms.

To counteract this cellular alarm system, many if not most viruses have evolved mechanisms to counteract this effect and repress apoptosis:

- *Bcl-2 homologs*: A number of viruses encode Bcl-2 (a negative regulator of apoptosis) homologues (e.g. adenovirus E1B-19k, HHV-8 KSbcl-2).
- *Caspase inhibition*: Caspases are a family of cysteine proteases which are important inducers of apoptosis. Inhibiting these enzymes is an effective way of preventing apoptosis (e.g. baculovirus p35, serpins, vIAPs – 'inhibitors of apoptosis').
- *Fas/TNF inhibition*: Viruses have evolved several mechanisms to block the effects of Fas/TNF, including blocking signalling through the plasma membrane (e.g. adenovirus E3), tumour necrosis factor receptor (TNFR) mimics (e.g. poxvirus crmA), mimics of death signalling factors (vFLIPs) and interactions with signalling factors such as FADD and TRADD (e.g. HHV-4 (EBV) LMP-1).
- *p53 inhibition*: A number of viruses which interact with p53 have evolved proteins to counteract possible triggering of apoptosis (e.g. adenovirus E1B-55k and E4, SV40 T-antigen and papillomavirus E6).
- *Miscellaneous*: Many other mechanisms are now being described in a variety of viruses (e.g. HIV, influenza, reovirus, etc.).

Without such inhibitory mechanisms, most viruses would simply not be able to replicate due to the death of the host cell before the replication cycle was complete. However, there is evidence that at least some viruses use apoptosis to their benefit. (+)sense RNA viruses with lytic replication cycles, such as poliovirus, hepatitis A virus and Sindbis virus, appear to be able regulate apoptosis, initially repressing it to allow replication to take place, then inducing it to allow the release of virus particles from the cell.

INTERFERONS

By the 1950s, interference (i.e. the blocking of a virus infection by a competing virus) was a well-known phenomenon in virology. In some cases, the mechanism responsible is just that; for example, avian retroviruses are grouped into nine interference groups, A–I, based on their ability to infect various strains of chickens, pheasants, partridges, quail, etc., or cell lines derived from these species. In this case, the inability of particular viruses to infect the cells of some strains is due to the expression of the envelope glycoprotein of an endogenous provirus present in the cells, which sequesters the cellular receptor needed by the exogenous virus for infection. In other cases, the mechanism of virus interference is less clear.

In 1957, Alick Issacs and Jean Lindenmann were studying this phenomenon and performed the following experiment. Pieces of chick chorioallantoic membrane were exposed to UV-inactivated (non-infectious) influenza virus in tissue culture. The 'conditioned' medium from these experiments (which did not contain infectious virus) was found to inhibit the infection of fresh pieces of chick chorioallantoic membrane by (infectious) influenza virus in separate cultures. Their conclusion was that a soluble factor, which they called 'interferon', was produced by cells as a result of virus infection and that this factor could prevent the infection of other cells. As a result of this provocative observation interferon became the great hope for virology and was thought to be directly equivalent to the use of antibiotics to treat bacterial infections.

The true situation has turned out to be far more complex than was first thought. Interferons do have antiviral properties, but by and large their effects are exerted indirectly via their major function as cellular regulatory proteins. Interferons are immensely potent; less than 50 molecules per cell show evidence of antiviral activity. Hence, following Isaacs and Lindenmann's initial discovery, many fairly fruitless years were spent trying to purify minute amounts of naturally produced interferon. This situation changed with the development of molecular biology and the cloning and expression of interferon genes, which has led to rapid advances in our understanding over the last 15 years. There are three types of interferon: α, β and γ.

- *Interferon-α*: There are at least 15 molecular species of interferon-α, all of which are closely related; some species differ by only one amino acid. They are synthesized predominantly by lymphocytes. The mature proteins contain 143 amino acids, with a minimum homology of 77% between the different types. All the genes encoding interferon-α are located on human chromosome 9 and gene duplication is thought to be responsible for this proliferation of genes.
- *Interferon-β*: There is a single gene for interferon-β, also on human chromosome 9. The mature protein contains 145 amino acids and, unlike interferon-α, is glycosylated, with approximately 30% homology to other interferons. It is synthesized predominantly by fibroblasts.
- *Interferon-γ*: There is a single gene for interferon-γ, on human chromosome 12. The mature protein contains 146 amino acids, is glycosylated, has very low sequence homology to other interferons. It is synthesized predominantly by lymphocytes.

Since there are clear biological differences between them, IFN-α and IFN-β are known as type I IFN, and IFN-γ as type II IFN. Induction of interferon synthesis results from upregulation of transcription from the interferon gene **promoters** There are three main mechanisms involved:

1 *Virus infection*: This mechanism is thought to act by the inhibition of cellular protein synthesis which occurs during many virus infections, resulting in a reduction in the concentration of intracellular repressor proteins and hence in increased interferon gene transcription. In general, RNA viruses are potent inducers of interferon while DNA viruses are relatively poor inducers. However, there are exceptions to this rule (e.g. poxviruses are very potent inducers). The molecular events in the induction of interferon synthesis by virus infection are not clear. In some cases (e.g. influenza virus), UV-inactivated virus is a potent inducer.

Therefore, virus replication is not necessarily required. Induction by viruses might involve perturbation of the normal cellular environment and/or production of small amounts of double-stranded RNA (see below).

2 *Double-stranded (**ds**) RNA*: All naturally occurring double-stranded RNAs (e.g. reovirus **genomes**) are potent inducers of interferon, as are synthetic molecules (e.g. poly I: C). Therefore, this process is independent of nucleotide sequence. Single-stranded RNA and double-stranded DNA are not inducers, hence the mechanism of induction is thought to depend on the secondary structure of the RNA rather than any particular nucleotide sequence.

3 *Metabolic inhibitors*: Compounds which inhibit cellular transcription (e.g. actino-mycin D) or translation (e.g. cycloheximide) result in induction of interferon. Tumour promoters such as TPA (tetradecanoyl phorbol acetate) or DMSO (dimethyl sulfoxide) are also inducers. Their mechanism of action remains unknown but they almost certainly act at the level of transcription.

The effects of IFNs are exerted via specific receptors which are ubiquitous on nearly all cell types (therefore, nearly all cells are potentially IFN-responsive). There are distinct receptors for type I and type II IFNs, each of which consists of two polypeptide chains. Binding of IFN to the type I receptor activates a specific cytoplasmic tyrosine kinase (Janus kinase, Jak1), which phosphorylates another cellular protein STAT2 (signal transducer and activator of transcription). This is transported to the nucleus and turns on transcriptional activation of IFN-responsive genes (including *IFN*, resulting in amplification of the original signal). Binding of IFN to the type II receptor activates a different cytoplasmic tyrosine kinase (Jak2), which phosphorylates the cellular protein STAT1, leading to transcriptional activation of a different set of genes.

The main action is on cellular regulatory activities and is rather complex. Interferon affects both cellular proliferation and immunomodulation. These effects result from the induction of transcription of a wide variety of cellular genes, including other cytokines. The net result is complex regulation of a cell's ability to proliferate, differentiate and communicate. This cell regulatory activity itself has indirect effects on virus replication (see below). All interferons have similar antiviral capacities, but IFN-γ is by far the most potent cellular regulator.

The effect of interferons on virus infections *in vivo* is extremely important. Animals experimentally infected with viruses and injected with anti-interferon antibodies experience much more severe infections than control animals infected with the same virus. This is because interferons protect cells from damage and death. However, they do not appear to play a major role in the clearance of virus infections – the other parts of the immune response are necessary for this. Interferon is a 'firebreak' which inhibits virus replication in its earliest stages by several mechanisms. Two of these are understood in some detail (below), but there are a number of others (in some cases specific to certain viruses) which are less well understood.

Figure 6.6 Mechanism of induction of 2′,5′-oligo A synthetase by interferons.

Interferons induce transcription of a cellular gene encoding 2′,5′-oligo A synthetase (Figure 6.6). There are at least four molecular species of 2′,5′-oligo A, induced by different forms of interferon. This compound activates an RNA-digesting enzyme, RNAse L, which digests virus genomic RNAs, virus and cellular mRNAs and cellular ribosomal RNAs. The end result of this mechanism is a reduction in protein synthesis (due to the degradation of mRNAs and rRNAs) and therefore, the cell is protected from virus damage. The second method relies on the activation of a 68 kDa protein called PKR (RNA-activated protein kinase) (Figure 6.7). PKR phosphorylates a cellular factor, eIF2α, which is required by ribosomes for the initiation of translation. Therefore, the net result of this mechanism is also the inhibition of protein synthesis and this reinforces the 2′,5′-oligo A mechanism. A third, well-established mechanism depends on the M_x gene, a single-copy gene located on human chromosome 21, whose transcription is induced by IFN-α and IFN-β but not IFN-γ. The product of this gene inhibits the primary transcription of influenza virus but not of other viruses. Its method of action is unknown.

Figure 6.7 Mechanism of induction of PKR by interferons.

In addition to the three mechanisms above, there are many additional recorded effects of interferons. They inhibit the **penetration** and **uncoating** of SV40 and some other viruses, possibly by altering the composition/structure of the cell membrane; they inhibit the primary transcription of many virus **genomes** (e.g. SV40, HSV) and also cell **transformation** by retroviruses. None of the molecular mechanisms by which these effects are mediated have been fully explained.

In conclusion, it can be stated that interferons are a powerful weapon against virus infection, but that they act as a blunderbuss, rather than a 'magic bullet'! The severe side-effects (fever, nausea, malaise) which result from the powerful cell-regulatory action of interferons means that they will never be widely used for the treatment of trivial virus infections – they are not the cure for the common cold. However, as the cell-regulatory potential of interferons is becoming better understood, they are finding increasing use as a treatment for certain cancers (e.g. the use of IFN-α in the treatment of hairy cell leukaemia). Current therapeutic uses of interferons are summarized in Table 6.1. The long-term prospects for their use as antiviral compounds are less certain, except for possibly in life-threatening infections where there is no alternative therapy, e.g. chronic viral hepatitis.

EVASION OF IMMUNE RESPONSES BY VIRUSES

In total, the many innate and adaptive components of the immune system present a powerful barrier to virus replication. Simply by virtue of their continued existence, it is obvious that viruses have, over millennia, evolved various effective 'counter-surveillance' mechanisms in this molecular arms race:

■ *Inhibition of MHC class I-restricted antigen presentation*: As described above, CTLs can only respond to foreign antigens presented by MHC I complexes on the target cell. A number of viruses interfere with MHC I expression or function to disrupt this process and evade the CTL response. Such mechanisms include downregula-

Table 6.1 Therapeutic uses of interferons

Condition	Virus
Chronic active hepatitis	HBV, HCV
Condylomata accuminata (genital warts)	Papillomaviruses
Tumours	
Hairy cell leukaemia	---
Kaposi's sarcoma (in AIDS patients)	HHV-8 (?)
Congenital diseases	
Chronic granulomatous disease - IFN-γ reduces bacterial infections.	---

tion of MHC I expression by adenoviruses and interference with the antigen processing required to form an MHC I/antigen complex by herpesviruses.

■ *Inhibition of MHC II restricted-antigen presentation*: MHC-II antigens are essential in the adaptive immune response in order to stimulate the development of antigen-responsive clones of effector cells. Again, herpesviruses and papillomaviruses interfere with the processing and surface expression of MHC II/antigen complexes, inhibiting the CTL response.

■ *Inhibition of natural killer cell lysis*: The poxvirus *Molluscum contagiosum virus* encodes a homologue of MHC I which is expressed on the surface of infected cells but is unable to bind an antigenic peptide, thus avoiding killing by NK cells which would be triggered by the absence of MHC I on the cell surface. Similar proteins are made by other viruses such as HHV-5 (CMV), and herpesviruses in general appear to have a number of sophisticated mechanisms to avoid NK cell killing.

■ *Interference with apoptosis*: See above.

■ *Inhibition of cytokine action*: Cytokines are secreted polypeptides that co-ordinate important aspects of the immune response, including inflammation, cellular activation, proliferation, differentiation and chemotaxis. Some viruses are able to inhibit the expression of certain chemokines directly. Alternatively, herpesviruses and poxviruses encode 'viroceptors' – virus homologues of host cytokine receptors which compete with cellular receptors for cytokine binding but fail to give transmembrane signals. High-affinity binding molecules may also neutralize cytokines directly, and molecules known as 'virokines' block cytokine receptors, again without activating the intracellular signalling cascade.

Interferons are an effective means of curbing the worst effects of virus infections. Part of their wide-ranging efficacy results from their generalized, non-specific effects (e.g. the inhibition of protein synthesis in virus-infected cells). This lack of specificity means that it is very difficult for viruses to evolve strategies to counteract their effects. Nevertheless, there are instances where this has happened. The anti-interferon effect of adenovirus VA RNAs has already been described in Chapter 5. Other mechanisms of virus resistance to interferons include:

■ *Epstein-Barr virus* EBER RNAs are similar in structure and function to the adenovirus VA RNAs. The EBNA-2 protein also blocks interferon-induced signal transduction.

■ *Vaccinia virus* is known to show resistance to the antiviral effects of interferons. One of the early genes of this virus, *K3L*, encodes a protein which is homologous to $eIF2\alpha$ which inhibits the action of PKR. In addition, the E3L protein also binds ds RNA and inhibits PKR activation.

■ *Poliovirus* infection activates a cellular inhibitor of PKR in virus-infected cells.

■ *Reovirus* **capsid** protein $\sigma3$ is believed to sequester ds RNA and therefore prevent activation of PKR.

Evasion of humoral immunity

Although direct humoral immunity is less significant than cell-mediated immunity, the antiviral action of ADCC and complement make this a worthwhile target to inhibit. The most frequent means of subverting the humoral response is by high-frequency genetic variation of the B-cell epitopes on antigens to which antibodies bind. This is only possible for viruses which are genetically variable, e.g. influenza virus and HIV. Herpesviruses use alternative strategies, such as encoding viral Fc receptors to prevent Fc-dependent immune activation.

Evasion of the complement cascade

Poxviruses, herpesviruses and retrovirus families encode mimics of normal regulators of complement activation proteins, e.g. secreted proteins which block C3 convertase assembly and accelerate its decay. Poxviruses can also inhibit C9 polymerization, preventing membrane permeabilization.

VIRUS–HOST INTERACTIONS

At this point, it would be as well to state once again that virus pathogenesis is an abnormal situation of no value to the virus – the vast majority of virus infections are asymptomatic. However, for pathogenic viruses, there are a number of critical stages in replication which determine the nature of the disease they produce.

Control at site of entry

For all viruses, pathogenic or non-pathogenic, the first factor which influences the course of infection is the mechanism and site of entry into the body (Figure 6.8):

- *The skin*: Mammalian skin is a highly effective barrier against viruses. The outer layer (epidermis) consists of dead cells and therefore does not support virus replication. Very few viruses infect directly by this route unless there is prior injury such as minor trauma or puncture of the barrier, such as insect or animal bites or subcutaneous injections. Some viruses which do use this route are herpes simplex virus and papillomaviruses, although these viruses probably still require some form of disruption of the skin such as small abrasions or eczema.
- *Mucosal membranes*: The mucosal membranes of the eye and genitourinary (GU) tract are much more favourable routes of access for viruses to the tissues of the body. This is reflected by the number of viruses which can be sexually transmitted; virus infections of the eye are also quite common (Table 6.2).

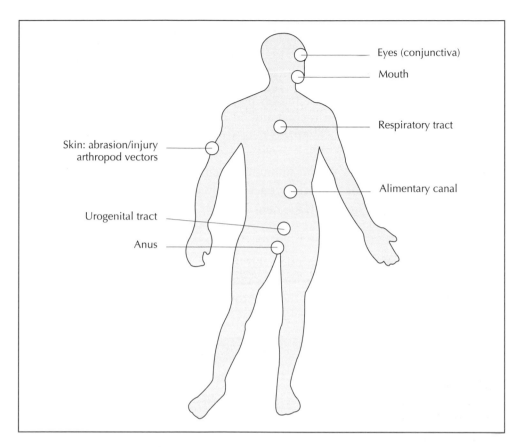

Figure 6.8 Schematic diagram to illustrate possible sites of virus entry into the body.

Table 6.2 Viruses which infect via mucosal surfaces	
Virus	**Site of infection**
Adenoviruses	Conjunctiva
Picornaviruses: Enterovirus 70	Conjunctiva
Papillomaviruses	Genitourinary tract
Herpesviruses	Genitourinary tract
Retroviruses: HIV, HTLV	Genitourinary tract

■ *Alimentary canal*: Viruses may infect the alimentary canal via the mouth, oropharynx, gut or rectum, although viruses which infect the gut via the oral route must survive passage through the stomach, an extremely hostile environment with a very low pH and high concentrations of digestive enzymes. Nevertheless, the gut is a highly valued prize for viruses – the intestinal epithelium is constantly replicating and there is a good deal of lymphoid tissue associated with the gut which provides many opportunities for virus replication. Moreover, the constant intake of food and fluids provides ample opportunity for viruses to infect these tissues (Table 6.3). To counteract this problem, the gut has many specific (e.g. secretory antibodies) and non-specific (e.g. stomach acids and bile salts) defence mechanisms.

■ *Respiratory tract*: The respiratory tract is probably the most frequent site of virus infection. As with the gut, it is constantly in contact with external virus particles which are taken in during respiration. As a result, the respiratory tract also has defences aimed at virus infection − filtering of particulate matter in the sinuses, and cells and antibodies of the immune system present in the lower regions. Viruses which infect the respiratory tract usually come directly from the respiratory tract of others, since aerosol spread is very efficient: 'coughs and sneezes spread diseases' (Table 6.4).

The natural environment is a considerable barrier to virus infections. Most viruses are relatively sensitive to heat, drying, ultraviolet light (sunlight), etc., although a few types are quite resistant to these factors. This is particularly important for

Table 6.3 Viruses which infect via the alimentary canal

Virus	Site of infection
Herpesviruses	Mouth and oropharynx
Adenoviruses	Intestinal tract
Caliciviruses	Intestinal tract
Coronaviruses	Intestinal tract
Picornaviruses: enteroviruses	Intestinal tract
Reoviruses	Intestinal tract

Table 6.4 Viruses which infect via the respiratory tract

Virus	Localized infections
Adenoviruses	Upper respiratory tract
Coronaviruses	Upper respiratory tract
Orthomyxoviruses	Upper respiratory tract
Picornaviruses: rhinoviruses	Upper respiratory tract
Paramyxoviruses: parainfluenza, respiratory syncytial virus (RSV)	Lower respiratory tract
Virus	**Systemic infections**
Herpesviruses	Varicella-Zoster (VZV)
Paramyxoviruses	Measles, mumps
Poxviruses	Smallpox
Togaviruses	Rubella

viruses which are spread via contaminated water or foodstuffs – not only must they be able to survive in the environment until they are ingested by another host, but as most are spread by the faecal–oral route, they must also be able to pass through the stomach to infect the gut before being shed in the faeces. One way of overcoming environmental stress is to take advantage of a secondary vector for transmission between the primary hosts (Figure 6.9). As with plant viruses (above), the virus may or may not replicate while in the vector. Viruses without a secondary vector must rely on continued host-to-host transmission, and have evolved various strategies to do this (Table 6.5):

- *Horizontal transmission*: The direct host-to-host transmission of viruses. This strategy relies on a high rate of infection to maintain the virus population.
- *Vertical transmission*: The transmission of the virus from one generation of hosts to the next. This may occur by infection of the fetus before, during, or shortly after birth (e.g. during breastfeeding). More rarely, it may involve direct transfer of the virus via the germline itself, e.g. retroviruses. In contrast to horizontal transmission, this strategy relies on long-term persistence of the virus in the host rather than rapid propagation and dissemination of the virus.

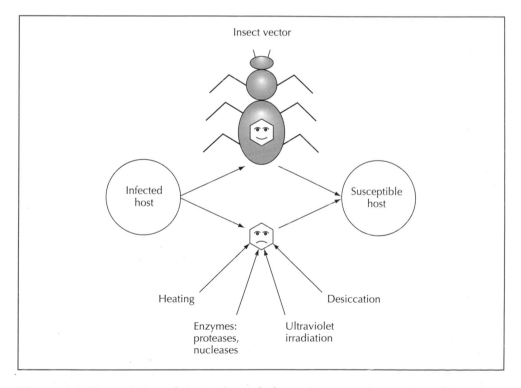

Figure 6.9 Transmission of viruses through the environment. Some viruses have adopted the use of vectors such as insects or other arthropods to avoid environmental stress.

Table 6.5 Virus transmission patterns

Pattern	Example
Horizontal transmission	
Human–human (aerosol)	Influenza
Human–human (faecal–oral)	Rotaviruses
Animal–human (direct)	Rabies
Animal–human (vector)	Bunyaviruses
Vertical transmission	
Placental–fetal	Rubella
Mother–child (birth)	HSV, HIV
Mother–child (breastfeeding)	HIV, HTLV
Germline	In mice, retroviruses; In humans ?

Control of spread through the host

Having gained entry to a potential host, the virus must initiate an infection by entering a susceptible cell (primary replication). This initial interaction frequently determines whether the infection will remain localized at the site of entry or spread to become a **systemic infection** (Table 6.6). In some cases, virus spread is controlled by infection of polarized epithelial cells and the preferential **release** of virus from either the apical (e.g. influenza virus – a localized infection in the upper respiratory tract) or basolateral (e.g. rhabdoviruses – a systemic infection) surface of the cells (Figure 6.10).

Following primary replication at the site of infection, the next stage may be spread throughout the host. In addition to direct cell-to-cell contact, there are two main mechanisms for spread throughout the host:

Table 6.6 Examples of localized and systemic virus infections

Virus	Primary replication	Secondary replication
Localized infections		
Papillomaviruses	Dermis	---
Rhinoviruses	Upper respiratory tract	---
Rotaviruses	Intestinal epithelium	---
Systemic infections		
Enteroviruses	Intestinal epithelium	Lymphoid tissues, CNS
Herpesviruses	Oropharynx or GU tract	Lymphoid cells, CNS

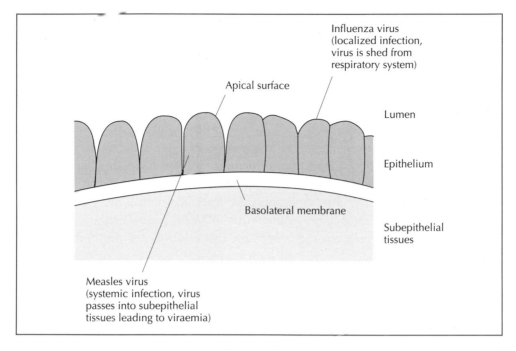

Figure 6.10 Virus infection of polarized epithelial cells.

1 *Via the bloodstream*: Viruses may get into the bloodstream by direct inoculation, for example, by arthropod vectors, blood transfusion or intravenous drug abuse (sharing of non-sterilized needles). The virus may travel free in the plasma (e.g. togaviruses, enteroviruses), or in association with red cells (orbiviruses), platelets (HSV), lymphocytes (EBV, CMV), or monocytes (lentiviruses). Primary viraemia usually precedes and is necessary for the spread of virus to other parts of the body via the bloodstream and is followed by a more generalized, higher **titre** secondary viraemia as the virus reaches the other target tissues or replicates directly in blood cells.

2 *Via the nervous system*: As above, spread of virus to the nervous system is usually preceded by primary viraemia. In some cases, spread occurs directly by contact with neurones at the primary site of infection, in other cases it occurs via the bloodstream. Once in peripheral nerves, the virus can spread to the CNS by axonal transport along neurones. The classic example of this is herpes simplex virus (see Latent Infection, below). Viruses can cross synaptic junctions since these frequently contain virus **receptors**, allowing the virus to 'jump' from one cell to another.

The spread of the virus to various parts of the body is controlled to a large extent by its cell or tissue **tropism**. Tissue tropism is controlled partly by the route of infection, but largely by the interaction of a **virus attachment protein** with a specific receptor molecule on the surface of a cell (as discussed in Chapter 4), and has considerable effect on pathogenesis.

At this stage, following significant virus replication and the production of virus antigens, the host immune response comes into play. This has already been discussed (above) and obviously has a major impact on the outcome of an infection. To a large extent, the efficiency of the immune response determines the amount of secondary replication which occurs and hence, the spread to other parts of the body. If a virus can be prevented from reaching tissues where secondary replication can occur, generally no disease results, although there are some exceptions to this. The immune response also plays a large part in determining the amount of cell and tissue damage that occurs as a result of virus replication. As described above, the production of interferons is a major factor in preventing virus-induced tissue damage.

The immune system is not the only factor that controls cell death, the amount of which varies considerably for different viruses. Viruses may replicate widely throughout the body without any disease symptoms if they do not cause significant cell damage or death. Retroviruses do not generally cause cell death, being released from the cell by budding rather than by cell lysis, and cause persistent infections, even being passed vertically to the offspring if they infect the germline. All vertebrate genomes, including humans, are littered with retrovirus **genomes** which have been with us for millions of years (Chapter 3). At present, these ancient virus genomes are not known to cause any disease in humans, although there are examples of tumours caused by them in rodents. Conversely, picornaviruses cause lysis and death of the cells in which they replicate, leading to fever and increased mucus secretion in the case of rhinoviruses, and paralysis or death (usually due to respiratory failure due to damage to the central nervous system resulting, in part, from virus replication in these cells) in the case of poliovirus.

Balance between clearance and persistence

The eventual outcome of any virus infection depends on a balance between clearance by the host organism and persistence by the virus. Clearance is mediated by the immune system (as discussed previously). However, the virus is a moving target which rapidly responds to pressure from the immune system by altering its antigenic composition (whenever possible). The classic example of this phenomenon is influenza virus, which displays two genetic mechanisms, called antigenic drift and antigenic shift, that allow the virus to alter its antigenic constitution.

Antigenic drift involves the gradual accumulation of minor mutations (e.g. nucleotide substitutions) in the virus **genome** which result in subtly altered coding potential and therefore altered antigenicity, leading to decreased recognition by the immune system. This process occurs in all viruses all the time, but at greatly different rates; for example, it is much more frequent in RNA viruses than in DNA viruses. In response, the immune system constantly adapts by recognition of and response to novel antigenic structures – but it is always one step behind. In most cases, however, the immune system is eventually able to overwhelm the virus, resulting in clearance.

In antigenic shift, a sudden and dramatic change in the antigenicity of a virus occurs owing to reassortment of the segmented virus genome with another genome of a different antigenic type (see Chapter 3). This results initially in the failure of the immune system to recognize a new antigenic type, giving the virus the upper hand (Figure 6.11).

The occurrence of past antigenic shifts in influenza virus populations is recorded by **pandemics** (worldwide epidemics; Figure 6.12). These events are marked by the sudden introduction of a new antigenic type of haemagglutinin and/or neuraminidase into the circulating virus, overcoming previous immunity in the human population. Previous haemagglutinin/neuraminidase types become resurgent when a sufficiently high proportion of the people who have 'immunological memory' of that type have died, thus overcoming the effect of 'herd immunity'.

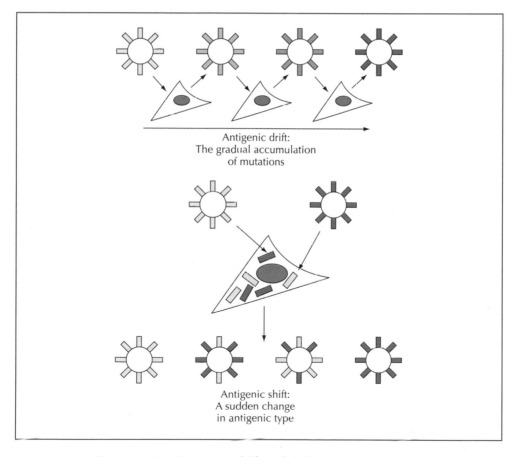

Figure 6.11 Antigenic shift and drift in influenza virus.

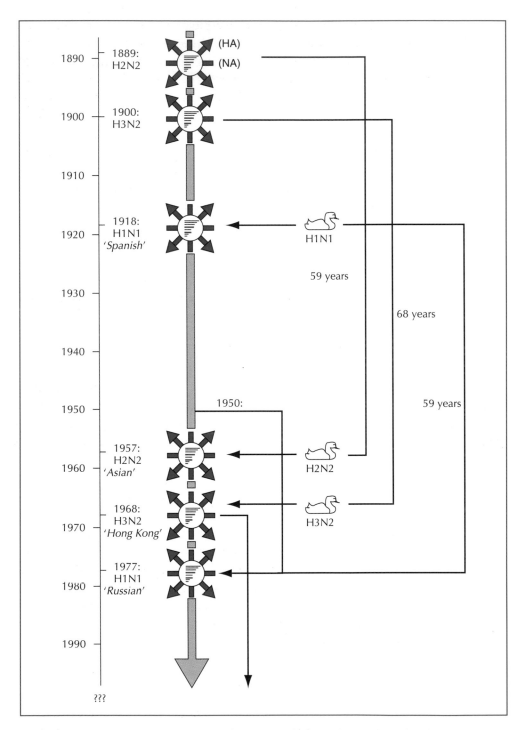

Figure 6.12 Influenza pandemics.

The other side of the relationship that determines the eventual outcome of a virus infection is the ability of the virus to persist in the host. Long–term persistence of viruses results from two main mechanisms. The first is the regulation of **lytic** potential. The strategy followed here is to achieve the continued survival of a critical number of virus infected cells, i.e. sufficient to continue the infection without killing the host organism. For viruses which do not usually kill the cells in which they replicate, this is not usually a problem; hence these viruses tend naturally to cause persistent infections, e.g. retroviruses. For viruses that undergo lytic infection, e.g. herpesviruses, it is necessary to develop mechanisms which restrict virus gene expression, and consequently, cell damage (see below). The second aspect of persistence is the evasion of immune surveillance, discussed above.

THE COURSE OF VIRUS INFECTIONS

Patterns of virus infection can be divided into a number of different types, according to how long their effects last.

Abortive infection

Abortive infection occurs when a virus infects a cell (or host), but cannot complete the full replication cycle. Therefore, this is a non-productive infection. However, the outcome of such infections is not necessarily insignificant; for example, SV40 infection of non-permissive rodent cells sometimes results in **transformation** of the cells (see Chapter 7).

Acute infection

This pattern is familiar for many common virus infections (e.g. 'colds'). In these relatively brief infections, the virus is usually eliminated completely by the immune system. Typically, in acute infections, much virus replication occurs before the onset of any symptoms (e.g. fever), which are the result not only of virus replication but of the activation of the immune system. Therefore, acute infections present a serious problem for the epidemiologist and are the pattern most frequently associated with **epidemics** (e.g. influenza, measles, etc.).

Chronic infection

These are the converse of acute infections, i.e. they are prolonged and stubborn. To cause this type of infection, the virus must persist in the host for a significant period. To the clinician, there is no clear distinction between chronic, persistent and latent infections and the terms are often used interchangeably. They are listed separately here because to virologists, there are significant differences in the events which occur during these infections.

Persistent infection

These infections result from a delicate balance between the virus and the host organism, in which ongoing virus replication occurs, but the virus adjusts its replication and pathogenicity to avoid killing the host. They differ from chronic infections in that whereas in chronic infections the virus is usually eventually cleared by the host (unless the infection proves fatal), in persistent infections, the virus may continue to be present and to replicate in the host for its entire lifetime.

The best-studied example of such a system is lymphocytic choriomeningitis virus (LCMV, an arenavirus) infection in mice (Figure 6.13). Mice can be experimentally infected with this virus either at a peripheral site (e.g. a footpad or the tail) or by direct inoculation into the brain. Adult mice infected in the latter way are killed by the virus, but if infected by a peripheral route, there are two possible outcomes to the infection: some mice die, whereas others survive, having cleared the virus from the body completely. It is not clear what factors determine the survival or death of LCMV-infected mice, but other evidence shows that this is related to the immune response to the virus. In immunosuppressed adult mice which are infected via the CNS route, a persistent infection is established in which the virus is not cleared (due to the non-functional immune system), but remarkably, these mice are not killed by

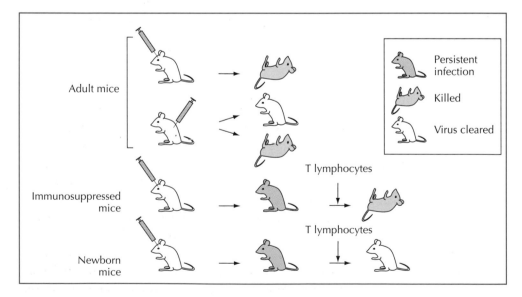

Figure 6.13 Persistent infection of mice by *Lymphocytic choriomeningitis virus* (LCMV).

the virus. If, however, syngeneic LCMV-specific T lymphocytes (i.e. of the same MHC type) are injected into these persistently infected mice, the animals develop the full pathogenic symptoms of LCMV infection and are killed. Newborn mice, whose immune systems are immature, infected via the CNS route also develop a persistent infection, but in this case, if subsequently injected with syngeneic LCMV-specific T lymphocytes, they clear the virus and survive the infection. The mechanisms which control these events are not completely understood, but evidently there is a delicate balance between the virus and the host animal and that the immune response to the virus is partly responsible for the pathology of the disease and the death of the animals.

Not infrequently, persistent infections may result from the production of **defective-interfering (D.I.) particles** (see Chapter 3). Such particles contain a partial deletion of the virus **genome** and are replication defective, but are maintained and may even tend to accumulate during infections because they can replicate in the presence of replication-competent helper virus. The production of D.I. particles is a common consequence of virus infection of animals, particularly by RNA viruses, but also occurs with DNA viruses and plant viruses and can be mimicked *in vitro* by continuous high **titre** passage of virus. Although not able to replicate themselves independently, D.I. particles are not necessarily genetically inert and may alter the course of an infection by **recombination** with the genome of a replication-competent virus. The presence of D.I. particles can profoundly influence the course and the outcome of a virus infection. In some cases, they appear to moderate pathogenesis, whereas in others they potentiate it, making the symptoms of the disease much more severe. Moreover, as D.I. particles effectively cause restricted gene expression (because they are genetically deleted), they may also result in a persistent infection by a virus which normally causes an acute infection and is rapidly cleared from the body.

Latent infection

This is the ultimate infection! In latent infection the virus is able to downregulate its gene expression and establish an inactive state, i.e. with strictly limited gene expression and without ongoing virus replication. Latent virus infections typically persist for the entire life of the host. An example of such an infection in humans is *Herpes simplex virus* (HSV). Infection of sensory nerves serving the mucosa results in localized primary replication. Subsequently, the virus travels via axonal transport mechanisms further into the nervous system. There, it 'hides' in dorsal root ganglia, such as the trigeminal ganglion, establishing a truly latent infection. The nervous system is an immunologically privileged site and is not patrolled by the immune system in the same way as the rest of the body, but nevertheless, the major factor in latency is the ability of the virus to restrict its gene expression. This eliminates the possibility of recognition of infected cells by the immune system. Restricted gene expression is achieved by tight regulation of α-gene expression, which is an essential control point in herpesvirus replication (Chapter 5). There has been much interest in mRNAs which are made by HSV during latent infection; these are known as latency-associated transcripts or LATs and raise the possibility of parallels between HSV latency and **lysogeny** in **phage** λ. However, it has recently been shown that the LATs promote neuronal survival after HSV infection by inhibiting **apoptosis**. This anti-apoptosis function could promote reactivation by:

- providing more latently infected neurons for future reactivations,
- protecting neurons in which reactivation occurs, or
- protecting previously uninfected neurons during a reactivation.

When reactivated by some provocative stimulus, HSV travels down the sensory nerves to cause peripheral manifestations such as cold sores or genital ulcers. It is not altogether clear what constitutes a provocative stimulus but there are many possible alternatives, including psychological and physical factors. Periodic reactivation establishes the pattern of infection, with sporadic, sometimes very painful reappearance of disease symptoms for the rest of the host's life. Even worse than this, immunosuppression later in life can cause the latent infection to flare up (which indicates that the immune system normally has a role in helping to suppress these latent infections), resulting in a very severe, **systemic** and often life-threatening infection.

In a manner somewhat similar to herpesviruses, infection by retroviruses may result in a latent infection. Integration of the **provirus** into the host **genome** certainly results in the persistence of the virus for the lifetime of the host organism and may lead to an episodic pattern of disease. In some ways, acquired immune deficiency syndrome (AIDS), which results from HIV infection, shows aspects of this pattern of infection. The pathogenesis of AIDS is discussed in detail in Chapter 7.

PREVENTION AND THERAPY OF VIRUS INFECTION

There are two aspects of the response to the threat of virus diseases: first, prevention of infection, and second, treatment of the disease. The former strategy relies on two approaches: public and personal hygiene, which perhaps plays the major role in preventing virus infection (e.g. provision of clean drinking water and disposal of sewage; good medical practice such as the sterilization of surgical instruments) and **vaccination**, which makes use of the immune system to combat virus infections. Most of the damage to cells during virus infections occurs very early, often before the clinical symptoms of disease appear. This makes the treatment of virus infection very difficult, and therefore, in addition to being cheaper, prevention of virus infection is undoubtedly better than cure.

To design effective **vaccines**, it is important to understand both the immune response to virus infection (above) and the stages of virus replication that are appropriate targets for immune intervention. To be effective, vaccines must stimulate as many of the body's defence mechanisms as possible. In practice, this usually means trying to mimic the disease, without of course causing pathogenesis – for example, the use of nasally administered influenza vaccines and orally administered poliovirus vaccines. To be effective, it is not necessary to get 100% uptake of vaccine. 'Herd immunity' results from the break in transmission of a virus which occurs when a sufficiently high proportion of a population has been vaccinated. This strategy is most effective where there is no alternative host for the virus, e.g. measles, and in practice is the situation that usually occurs since it is impossible to achieve 100% coverage with any vaccine. However, this is a risky business. If protection of the population falls below a critical level, **epidemics** can easily occur.

There are four basic types of vaccine: subunit vaccines, inactivated vaccines and live virus vaccines.

DNA vaccines

These are the newest type of vaccine and consist of only a DNA molecule encoding the antigen(s) of interest and possibly, co-stimulatory molecules such as cytokines. The concept behind these vaccines is that the DNA component will be expressed *in vivo*, creating small amounts of antigenic protein which serve to prime the immune response so that a protective response can be rapidly generated when the real antigen is encountered. In theory, these vaccines could be manufactured quickly and should efficiently induce both humoral and cell-mediated immunity. Initial clinical studies have indicated that there is still some way to go until this experimental technology becomes a practical proposition.

Subunit vaccines

These consist of only some components of the virus, sufficient to induce a protective immune response but not enough to allow any danger of infection. In general terms, they are completely safe, except for very rare cases in which adverse immune reactions may occur. Unfortunately, at present, they are also the least effective and most expensive type of vaccines. The major technical problems associated with subunit vaccines are their relatively poor antigenicity and the need for new delivery systems, such as improved carriers and **adjuvants**. There are several categories of such vaccines:

■ *Synthetic vaccines*, such as short, chemically synthesized peptides. The major disadvantage with these molecules is that they are not usually very effective immunogens and are very costly to produce. However, because they can be made to order for any desired sequence, they have great potential for the future. None are currently in use.

■ *Recombinant vaccines*, produced by genetic engineering. Such vaccines have been already produced and are better than the above type because they tend to give rise to a more effective immune response. Some practical success has already been achieved with this type of vaccine. For example, vaccination against *Hepatitis B virus* (HBV) used to rely on the use of 'Australian antigen' (HBsAg) obtained from the serum of chronic HBV carriers. This was a very risky practice indeed (because HBV carriers are often also infected with HIV). A completely safe recombinant HBV vaccine produced in yeast is now widely used.

■ *Virus vectors*, i.e. recombinant virus **genomes** genetically manipulated to express protective antigens from (unrelated) pathogenic viruses. The idea here is to utilize the genome of a well-understood, attenuated virus to express and present antigens to the immune system. Many different viruses offer possibilities for this type of approach, but the most highly developed system so far is based on the *Vaccinia virus* (VV) genome. This virus has been used to vaccinate millions of people worldwide in the campaign to eradicate smallpox (see below), and is generally a safe and effective vehicle for antigen delivery. Recombinant vaccines are difficult to produce and no human example is clearly successful yet, although many different trials are currently underway. VV-rabies recombinants have been used to eradicate rabies in European fox populations. Although vaccinia-based vaccines have many advantages, there are also disadvantages for use in humans. For example, the high percentage of the human population which has already been vaccinated during the smallpox eradication campaign may result in a poor response to recombinant vaccines. Also, although generally safe, VV is dangerous in immunocompromised hosts, and thus cannot be used in HIV-infected individuals. A possible solution to these problems may be to use *Avipoxvirus* vectors, e.g. fowlpox or canarypox, as 'suicide vectors' which can only establish **abortive infections** of mammalian cells. These can express high levels of foreign proteins, present no danger of pathogenesis (abortive infection) and have no natural immunity in humans (avian virus).

Inactivated vaccines

Inactivated vaccines are produced by exposing the virus to a denaturing agent under precisely controlled conditions. The objective is to cause loss of virus infectivity without loss of antigenicity. Obviously, this involves a delicate balance. However, inactivated vaccines have certain advantages, such as generally being effective immunogens (if properly inactivated), being relatively stable, and carrying little or no risk of vaccine-associated virus infection (if properly inactivated, but accidents can and do occur). The disadvantage of these vaccines is that it is not possible to produce inactivated vaccines for all viruses, since denaturation of virus proteins may lead to loss of antigenicity, e.g. measles virus. Although relatively effective, 'killed' vaccines are sometimes not as effective at preventing infection as 'live' virus vaccines (see below), often because they fail to stimulate protective mucosal and cell-mediated immunity to the same extent. A more recent concern is that these vaccines contain virus nucleic acids, which may themselves be a source of infection, either of their own accord (e.g. (+)sense RNA virus **genomes**) or after **recombination** with other viruses.

Live (attenuated) virus vaccines

This strategy relies on the use of viruses with reduced pathogenicity to stimulate an immune response without causing disease. The vaccine strain may be a naturally occurring virus (e.g. the use of cowpox virus by Edward Jenner to vaccinate against smallpox) or artificially **attenuated** *in vitro* (e.g. the oral poliomyelitis vaccines produced by Albert Sabin). The advantage of attenuated vaccines is that they are good immunogens and induce long-lived, appropriate immunity. Set against this are their many disadvantages. They are often biochemically and genetically unstable and may either lose infectivity (when they become worthless) or revert to virulence unexpectedly. Despite intensive study, it is not possible to produce an attenuated vaccine to order, and there appears to be no general mechanism by which different viruses can be reliably and safely attenuated. Contamination of the vaccine stock with other, possibly pathogenic viruses is also possible – this was the way in which SV40 was first discovered in oral poliovirus vaccine in 1960. Inappropriate use of live virus vaccines, for example, in immunocompromised hosts or during pregnancy, may lead to vaccine-associated disease, whereas the same vaccine given to a healthy individual may be perfectly safe.

Despite these difficulties, vaccination against virus infection has been one of the great triumphs of medicine during the twentieth century. Most of the success stories result from the use of live attenuated vaccines; for example, the use of *Vaccinia virus* against smallpox. On 8 May 1980, the World Health Organization (WHO) officially declared smallpox to be completely eradicated, the first virus disease to be eliminated from the world. The WHO Expanded Programme on Immunization currently focuses on the prevention of selected childhood diseases and aims to eradicate poliomyelitis by the year 2005, reduce measles deaths and incidence, eliminate neonatal tetanus (a bacterial infection) and introduce hepatitis B vaccine worldwide. In 1999, wild poliovirus transmission still occurred in 22 countries, in central Africa, the Middle East and Asia, but the rest of the world was free of polio, including the entire Western Hemisphere, the Western Pacific Region (including China), most of the Middle East and large parts of southern and northern Africa. The vaccination campaign against measles virus is estimated to have reduced the total reported annual number of cases from 6 million to about half a million (still an underestimate) and considerably reduced the death total from the previous level of one million annually. It is certain that these advances will be continued by the development and application of vaccines produced by recombinant DNA technology.

Virus vaccines do not have to be based on **virion** structural proteins. For example, *Human papillomavirus* (HPV) infection is associated with cervical carcinoma (Chapter 7). Two HPV regulatory proteins, E6 and E7, are consistently expressed in tumour cells and vaccines based on live recombinant vaccinia viruses expressing the E6 and E7 proteins of HPV 16 and 18 are under development for the prevention and treatment of cervical cancer. This raises another important point. Although prevention of infection by prophylactic vaccination is much the preferred option, post-exposure therapeutic vaccines can be of great value in modifying the course of some virus infections. Examples of this are rabies virus, where the course of infection may be very long and there is time for post-exposure vaccination to generate an effective immune response and prevent the virus from carrying out secondary replication in the CNS, which is responsible for the pathogenesis of rabies. Other potential examples are in virus-associated tumours, such as HPV-induced cervical carcinoma, as described above.

VIRUS VECTORS AND GENE THERAPY

Viruses are being developed as gene delivery systems for the treatment of inherited and also acquired diseases. The first human trial to treat children with immunodeficiency resulting from a lack of the enzyme adenosine deaminase (ADA) began in September 1990 and showed encouraging although not completely successful results. Like most of the initial attempts, this trial used recombinant retrovirus **genomes** as vectors. A variety of different viruses are being tested as potential vectors (Table 6.7) and a large number of different trials are underway, e.g. the first human trial of gene therapy for cystic fibrosis began in 1993. Non-virus methods of gene delivery including liposome/DNA complexes, peptide/DNA complexes and direct injection of recombinant DNA are also under active investigation. It is important to note that such experiments are aimed at augmenting defective cellular genes in the somatic cells of patients to alleviate the symptoms of the disease and not at manipulating the human germline, which is a different issue. There can be no question that carefully applied, this new application of virology will change the treatment of inherited diseases in the future.

CHEMOTHERAPY OF VIRUS INFECTIONS

The alternative to **vaccination** is to attempt to treat virus infections using drugs which block virus replication (Table 6.8). Historically, discovery of antiviral drugs has been largely fortuitous. Spurred on by successes in the treatment of bacterial infections with antibiotics, drug companies launched huge blind-screening programmes to identify chemical compounds with antiviral activity, with relatively little success. The key to the success of any antiviral drug lies in its specificity. Almost any stage of virus replication can be a target for a drug, but the drug must be more toxic to the virus than the host. This is measured by the chemotherapeutic index, given by:

Table 6.7 Virus vectors in gene therapy

Virus	Advantages	Possible disadvantages
Adenoviruses	Relatively easily manipulated *in vitro* (cf. retroviruses); genes coupled to the major late promoter (MLP) are efficiently expressed in large amounts.	Possible pathogenesis associated with partly attenuated vectors (especially in the lungs); immune response makes multiple doses ineffective if gene needs to be administered repeatedly (virus does not integrate).
Parvoviruses (AAV)	Integrate into cellular DNA at high frequency to establish a stable latent state; not associated with any known disease; vectors can be constructed which will not express any viral gene products.	Only ~5 kb of DNA can be packaged into the parvovirus capsid and some viruses sequences must be retained for packaging; integration into host cells DNA may potentially have damaging consequences.
Herpesviruses	Relatively easy to manipulate *in vitro*; grows to high titres; long-term persistence in neuronal cells without integration.	(Long-term) pathogenic consequences?
Retroviruses	Integrate into cell genome giving long-lasting (life-long?) expression of recombinant gene.	Difficult to grow to high titre and purify for direct administration (patient cells need to be cultured *in vitro*); cannot infect non-dividing cells - most somatic cells (except lentiviruses?); insertional mutagenesis/activation of cellular oncogenes.

$$\frac{\text{Dose of drug which inhibits virus replication}}{\text{Dose of drug which is toxic to host}}$$

The smaller the value of the chemotherapeutic index, the better. In practice, a difference of several orders of magnitude between the two toxicity values is usually required to produce a safe and clinically useful drug. Modern technology, including

Table 6.8 Antiviral drugs

Drug	Viruses	Chemical type	Target
Vidarabine	Herpesviruses	Nucleoside analogue	Virus polymerase
Acyclovir	Herpes simplex virus (HSV)	Nucleoside analogue	Virus polymerase
Gancyclovir	Cytomegalovirus (CMV)	Nucleoside analogue	Virus polymerase (needs virus UL98 kinase for activation)
Nucleoside analogue reverse transcriptase inhibitors (NRTI), e.g. zidovudine (AZT = Retrovir, first approved in 1987), Didanosine (ddI), Zalcitabine (ddC), Stavudine (d4T), Lamivudine (3TC)	Retroviruses (HIV)	Nucleoside analogue	Reverse transcriptase
Non-nucleoside reverse transcriptase inhibitors (NNRTI): Nevirapine, Delavirdine	Retroviruses (HIV)	Nucleoside analogue	Reverse transcriptase
Protease inhibitors, e.g. Saquinavir, Ritonavir, Indinavir, Nelfinavir	HIV	Peptide analogue	HIV protease
Ribavirin	Broad spectrum: HCV, HSV, measles, mumps, Lassa fever	Triazole carboxamide	Virus replicase (complex action, direct or indirect)
Amantadine/ Rimantadine	Influenza A	Tricyclic amine	Matrix protein/ haemagglutinin
Neuraminidase inhibitors, e.g. Relenza	Influenza A and B	5–(Acetylamino)-4-[(aminoiminomethyl)-amino]-2,6-anhydro-3,4,5-trideoxy-D-glycero-D-galacto-non-2-enonic acid	Neuraminidase

molecular biology and computer–aided design of chemical compounds, allows the deliberate design of drugs, but to do this, it is necessary to 'know your enemy', i.e. to understand the key steps in virus replication which might be inhibited. Any of the stages of virus replication can be a target for antiviral intervention. The only requirements are:

1 That the process targeted be essential for replication.
2 That the drug is active against the virus but has 'acceptable toxicity' to the host organism.

What degree of toxicity is 'acceptable' clearly varies considerably, for example, between a cure for the common cold, which might be sold over the counter and taken by millions of people, and a drug used to treat fatal virus infections such as AIDS.

The attachment phase of replication can be inhibited in two ways: by agents which mimic the **virus-attachment protein** (VAP) and bind to the cellular **receptor**, or by agents which mimic the receptor and bind to the VAP. Synthetic peptides are the most logical class of compound to use for this purpose. While this is a promising line of research, there are considerable problems with clinical use of these substances, mostly the high cost of synthetic peptides and their poor pharmacokinetic properties.

It is difficult to target specifically the penetration/uncoating stages of virus replication as relatively little is known about them. Uncoating in particular is largely mediated by cellular enzymes and is therefore a poor target for intervention, although like penetration, it is often influenced by one or more virus proteins. Amantadine and rimantadine are two drugs that are active against influenza A viruses. The action of these closely related agents is to block cellular membrane ion channels. The target for both drugs is the influenza matrix protein (M_2), but resistance to the drug may also map to the haemagglutinin gene. This biphasic action results from the inability of drug-treated cells to lower the pH of the endosomal compartment (a function normally controlled by the M_2 gene product), which is essential to induce conformational changes in the haemagglutinin protein to permit membrane fusion (see Chapter 4).

Many viruses have evolved their own specific enzymes to replicate virus nucleic acids, preferentially at the expense of cellular molecules. There is often sufficient specificity in virus polymerases to provide a target for an antiviral agent, and this method has produced the majority of the specific antiviral drugs currently in use. Most of these drugs function as polymerase substrates (i.e. nucleoside/nucleotide) analogues, and their toxicity varies considerably from some which are well tolerated (e.g. acyclovir) to others which are quite toxic (e.g. AZT). There is a problem with the pharmacokinetics of these nucleoside analogues in that their typical serum half-life is 1–4 hours. Nucleoside analogues are, in fact, pro-drugs, since they need to be phosphorylated before becoming effective. This is the key to their selectivity:

■ Acyclovir is phosphorylated by HSV thymidine kinase 200 times more efficiently than by cellular enzymes.
■ Ganciclovir is 10 times more effective against CMV than acyclovir, but must be phosphorylated by a kinase encoded by CMV gene *UL97* before it becomes pharmaceutically active.

A series of other nucleoside analogues derived from these drugs and active against herpesviruses have been developed, e.g. valciclovir and famciclovir. These compounds have improved pharmacokinetic properties such as better oral bioavailability and longer half-lives. In addition to these, there are a number of non-nucleoside analogues which inhibit virus polymerases. Foscarnet is an analogue of pyrophosphate which interferes with the binding of incoming nucleotide triphosphates by virus DNA polymerases. Ribavirin is an interesting compound with a very wide spectrum of activity against many different viruses, especially against many (−)sense RNA viruses. The way in which these effects are caused are not entirely clear, but may include mechanisms such as the following:

- Ribavirin 5′ monophosphate inhibits inosine monophosphate dehydrogenase and decreases intracellular pools of guanosine triphosphate.
- Ribavirin 5′ triphosphate inhibits guanylyltransferase and the 5′ capping of mRNAs.
- Ribavirin 5′ triphosphate inhibits initiation and elongation by RNA polymerases.

Ribavirin is thus quite unlike the other nucleoside analogues described above and its use is likely to become much more widespread in future.

Virus gene expression is less amenable to chemical intervention than **genome** replication, because viruses are much more dependent on the cellular machinery for transcription, mRNA **splicing**, cytoplasmic export, and translation than for replication. To date, no clinically useful drugs which discriminate between virus and cellular gene expression have been developed. As with penetration and **uncoating**, for the majority of viruses, the processes of **assembly**, **maturation** and **release** are poorly understood, and therefore, have not yet become targets for antiviral intervention, with the exception of the anti-influenza drug Relenza, an inhibitor of influenza virus neuraminidase. Neuraminidase is involved in the release of virus particles budding from infected cells and this drug is believed to reduce the spread of virus to other cells.

The most striking aspect of antiviral chemotherapy is how few clinically useful drugs are available. As if this were not bad enough, there is also the problem of drug resistance to consider. In practice, the speed and frequency with which resistance arises when drugs are used to treat virus infections varies considerably and depends largely on the biology of the virus involved rather than on the chemistry of the compound. To illustrate this, two extreme cases – acyclovir and azidothymidine – are described.

Acyclovir used to treat *Herpes simplex virus* (HSV) infections is easily the most widely used antiviral drug. This is particularly true in the case of genital herpes, which causes painful recurrent ulcers on the genitals. It is estimated that 40–60 million people suffer from this condition in the USA. Fortunately, resistance to acyclovir arises infrequently. This is partly due to the high fidelity with which the DNA **genome** of HSV is copied (Chapter 3). Mechanisms which give rise to acyclovir resistance include:

- HSV *pol* gene mutants which do not incorporate acyclovir
- HSV thymidine kinase (TK) mutants in which TK activity is absent (TK⁻), reduced or shows altered substrate specificity.

Strangely, it is possible to find mutations which give rise to each of these phenotypes with a frequency of 10^{-3}–10^{-4} in clinical HSV isolates. The discrepancy between this and the very low frequency with which resistance is recorded clinically is probably explained by the observation that most *pol*/TK mutants appear to be attenuated (e.g. TK⁻ mutants of HSV do not reactivate from the latent state).

Conversely, azidothymidine (AZT) treatment of HIV infection is much less effective. In untreated HIV-infected individuals, AZT produces a rise in the numbers of CD4⁺ cells within 2–6 weeks. However, this beneficial effect is transient; after 20 weeks, CD4⁺ T-cell counts generally revert to baseline. This is due partly to the development of AZT resistance in treated HIV populations and to the toxicity of AZT on haematopoiesis, since the chemotherapeutic index of AZT is much worse than that of acyclovir. AZT resistance is initiated by the acquisition of a mutation in the HIV reverse transcriptase (RT) gene at codon 215. In conjunction with two to three additional mutations in the RT gene, a fully AZT-resistant phenotype develops. After 20 weeks of treatment, 40–50% of AZT-treated patients develop at least one of these mutations. This high frequency is due to the error-prone nature of reverse transcription (Chapter 3). Because of the large number of replicating HIV **genomes** in infected patients (Chapter 7), many mistakes occur continuously. It has been shown that the mutations which confer resistance already exist in untreated virus populations. Thus, treatment with AZT does not cause but merely selects these resistant viruses from the total pool.

With other anti-RT drugs, such as ddI, a resistant phenotype can result from a single base pair change. However, ddI has an even lower therapeutic index than AZT and relatively low levels of resistance can potentially render this drug useless. However, some combinations of resistant mutations may make it difficult for HIV to replicate and resistance to one RT inhibitor may counteract resistance to another. The current strategy for therapy of HIV infection is known as HAART (highly active antiretroviral therapy) and employs combinations of different drugs such as a protease inhibitor plus two nucleoside reverse transcriptase inhibitors. Molecular mechanisms of resistance and drug interactions are both important to consider in designing combination regimes:

- Combinations such as AZT + ddI or AZT + 3TC have antagonistic patterns of resistance and are effective.
- Combinations such as ddC + 3TC that show cross-reactive resistance should be avoided.
- Certain protease inhibitors affect liver function and can favourably affect the pharmacokinetics of RT inhibitors taken in combination.

Other potential benefits of combination antiviral therapy include lower toxicity profiles and the use of drugs that may have different tissue distributions or cell **tropisms**. Combination therapy may also prevent or delay the development of drug resistance. Combinations of drugs which can be employed include not only small synthetic molecules but also 'biological response modifiers' such as interleukins and interferons.

SUMMARY

Virus infection is a complex, multi-stage interaction between the virus and the host organism. The course and eventual outcome of any infection is the result of a balance between host and virus processes. Host factors involved include exposure to different routes of virus transmission and the control of virus replication by the immune response. Virus processes include the initial infection of the host, spread throughout the host and the regulation of gene expression to evade the immune response. Medical intervention against virus infections includes the use of vaccines to stimulate the immune response and drugs to inhibit virus replication. Molecular biology is stimulating the production of a new generation of antiviral drugs and vaccines.

FURTHER READING

Biron, C.A., Nguyen, K.B., Pien, G.C., Cousens, L.P. and Salazar-Mather, T.P. (1999). Natural killer cells in antiviral defense: function and regulation by innate cytokines. *Annual Review of Immunology* 17: 189–220.

Blair, E., Tisdale, M., Gough, G. and Rowlands, D. (1997). *Antiviral Therapy*. Springer-Verlag, New York. ISBN 1859960707.

Cox, N.J. and Subbarao, K. (2000). Global epidemiology of influenza: past and present. *Annual Review of Medicine* 51: 407–421.

Doherty, P. C. and Christensen, J.P. (2000). Accessing complexity: the dynamics of virus-specific T cell responses. *Annual Review of Immunology* 18: 561–592.

Goldsby, R.A., Kindt, T.J. and Osborne, B.A. (2000). *Kuby: Immunology* (4th edn). W.H. Freeman, New York. ISBN 0716733315.

Gurunathan, S., Klinman, D.M. and Seder, R.A. (2000). DNA vaccines: immunology, application, and optimization. *Annual Review of Immunology* 18: 927–974.

Lachmann, P. J. and Davies, A. (1997). Complement and immunity to viruses. *Immunological Reviews* 159: 69–77.

Lemoine, N.R. (Ed.) (2000). *Understanding Gene Therapy*. Springer-Verlag, Berlin. ISBN: 0387915125.

Stark, G.R., Kerr, I.M., Williams, B.R., Silverman, R.H. and Schreiber, R.D. (1998). How cells respond to interferons. *Annual Review of Biochemistry* 67: 227–264.

Tortorella D., Gewurz, B.E., Furman, M.H., Schust, D.J. and Ploegh, H.L. (2000).Viral subversion of the immune system. *Annual Review of Immunology* 18: 861–926.

Yewdell, J.W. and Bennink, J.R. (1999). Mechanisms of viral interference with MHC Class I antigen processing and presentation. *Annual Review of Cellular and Developmental Biology* 15: 579–606.

SELF-ASSESSMENT QUESTIONS

(6.1) Plant viruses (true or false?):

(a)   are responsible for an estimated US$60 000 000 worth of damage each year.

(b)   can be transmitted by infected seeds.

(c)   may be transmitted to new hosts as wind-blown dust or as rain-splashed mud.

(d)   never replicate in insect vectors.

(e)   always cause a systemic infection involving the whole plant.

(6.2) Are the following statements true or false?

(a)   Movement proteins allow plant viruses to be transmitted from insect vectors to plants.

(b)   Damage to virus-infected plants occurs through necrosis of cells, hypoplasia and hyperplasia.

(c)   The hypersensitive response in plants is functionally analogous to the production of interferons in animals.

(d)   The hypersensitive response in plants tends to limit the occurrence of systemic infection.

(e)   Virus-resistant plants have been created by genetic manipulation resulting in the endogenous expression of virus genes.

(6.3) Are the following statements true or false?

(a)   The major impact of the humoral immune response on virus infections is the eventual clearance of virus from the body.

(b)   Unlike bacteria, virus particles are not directly neutralized by antibodies or phagocytosed by white blood cells.

(c)   Overall, cell-mediated immunity is more important than humoral immunity in controlling virus infections.

(d)   Natural killer (NK) cells are the first cell-mediated defence mechanism to be activated against virus infection.

(e)   Cytotoxic T lymphocytes (CTLs) are not MHC-restricted.

(6.4) Are the following statements true or false?
(a)   Interferon was discovered in chickens in 1975.
(b)   Biochemical purification of interferons from natural sources was difficult because interferons were so abundant.
(c)   There are three distinct types of interferon: α, β and γ.
(d)   Interferons are synthesized only by fibroblasts.
(e)   Double-stranded DNA is a potent inducer of interferon synthesis.

(6.5) Are the following statements true or false?
(a)   All interferons have similar antiviral capacities, but act differently as cellular regulators.
(b) $2',5'$-oligo A activates RNAse L, which digests all RNAs.
(c)   PKR phosphorylates eIF2α, which is required for the initiation of translation.
(d)   Interferons are used to treat chronic viral hepatitis.
(e)   Several viruses have evolved mechanisms which enable them to resist the effects of interferons.

(6.6) Are the following statements true or false?
(a)   Mucosal membranes are favourable routes of access for viruses to the tissues of the body.
(b)   'Coughs and sneezes spread diseases.'
(c)   The natural environment is a considerable barrier to virus infections.
(d)   Primary systemic infection by viruses is frequently followed by localized secondary infection.
(e)   Spread of virus to the nervous system usually precedes primary viraemia.

(6.7) Viruses have evolved many tricks to fool the immune system (true or false?):
(a)   Antigenic variation.
(b)   Upregulation of MHC class I gene expression.
(c)   Upregulation of accessory molecules involved in immune recognition.
(d)   Infection of immunocompromised sites within the body.
(e)   Direct infection of the cells of the skin.

(6.8) Are the following statements true or false?
(a)   Abortive infection of cells can have significant pathological consequences.
(b)   In acute infections, much virus replication occurs before the onset of any symptoms.

(c)   In persistent infections, the virus adjusts its replication and patho-
        genicity to avoid killing the host.
(d)   Persistent infections may result from the production of defective-
        interfering (D.I.) particles.
(e)   Latent infections are typified by strictly limited gene expression
        without ongoing virus replication.

(6.9)   Are the following statements true or false?
(a)   Subunit vaccines are the most effective and least expensive virus
        vaccines.
(b)   No recombinant virus vaccines produced by genetic engineering are
        currently in use.
(c)   Inactivated virus vaccines are sometimes not as effective as 'live' virus
        vaccines because they fail to stimulate mucosal and cell–mediated
        immunity.
(d)   The majority of successful virus vaccines are based on attenuated
        viruses.
(e)   Retroviruses have been used successfully as vectors for gene therapy.

(6.10) Are the following statements true or false?
(a)   Prevention of virus infection by drug treatment is preferable to
        vaccination.
(b)   Any of the stages of virus replication can be a potential target for
        antiviral chemotherapy.
(c)   The majority of antiviral drugs in use are nucleoside/nucleotide
        analogues.
(d)   Ribavirin is active only against influenza A viruses.
(e)   The frequency with which viruses become resistant to antiviral
        drugs depends on the drug and the virus concerned.

Answers to Self-Assessment Questions are given in Appendix 4.

CHAPTER 7

PATHOGENESIS

Learning Objectives

On completing this chapter, you should be able to:
- Explain the concept of pathogenesis in the context of virus infection.
- Discuss the molecular basis for virus-induced immunodeficiency (including AIDS) and cell transformation by viruses.
- Understand the ways in which virus infection may result in cellular injury.

Pathogenicity, which is the capacity of one organism to cause disease in another, is a complex and variable phenomenon. For one thing, it is rather difficult to define. At the simplest level there is the question, what is disease? An all-embracing definition would be that it is a departure from the normal physiological parameters of an organism. This could range from a transient and very minor condition such as a slightly elevated temperature or rather subjective feelings of lethargy to chronic pathologic conditions which eventually result in death. Any of these conditions may result from a tremendous number of internal or external sources. However, there is rarely one single factor which 'causes' a disease. Most disease states are multi-factorial at one level or another.

Considering virus diseases only, there are two components involved: the direct effects of virus replication and the effects of bodily responses to the infection. The course of any virus infection is determined by a delicate and dynamic balance between the host and the virus, as described in Chapter 6. The extent and severity of virus pathogenesis is determined similarly. In some virus infections, most of the pathologic symptoms observed are attributable not to virus replication, but to the side-effects of the immune response. Inflammation, fever, headaches and skin rashes are not usually caused by viruses themselves, but by the cells of the immune system due to the release of potent chemicals such as interferons and interleukins. In the most extreme cases, it is possible that none of the pathologic effects of certain diseases are caused directly by the virus, except that its presence stimulates the activation of the immune system.

Virus pathogenesis is an abnormal and fairly rare situation. The majority of virus infections are silent and do not result in outward signs of disease. It is sometimes said that viruses would disappear if they killed their hosts. This is not necessarily true. It is perfectly possible to envisage viruses with a hit-and-run strategy, moving quickly from one dying host to the next and relying on continuing circulation for their survival. Nevertheless, there is a clear tendency for viruses not to injure their hosts if possible. A good example of this is the rabies virus. The symptoms of human rabies virus infections are truly dreadful, but thankfully rare. However, in its normal hosts (e.g. foxes), rabies virus infection produces a much milder disease which does not usually kill the animal. Humans are an unnatural, dead-end host for this virus and the severity of human rabies is extreme as the condition is rare. Ideally, a virus would not even provoke an immune response from its host, or at least be able to hide to avoid the effects. Herpesviruses and some retroviruses have evolved complex lifestyles which enable them to get close to this objective. Of course, fatal infections such as rabies and AIDS always grab the headlines. Much less effort has been devoted to isolating and studying the myriad viruses which have not (yet) caused well-defined diseases in humans, domestic animals or economically valuable crop plants.

In the past few decades, molecular genetic analysis has contributed enormously to our understanding of virus pathogenesis. Nucleotide sequencing and site-directed mutagenesis have been used to explore molecular determinants of virulence in many different viruses. Specific sequences and structures which are found only in disease-causing strains of virus and not in closely related attenuated or **avirulent** strains have been identified. Sequence analysis has also led to the identification of T-cell and B-cell epitopes on virus proteins responsible for their recognition by the immune system. Unfortunately, these advances do not automatically lead to an understanding of the mechanisms responsible for pathogenicity.

Unlike the rest of this book, this chapter is specifically about viruses which cause disease in animals. It does not discuss viruses that cause disease in plants, which have already been considered in Chapter 6. Three major aspects of virus pathogenesis are considered: direct cell damage resulting from virus replication, damage resulting from immune activation or suppression, and cell **transformation** caused by viruses.

MECHANISMS OF CELLULAR INJURY

Virus infection results in a number of changes which are detectable by visual or biochemical examination of infected cells. These changes result from the production of virus proteins and nucleic acids, but also from alterations to the biosynthetic capabilities of cells. Intracellular parasitism by viruses sequesters cellular apparatus such as ribosomes and raw materials which would normally be devoted to synthesizing molecules required by the cell. **Eukaryotic** cells must carry out constant macromolecular synthesis, whether they are growing and dividing or in a state of quiescence. A growing cell clearly needs to manufacture more proteins, more nucleic acids and more of all of its myriad components to increase its size before dividing. However, there is a much more fundamental requirement for such activity. The function of all cells is regulated by controlled expression of their genetic information and the subsequent degradation of the molecules produced. Such control relies on a delicate and dynamic balance between synthesis and decay, which determines the intracellular levels of all the important molecules in the cell. This is particularly true of the control of the cell cycle, which determines the behaviour of dividing cells (see Cell Transformation by DNA Viruses). In general terms, a number of common phenotypic changes can be recognized in virus-infected cells. These changes are often referred to as the **cytopathic effects** (**c.p.e.**) of a virus, and include:

- *Altered shape:* Adherent cells, which are normally attached to other cells (*in vivo*) or an artificial substrate (*in vitro*), may assume a rounded shape different from their normal flattened appearance. The extended 'processes' (extensions of the cell surface resembling tendrils) involved in attachment or mobility are withdrawn into the cell.
- *Detachment from the substrate:* For adherent cells, this is the stage of cell damage which follows that above. Both of these effects are caused by partial degradation or disruption of the cytoskeleton which is normally responsible for maintaining the shape of the cell.
- *Lysis:* This is the most extreme case, where the entire cell breaks down. Membrane integrity is lost and the cell may swell due to the absorption of extracellular fluid and finally, break open. This is an extreme case of cell damage and it is important to realize that not all viruses induce this effect, although they may cause other cytopathic effects. Lysis is beneficial to a virus in that it provides an obvious method of releasing new virus particles from an infected cell. However, there are alternative ways of achieving this, such as **release** by **budding** (Chapter 4).
- *Membrane fusion:* The membranes of adjacent cells fuse, resulting in a mass of cytoplasm containing more than one nucleus, known as a **syncytium**, or, depending on the number of cells which merge, a giant cell. Fused cells are short lived and subsequently lyse – apart from direct effects of the virus, they cannot tolerate more than one non-synchronized nucleus per cell.
- *Membrane permeability:* A number of viruses cause an increase in membrane permeability, allowing an influx of extracellular ions such as sodium. Translation of some virus mRNAs is resistant to high concentrations of sodium ions, permitting the expression of virus genes at the expense of cellular messages.

- **Inclusion bodies:** These are areas of the cell where virus components have accumulated. They are frequently sites of virus assembly, and some cellular inclusions consist of crystalline arrays of virus particles. It is not clear how these structures damage the cell, but they are frequently associated with viruses which cause cell lysis, such as herpesviruses and rabies virus.
- **Apoptosis:** Virus infection may trigger apoptosis ('programmed cell death'), a highly specific mechanism involved in the normal growth and development of organisms (see Chapter 6).

In some cases, a great deal of detail is known about the molecular mechanisms of cell injury. A number of viruses which cause cell lysis exhibit a phenomenon known as **shutoff** early in infection. Shutoff is the sudden and dramatic cessation of most host cell macromolecular synthesis. In poliovirus-infected cells, this is the result of production of the virus 2A protein. This molecule is a protease which cleaves the p220 component of eIF-4F, a complex of proteins required for cap-dependent translation of messenger RNAs by ribosomes. Since poliovirus RNA does not have a 5' methylated cap, but is modified by the addition of the VPg protein, virus RNA continues to be translated. In poliovirus-infected cells, the dissociation of mRNAs and polyribosomes from the cytoskeleton can be observed and this is the reason for the inability of the cell to translate its own messages. A few hours after translation ceases, lysis of the cell occurs.

In other cases, cessation of cellular macromolecular synthesis results from a different molecular mechanism. For many viruses, the sequence of events that occurs is not known. In the case of adenoviruses, the penton protein (part of the virus **capsid**) has a toxic effect on cells. Although its precise action on cells is not known, addition of purified penton protein to cultured cells results in their rapid death. Toxin production by pathogenic bacteria is a common phenomenon, but this is the only well-established case of a virus-encoded molecule with a toxin-like action. However, some of the normal contents of cells released on lysis may have toxic effects on other cells, and antigens which are not recognized as 'self' by the body (e.g. nuclear proteins) may result in immune activation and inflammation. The adenovirus E3-11.6K protein is synthesized in small amounts from the E3 promoter at early stages of infection and in large amounts from the major late promoter at late stages of infection (Chapter 5). It has recently been shown that E3-11.6K is required for the lysis of adenovirus-infected cells and the **release** of virus particles from the nucleus.

Membrane **fusion** is the result of virus-encoded proteins required for infection of cells (see Chapter 4), typically, the glycoproteins of **enveloped viruses**. One of the best-known examples of such a protein comes from Sendai virus (a paramyxovirus), which has been used to induce cell fusion during the production of monoclonal antibodies (Chapter 1). At least nine of the eleven known herpes simplex virus (HSV/HHV-1) glycoproteins have been characterized with regard to their role in virus replication. A number of these proteins are involved in fusion of the virus envelope with the cell membrane and also in cell **penetration**. Production of fused **syncytia** is a common feature of HSV infection.

Another virus which causes cell fusion is *Human immunodeficiency virus* (HIV). Infection of CD4$^+$ cells with some but not all isolates of HIV causes cell–cell fusion and the production of syncytia or giant cells (Figure 7.1). The protein responsible for this is the transmembrane envelope glycoprotein of the virus (gp41) and the domain near the amino-terminus responsible for this fusogenic activity has been identified by molecular genetic analysis. Because HIV infects CD4$^+$ cells and it is the reduction in the number of these crucial cells of the immune system which is the most obvious defect in AIDS, it was initially believed that direct killing of these cells by the virus was the basis for the pathogenesis of AIDS. Although direct cell killing by HIV undoubtedly occurs *in vivo*, it is now believed that the pathogenesis of AIDS is considerably more complex (see Viruses and Immunodeficiency). Many animal retroviruses also cause cell killing, and in most cases it appears that the envelope protein of the virus is required, although there may be more than one mechanism involved.

VIRUSES AND IMMUNODEFICIENCY

At least two groups of viruses, herpesviruses and retroviruses, directly infect the cells of the immune system. This has important consequences for the outcome of the infection and for the immune system of the host. *Herpes simplex virus* (HSV) establishes a **systemic infection**, spreading via the bloodstream in association with platelets, but does not show particular **tropism** for cells of the immune system. However, *Herpes saimirii* and *Marek's disease virus* are herpesviruses which cause lymphoproliferative diseases (but not clonal tumours) in monkeys and chickens, respectively. The most recently discovered human herpesviruses, human herpesvirus 6 (HHV-6), HHV-7 and HHV-8 all infect lymphocytes (Chapter 8).

Epstein–Barr virus (HHV-4, EBV) infection of B cells leads to their immortalization and proliferation, resulting in 'glandular fever' or mononucleosis, a debilitating but benign condition. EBV was first identified in a lymphoblastoid cell line derived from Burkitt's lymphoma and, in rare instances, EBV infection may lead to the formation of a malignant tumour (see Cell Transformation by DNA Viruses). While some herpesviruses such as HSV are notably cytopathic, most of the lymphotropic herpesviruses do not cause a significant degree of cellular injury. However, infection of the delicate cells of the immune system may perturb their normal function. Because the immune system is internally regulated by complex networks of interlinking signals, relatively small changes in cellular function can result in its collapse. Alteration of the normal pattern of production of cytokines could have profound effects on immune function. The *trans*-regulatory proteins involved in the control of herpesvirus gene expression may also affect the transcription of cellular

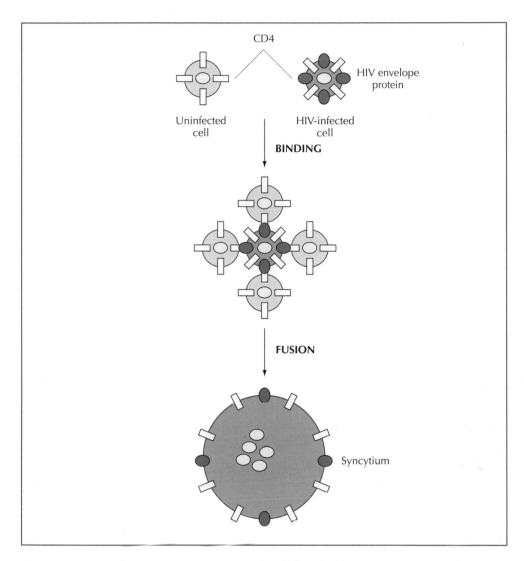

Figure 7.1 Mechanisim of HIV-induced cell fusion. The virus envelope glycoprotein, whose role on virus particles is in receptor-binding and membrane fusion, is expressed on the surface of infected cells. Uninfected cells CD4$^+$ cells coming into contact with these infected cells are fused together to form a multi-nucleate syncytium.

genes. Therefore, the effects of herpesviruses on immune cells are more complex than just cell killing.

Retroviruses cause a variety of pathogenic conditions including paralysis, arthritis, anaemia and malignant cellular **transformation**. A significant number of retroviruses infect the cells of the immune system. Although these infections may lead to a diverse array of diseases and haematopoietic abnormalities such as anaemia and lymphoproliferation, the most commonly recognized consequence of retrovirus infection is the formation of lymphoid tumours (see Cell Transformation by RNA Viruses). However, some degree of immunodeficiency, ranging from very mild to quite severe, is a common consequence of the interference with the immune system resulting from the presence of a lymphoid or myeloid tumour.

The most prominent aspect of virus-induced immunodeficiency is acquired immune deficiency syndrome (AIDS), a consequence of infection with *Human immunodeficiency virus* (HIV), a member of the genus *Lentivirus* of the *Retroviridae*. There are a number of similar lentiviruses which cause immunodeficiency diseases in animals. Unlike infection by other types of retrovirus, HIV infection does not directly result in the formation of tumours. Some tumours, such as B-cell lymphomas, are sometimes seen in AIDS patients but these are consequence of the lack of immune surveillance which is responsible for the destruction of tumours in healthy individuals. The clinical course of AIDS is long and very variable. A great number of different abnormalities of the immune system are seen in AIDS (Table 7.1). As a result of the biology of lentivirus infections, the pathogenesis of AIDS is highly complex.

It is still not clear how much of the pathology of AIDS is caused directly by the virus and how much is caused by the immune system. There are numerous models that have been suggested to explain how HIV causes immunodeficiency. These mechanisms are not mutually exclusive and indeed it is probable that the underlying loss of CD4+ cells in AIDS is multi-factorial, as described below.

Direct cell killing

This was the earliest mechanism suggested, based on the behaviour of laboratory isolates of HIV. Cell **fusion** resulting in **syncytium** formation is one of the major mechanisms of cell killing by HIV *in vitro* (Figure 7.1). However, different isolates of HIV vary considerably in the extent to which they promote the fusion of infected cells. Subsequent experiments suggested there may not be sufficient virus present in AIDS patients to account for all the damage seen, although killing of CD4+ cells may

Table 7.1 Immune abnormalities in HIV infection

Altered cytokine expression
Decreased CTL and NK cell function
Decreased humoral and proliferative response to antigens and mitogens
Decreased MHC-II expression
Decreased monocyte chemotaxis
Depletion of CD4+ cells
Impaired delayed type hypersensitvity (DTH) reactions
Lymphopaenia
Polyclonal B-cell activation

contribute to the overall pathogenesis of AIDS in some circumstances. Recently, it has become clear that up to half of the $CD4^+$ cells in the body may be infected with HIV, so the idea of direct cell killing has been re-examined, but in light of induction of apoptosis (see below) rather than by cell fusion.

Indirect killing of HIV-infected cells

Indirect effects of infection, e.g. disturbances in cell biochemistry and cytokine production, may also affect the regulation of the immune system. However, the expression of virus antigens on the surface of infected cells leads to indirect killing by the immune system – effectively a type of autoimmunity. The extent of this activity is dependent on the virus load and replication kinetics in infected individuals (see below).

Antigenic diversity

This theory proposes that the continual generation of new antigenic variants eventually swamps and overcomes the immune system, leading to its collapse. There is no doubt that new antigenic variants of HIV constantly arise during the long course of AIDS because of the low fidelity of reverse transcription (Chapter 3). It is envisaged that there might be a 'ratchet' effect, with each new variant contributing to the slight but irreversible decline in immune function (as described in the sections on T-cell Anergy and Apoptosis below) (Figure 7.2). Because of the way virus infections are handled by the immune system, it is probable that variation of T-cell epitopes on target proteins recognized by CTLs are more important than B-cell epitopes which generate the antibody response to a foreign antigen (Chapter 6). Mathematical models have been constructed which simulate antigenic variation during the course of infection. When primed with known data about the state of immune system during HIV infection, these provide an accurate depiction of the course of AIDS. Recently, it has been shown that there is a simple relationship between virus load and survival time, and that a patient can withstand only ~1300 'viral years' of HIV (i.e. copies of the virus genome/ml $\times$ survival time in years).

T-cell anergy

Anergy is an immunologically unresponsive state in which lymphocytes are present but not functionally active. This is usually due to incomplete activation signals and may be an important regulatory mechanism in the immune system, e.g. tolerance of 'self' antigens. In AIDS, anergy could be induced due to HIV infection, e.g. interference with cytokine expression. There is experimental *in vitro* evidence that gp120–CD4 interactions result in anergy due to interference with signal transduction. Many AIDS patients are anergic, i.e. fail to mount a delayed-type hypersensitivity (DTH)

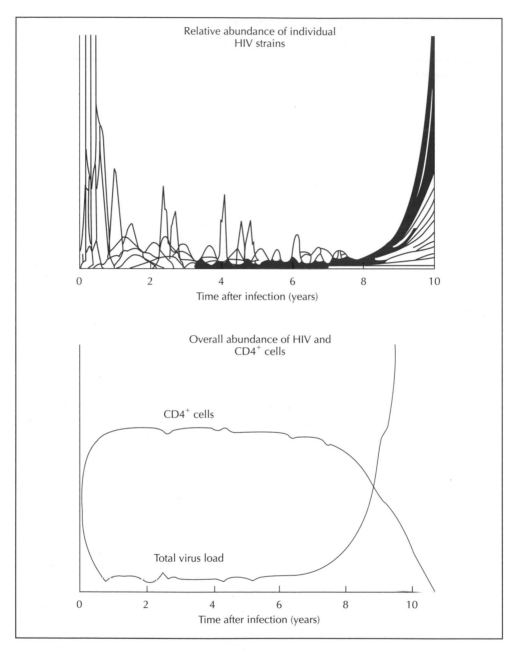

Figure 7.2 Antigenic diversity threshold theory of AIDS pathogenesis. Each line on the upper graph shows the (theoretical) relative abundance of an individual HIV strain (antigenic type) in a single case of AIDS. The lower graph shows the total virus load (i.e. total number of HIV strains) and number of CD4⁺ cells predicted by a computer model.

response to skin-test antigens. Impaired DTH responses are directly related to decreasing CD4$^+$ T lymphocyte counts. However, there is no strong evidence that this phenomenon is directly related to any aspect of HIV infection *in vivo* rather than to general depletion of immune functions.

Apoptosis

Apoptosis or 'programmed cell death' is believed to be a normal part of T-cell maturation, e.g. the elimination of self-responsive clones. Many unrelated viruses are known to induce apoptosis in infected cells (Chapter 6). Like T-cell anergy, apoptosis could potentially be induced in large numbers of uninfected cells by factors released from a much smaller number of HIV-infected cells. In addition to clonal deletion as a normal part of the evolution of the T-cell repertoire, apoptosis may be induced following T-cell activation as a negative regulatory mechanism to control the strength and duration of the immune response. This is relevant, since HIV infection of T cells induces an activated phenotype, e.g. surface expression of CD45 and HLA-DR markers, which suggests that these cells may be inevitably doomed due to activation of the apoptosis pathway. Because HIV establishes a persistent infection, it is by no means clear that apoptosis has an entirely negative effect – induction of cell death may well limit virus production and slow down the course of infection. The present situation is rather confused, with several HIV proteins having been identified as both inducers and repressors of apoptosis under various circumstances (Table 7.2). However, the proportion of CD4$^+$ T cells in the later stages of apoptosis is about twofold higher in HIV-1 infected individuals than in uninfected people.

Table 7.2 HIV and apoptosis	
Virus gene	**Effects** **Induction**
Tat	Increased FasL synthesis; downregulating expression of manganese-dependent superoxide dismutase; activation of cyclin-dependent kinases.
gp160	Increases intracellular calcium levels; CD4 cross-linking; CXCR4 chemokine receptor signalling.
Vpr	Causes cell cycle arrest in G$_2$ phase.
	Repression
Tat	Induction of Bcl-2
Vpr	Supresion of transcription factor NF-κB activity.

Superantigens

Superantigens are molecules which short-circuit the immune system, resulting in massive activation of T cells rather than the usual, carefully controlled response to foreign antigens. It is believed that they do this by binding to both the variable region of the β-chain of the T-cell receptor (Vβ) and to MHC class II molecules, cross-linking them in a non-specific way (Figure 7.3). This results in polyclonal T-cell activation rather than the usual situation where only the few clones of T cells responsive to a particular antigen presented by the MHC class II molecule are activated. The over-response of the immune system produced results in autoimmunity as whole families of T cells which bind superantigens are activated, and immunosuppression as the activated cells are killed by other activated T cells or undergo **apoptosis**. However, unlike other retroviruses (e.g. mouse mammary tumour virus and the murine leukaemia virus responsible for murine acquired immunodeficiency syndrome), no superantigen has been conclusively identified in HIV, despite intensive investigation. Thus the practical relevance of superantigens in AIDS is thus in doubt. However, it is possible that exposure to superantigens produced by opportunistic infection(s) might play a role in AIDS.

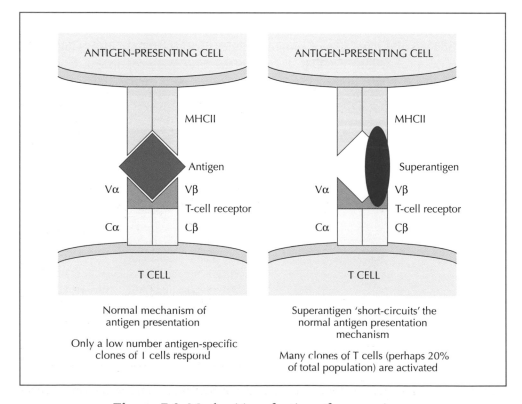

Figure 7.3 Mechanisim of action of superantigens

T_H1/T_H2 imbalance

Regulation of the immune system depends on a complex network of cells, but central to the process is the role of CD4$^+$ T-helper (T_H) cells. Immunological theory suggests that there are two types of these: T_H1 cells, which promote the cell-mediated response, and T_H2 cells, which promote the humoral response (Figure 7.4). This theory suggests that early in HIV infection, T_H1-responsive T cells predominate and are effective in controlling (but not eliminating) the virus. At some point, a (relative) loss of the T_H1 response occurs and T_H2 HIV-responsive cells predominate. It has been reported that at least some virus variants can inhibit the CTL response to HIV. The hypothesis is therefore that the T_H2-dominated humoral response is not effective at maintaining HIV replication at a low level and the virus load builds up, resulting in AIDS. Although this is largely a theoretical proposal which has not been proved, this thinking is shaping our understanding of the immune response to many different pathogens, not just HIV. However, no experimental study has demonstrated an actual switch from the T_H1 to T_H2 pattern of cytokine expression and secretion that is associated with disease progression, hence there is no evidence for the involvement of these mechanisms in AIDS.

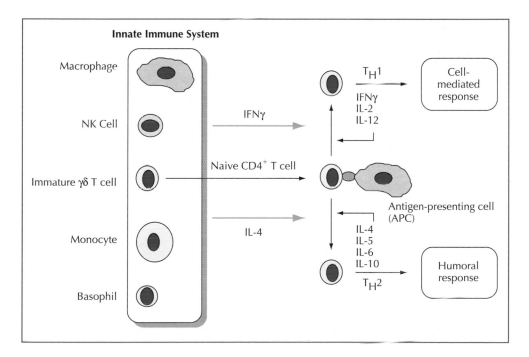

Figure 7.4 Regulation of the cell-mediated and humoral immune responses. IFN, interferon; IL, interleukin; T_H, T-helper cell.

Virus load and replication kinetics

Experiments involving accurate quantitation of the amount of virus in infected individuals have revealed that much higher virus loads are present than was originally measured by less sensitive techniques. Using quantitative polymerase chain reaction (PCR) methods to accurately measure the amount of virus present and determine how these levels change when patients are treated with drugs which inhibit HIV replication, it has been shown that:

- Continuous and highly productive replication of HIV occurs in all infected individuals, although the rates of virus production vary by up to 70-fold in different individuals.
- The average half-life of an HIV particle *in vivo* is 2.1 days.
- Up to $10^9 - 10^{10}$ HIV particles are produced each day.
- An average of 2×10^9 new CD4$^+$ cells are produced each day.

Thus contrary to what was initially believed, there is a very dynamic situation in HIV-infected people involving continuous infection, destruction and replacement of CD4$^+$ cells. Billions of new CD4$^+$ cells are produced, infected and killed each day. These data suggest a return to cellular killing (although predominantly through apoptosis and immune-mediated killing rather than cell fusion) as a direct cause of the CD4$^+$ cell decline in AIDS.

These new ideas are informing future thinking about possible therapeutic intervention in HIV-infected individuals. What is clear is that the presence of HIV is necessary for the development of AIDS and that it is vital that the worldwide spread of HIV infection is halted and reversed. Work on developing anti-HIV **vaccines** is continuing but because of the complex biology of the virus, is proving to be formidably difficult. A better understanding of the pathogenesis of AIDS and, in particular, the role of the immune system in the early stages of the disease is vital to permit the development of more appropriate therapies for AIDS. Highly active antiretroviral therapy (HAART – Chapter 6) has a dramatic effect on suppressing virus production and temporarily restores CD4 cell populations. Unfortunately, because of the long half-life of latently infected cells, the estimated time to completely eradicate HIV from the body is roughly 12–60 years – something which is not presently achievable due to the failure of therapy as a result of drug toxicity and virus resistance.

VIRUS-RELATED DISEASES

There are a number of human disease syndromes for which virus infections are believed to be a necessary prerequisite. In some instances, the link between a particular virus and a pathological condition is well established, but it is clear that the pathogenesis of the disease is complex and also involves the immune system of the host. In other cases, the pathogenic involvement of a particular virus is less certain, and in a few instances, rather speculative.

Although the incidence of measles virus infection has been reduced sharply by **vaccination** (Chapter 6), measles still causes hundreds of thousands of deaths each year. The normal course of measles virus infection is an acute febrile illness, during which the virus spreads throughout the body, infecting many tissues. The vast majority of people spontaneously recover from the disease without any lasting harm. In rare cases (about 1 in 2000), measles may progress to a severe encephalitis. This is still an acute condition which either regresses or kills the patient within a few weeks. There is however, another, much rarer late consequence of measles virus infection which occurs many months or years after initial infection of the host. This is the condition known as subacute sclerosing panencephalitis (SSPE). Evidence of prior measles virus infection (antibodies or direct detection of the virus) is found in all patients with SSPE, whether they can recall having had a symptomatic case of measles or not. In about 1 in 300 000 cases of measles, the virus is not cleared from the body by the immune system, but establishes a persistent infection in the CNS. In this condition, virus replication continues at a low level, but defects in the **envelope protein** genes prevent the production of extracellular infectious virus particles. The lack of envelope protein production causes the failure of the immune system to recognize and eliminate infected cells. However, the virus is able to spread directly from cell to cell, bypassing the usual route of infection. It is not known to what extent damage to the cells of the brain is caused directly by virus replication, or whether there is any contribution by the immune system to the pathogenesis of SSPE. Vaccination against measles virus and the prevention of primary infection should ultimately eliminate this condition.

Another well-established case where the immune system is implicated in pathogenesis concerns dengue virus infections. *Dengue virus* is a flavivirus which is transmitted from one human host to another via mosquitoes. The primary infection may be asymptomatic, or may result in dengue fever. Dengue fever is normally a self-limited illness from which patients recover after 7–10 days without further complications. Following primary infections, patients carry antibodies to the virus. Unfortunately, there are four serotypes of dengue virus (DEN-1, -2, -3 and -4) and the presence of antibody directed against one type does not give cross-protection against the other three; worse still is the fact that antibodies can enhance the infection of peripheral blood mononuclear cells by Fc-receptor mediated uptake of antibody-coated dengue virus particles (see Chapter 4). In a few cases, the consequences of dengue virus infection are much more severe than the usual fever. Dengue haemorrhagic fever (DHF) is a life-threatening disease. In the most extreme cases, so much internal haemorrhaging occurs that hypovolaemic shock (dengue shock syndrome, DSS) occurs. DSS is frequently fatal. The occurrence of shock in dengue and other haemorrhagic fevers is partly due to the virus, but is largely due to immune-mediated damage to virus-infected cells (Figure 7.5). DHF and DSS following primary dengue virus infections occur in approximately 1 in 14 000 and 1 in 500 patients respectively. However, after secondary dengue virus infections, the incidence of DHF is 1 in 90 and DSS 1 in 50, since cross-reactive but non-neutralizing antibodies to the virus are now present. These figures show the problems of cross-infection with different serotypes of Dengue virus, and the difficulties which must be faced in developing a safe **vaccine** against the virus. *Dengue virus* is discussed further later in this chapter (New and Emergent Viruses).

Another instance where virus vaccines have resulted in increased pathology rather than the prevention of disease is the occurrence of post-vaccination Reye's syndrome. Reye's syndrome is a neurological condition involving acute cerebral oedema and occurs almost exclusively in children. It is well known as a rare post-infection complication of a number of different viruses, but most commonly influenza virus and VZV (chicken pox). Symptoms include frequent vomiting, painful headaches, behavioural changes, extreme tiredness and disorientation. The chances of contracting Reye's syndrome are increased if aspirin is administered during the initial illness. The basis for the pathogenesis of this condition is completely unknown, but some of the most unfortunate cases have followed the administration of experimental influenza virus vaccines.

Guillain–Barré syndrome is a similarly mysterious condition in which demyeli-

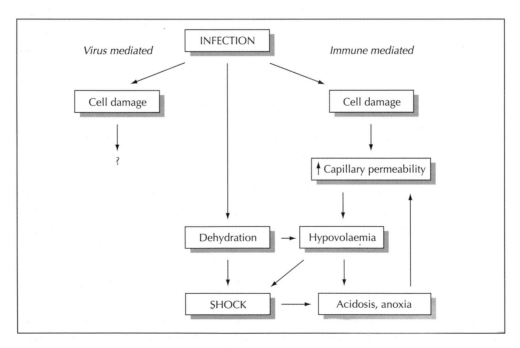

Figure 7.5 Causes of shock in haemorrhagic fevers.

nation of nerves results in partial paralysis and muscle weakness. The onset of Guillain–Barré syndrome usually follows an acute 'virus-like' infection, but no single agent has ever been firmly associated with this condition. Kawasaki disease is similar to Reye's syndrome in that it occurs in children, but distinct in that it results in serious damage to the heart. Like Guillain–Barré syndrome, Kawasaki disease appears to follow acute infections. The disease itself is not infectious but does appear to occur in **epidemics**, which suggests an infectious agent as the cause. A large number of bacterial and virus pathogens have been suggested to be associated with the induction of Kawasaki disease, but once again the underlying cause of the pathology is unknown. It would appear that acute infection itself rather than a particular pathogen may be responsible for the onset of these diseases.

In recent years, there has been a search for an agent responsible for a newly diagnosed disease called chronic fatigue syndrome (CFS) or myalgic encephalomyelitis (ME). Unlike the other conditions described above, CFS is a rather ill-defined disease and is not recognized by all physicians. Recent research has discounted the earlier idea that EBV might cause CFS but a variety of other possible virus causes including other herpesviruses, enteroviruses and retroviruses have also been suggested. Several recent reports have suggested that measles infection before full immunological competence (e.g. younger then 2 years) may be linked to ulcerative colitis and Crohn's disease. This idea is plausible since *Measles virus* can infect and persist in endothelial cells in the gastrointestinal tract and cause an immune response with giant cell formation. However, more evidence needs to be obtained before this can be verified.

All these various conditions and syndromes illustrate the complexity of virus pathogenesis and show that the direct effects of virus replication and self-inflicted damage resulting from poor control of the immune system are sometimes hard to differentiate.

BACTERIOPHAGES AND HUMAN DISEASE

Can **bacteriophages**, viruses which are only capable of infecting **prokaryotic** cells, play a role in human disease? Surprisingly, the answer is yes. Shiga toxin (Stx)-producing *Escherichia coli* (STEC) are able to cause intestinal foodborne diseases such as diarrhoea and haemorrhagic colitis. STEC serotype O157:H7, 'the hamburger bug', has received much attention in recent years. STEC infections can lead to fatal complications such as haemolytic–uraemic syndrome, and neurological disorders. The major virulence characteristics of these strains of bacteria are the ability to colonize the bowel (a natural trait of *Escherichia coli*) and the production of secreted 'Shiga toxins', which can damage endothelial and tubular cells and may result in acute kidney failure. At least 100 different *E. coli* serotypes produce Shiga toxins, and STEC bacteria occur frequently in the bowels of cattle and other domestic animals such as sheep, goats, pigs and horses. Meat is infected by faecal contamination, usually at the time of slaughter. Ground meat such as hamburger is particularly dangerous since surface bacterial contamination may become buried deep within the meat, where it may not be inactivated by cooking.

What has this got to do with bacteriophages? Various types of Stx are known, but they fall into two main types, Shiga toxin 1 (Stx1) and Shiga toxin 2 (Stx2). The Stx1 and Stx2 toxin genes are encoded in the genome of **lysogenic** lambda-like prophages within the bacteria. Stimuli such as UV light or mitomycin C are known to induce these prophages to release a crop of phage particles which can infect and lysogenize other susceptible bacteria within the gut, accounting for the high prevalence of STEC bacteria (up to 50% of cattle in some herds). Recent research has shown that the scandalous overuse of antibiotics as 'growth promoters' in animal husbandry and even antibiotic treatment of infected people can stimulate the production of phage particles and contributes to the increased prevalance of STEC bacteria and growing human death toll. Other bacterial virulence determinants are also encoded by lysogenic phages (e.g. *Diphtheria* toxin, *Streptococcus* erythrogenic toxins, *Staphylococcus* enterotoxins), although the selective pressures that maintain these arrangements are not yet understood. Emerging bacterial genome sequence data strongly indicates that phages have been responsible for spreading virulence determinants across a wide range of pathogens.

The other area where bacteriophages may influence human illness is phage therapy – the use of bacteriophages as antibiotics. This is not a new idea, initial experiments having been performed (unsuccessfully) shortly after the discovery of bacteriophages almost 100 years ago (Appendix 3 ✍). However, with increasing resistance of bacteria to antibiotics and the emergence of 'superbugs' immune to all effective treatments, this idea has undergone a resurgence of interest. Although attractive in theory, the approach suffers from a number of defects:

- Bacteriophages are quite specific in their receptor usage and hence the strains of bacteria they can infect. Thus they are 'narrow spectrum' antibacterial agents.
- Bacteria exposed to bacteriophages rapidly develop resistance to infection by downregulating or mutating the phage receptor.
- Liberation of endotoxin as a consequence of widespread lysis of bacteria within the body can lead to toxic shock.
- Repeated administration of bacteriophages results in an immune response which neutralizes the phage particles before they can act.

Nevertheless, it may be that this is a useful therapy for certain bacterial infections which cannot be treated by conventional means.

CELL TRANSFORMATION BY VIRUSES

Transformation is a change in the morphological, biochemical or growth parameters of a cell. Transformation may or may not result in cells able to produce tumours in experimental animals, which is properly known as neoplastic transformation. Therefore, transformed cells do not automatically result in the development of 'cancer'. Carcinogenesis (or more properly, oncogenesis) is a complex, multi-step process in which cellular transformation may be only the first, although essential, step along the way. Transformed cells have an altered phenotype, which is displayed as one (or more) of the following characteristics:

■ *Loss of anchorage dependence:* Normal (i.e. non-transformed) adherent cells such as fibroblasts or epithelial cells require a surface to which they can adhere. In the body, this requirement is supplied by adjacent cells or structures. *In vitro*, it is met by the glass or plastic vessels in which the cells are cultivated. Some transformed cells lose the ability to adhere to solid surfaces and float free (or in clumps) in the culture medium without loss of viability.

■ *Loss of contact inhibition:* Normal adherent cells in culture divide and grow until they have coated all the available surface for attachment. At this point, when adjacent cells are touching each other, cell division stops – the cells do not continue to grow and pile up on top of one another. Many transformed cells have lost this characteristic. Single transformed cells in a culture dish become visible as small thickened areas of growth called 'transformed foci' – clones of cells all derived from a single original cell.

■ *Colony formation in semi-solid media:* Most normal cells (both adherent and non-adherent cells such as lymphocytes) will not grow in media that are partially solid owing to the addition of substances such as agarose or hydroxymethyl cellulose. However, many transformed cells will grow under these conditions, forming colonies since movement of the cells is restricted by the medium.

■ *Decreased requirements for growth factors:* All cells require multiple factors for growth. In a broad sense, these include compounds such as ions, vitamins and hormones, which cannot be manufactured by the cell. More specifically, it includes regulatory peptides such as epidermal growth factor (EGF) and platelet-derived growth factor (PDGF) which regulate the growth of cells. These are potent molecules that have powerful effects on cell growth. Some transformed cells may have decreased or may even have lost their requirement for particular factors. The production by a cell of a growth factor which is required for its own growth is known as **autocrine** stimulation and is one route by which cells may be transformed.

Cell transformation is a single-hit process, i.e. a single virus transforms a single cell (cf. oncogenesis, i.e. the formation of tumours, which is a multi-step process). All or part of the virus **genome** persists in the transformed cell and is usually (but not always) integrated into the host cell **chromatin**. Transformation is usually accompanied by continued expression of a limited repertoire of virus genes, or rarely by **productive infection**. Virus genomes found in transformed cells are frequently replication–defective and contain substantial deletions.

Transformation is mediated by proteins encoded by **oncogenes**. These regulatory genes can be grouped in several ways, for example, by their origins, biochemical function or subcellular locations (Table 7.3). Cell-transforming viruses may have RNA or DNA genomes, but all have at least a DNA stage in their replication cycle, i.e. the only RNA viruses directly capable of cell transformation are the retroviruses (Table 7.4). Certain retroviruses carry homologues of c-*oncs* derived originally from the cellular genes and known as v-*oncs*. In contrast, the oncogenes of cell-transforming DNA viruses are unique to the virus genome – there are no homologous sequences present in normal cells.

Genes involved in the formation of tumours can be grouped by their biochemical functions:

Table 7.3 Categories of oncogenes

Type	Example
Extracellular growth factors: (homologues of normal growth factors)	c-*sis*: encodes the PDGF B (v-*sis* in *Simian sarcoma virus*). *int-2*: encodes an FGF-related growth factor (common site of integration for *Mouse mammary tumour virus*).
Receptor tyrosine kinases: (associated with the inner surface of the cell membrane)	c-*fms*: encodes the colony stimulating factor-1 (CSF-1) receptor – first identified as a retrovirus oncogene. c-*kit*: encodes the mast cell growth factor receptor.
Membrane associated non-receptor tyrosine kinases: (signal transduction)	c-*src*: v-src was the first identified oncogene (*Rous sarcoma virus*) *lck*: associated with the CD4 and CD8 antigens of T-cells.
G-protein coupled receptors: (signal transduction)	*mas*: encodes the angiotensin receptor.
Membrane associated G-proteins:	c-*ras*: there are three different homologues of c-*ras* gene, each identified in a different type of tumour and each transduced by a different retrovirus.
Serine/theonine kinases: (signal transduction)	c-*raf*: involved in the signalling pathway – responsible for theonine phosphorylation of MAP kinase following receptor activation.
Nuclear DNA-binding/transcription factors:	c-*myc*: (v-*myc* in *Avian myelocytomatosis virus*) – disruption of c-*myc* by retroviral integration or chromosomal rearrangements results in sarcomas. c-*fos*: (v-*fos* in *Feline osteosarcoma virus*) – interacts with a second proto-oncogene protein, *Jun* to form a transcriptional regulatory complex.

Virus type	Time to tumour formation	Efficiency of tumour formation	Type of oncogene
Transducing (acutely transforming)	Short (e.g. weeks)	High - up to 100%	c-*onc* transduced by virus, i.e. v-*onc* present in virus genome (usually replication defective)
Cis-activating (chronic transforming)	Intermediate (e.g. months)	Intermediate	c-*onc* in cell genome activated by provirus insertion – no oncogene present in virus genome (replication competent)
Trans-activating	Long (e.g. years)	Low (<1%)	Activation of cellular genes by *trans*-acting virus proteins (replication competent)

Table 7.4 Cell-transforming retroviruses

- *Oncogenes and proto-oncogenes:* Oncogenes are mutated forms of proto-oncogenes, cellular genes whose normal function is to promote the normal growth and division of cells.
- *Tumour suppressor genes:* These are genes which normally function to inhibit the cell cycle and cell division.
- *DNA repair genes:* These genes ensure that each strand of genetic information is accurately copied during cell division of the cell cycle. Mutations in these genes lead to an increase in the frequency of other mutations, e.g. in conditions such as ataxia–telangiectasia and xeroderma pigmentosum.

The functions of **oncogene** products depend on their cellular location (Figure 7.6). Several classes of oncogenes are associated with the process of signal transduction, i.e. the transfer of information derived from the binding of extracellular ligands to cellular receptors to the nucleus (Figure 7.7). Many of the kinases in these groups have a common type of structure with conserved functional domains representing the hydrophobic transmembrane and hydrophilic intracellular kinase regions (Figure 7.8). These proteins are associated with the cell membranes or are present in the cytoplasm. Other classes of oncogenes located in the nucleus are normally involved with the control of the cell cycle (Figure 7.9). The products of these genes overcome the restriction between the G_1 and S phases of the cell cycle, which is the key control point in preventing uncontrolled cell division. Some virus oncogenes are not sufficient on their own to produce a fully transformed phenotype in cells. However, in some instances, they may cooperate with another oncogene of complementary function to produce a fully transformed phenotype. For example, the adenovirus *E1A* gene plus either the *E1B* gene or the c-*ras* gene transforms NIH 3T3 cells (a mouse

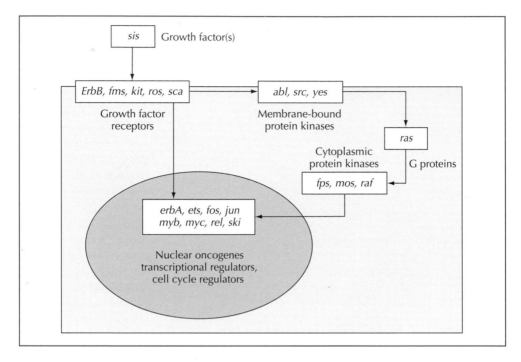

Figure 7.6 Subcellular location of oncoproteins.

fibroblast cell line). This further underlines the fact that oncogenesis is a complex, multi-step process.

Cell transformation by retroviruses

Not all retroviruses are capable of transforming cells; for example, lentiviruses such as HIV do not transform cells, although they are cytopathic. The retroviruses which can transform cells fall into three groups: transducing, *cis*-activating and *trans*-activating. The characteristics of these groups are given in Table 7.4.

If **oncogenes** are present in all cells, why does transformation occur as a result of virus infection? The reason is that oncogenes may become activated in one of two ways, either by subtle changes to the normal structure of the gene, or by interruption of the normal control of expression. The transforming genes of the acutely transforming retroviruses (v-*oncs*) are derived from and are highly homologous to c-*oncs* and are believed to have been transduced by viruses. However, most v-*oncs* possess slight alterations from their c-*onc* progenitors. Many contain minor sequence alterations which alter the structure and the function of the oncoprotein produced. Others contain short deletions of part of the gene. Most oncoproteins from replication-defective, acutely transforming retroviruses are **fusion proteins**, containing additional sequences derived from virus genes, most commonly virus *gag* sequences at the amino–terminus of the protein. These additional sequences may alter the func-

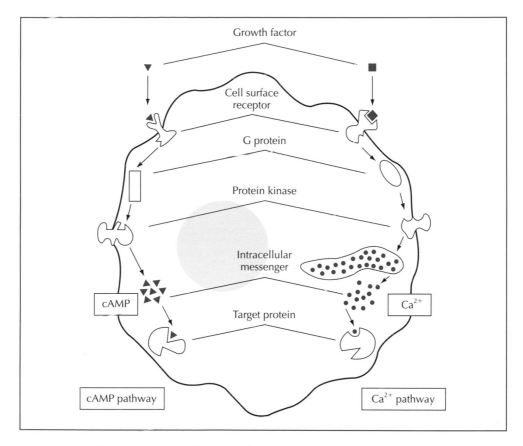

Figure 7.7 Cellular mechanisim of signal transduction.

tion or the cellular localization of the protein and these abnormal attributes result in transformation.

Alternatively, viruses may result in abnormal expression of an unaltered onco-protein. This might be either the overexpression of an oncogene under the control of a virus **promoter** rather than its normal promoter in the cell, or the inappropri-ate temporal expression of an oncoprotein which disrupts the cell cycle. Chronic transforming retrovirus **genomes** do not contain oncogenes. These viruses activate c-*oncs* by a mechanism known as insertional activation. A **provirus** which integrates into the host cell genome close to a c-*onc* sequence may indirectly activate the expression of the gene in a way analogous to that in which v-*oncs* have been activated by transduction (Figure 7.10). This can occur if the provirus is integrated upstream of the c-*onc* gene, which might be expressed via a read-through transcript of the virus genome plus downstream sequences. However, insertional activation can also occur when a provirus integrates downstream of a c-*onc* sequence or upstream but in an inverted orientation. In these cases, activation results from **enhancer elements** in the virus promoter (see Chapter 5). These can act even if the provirus integrates at

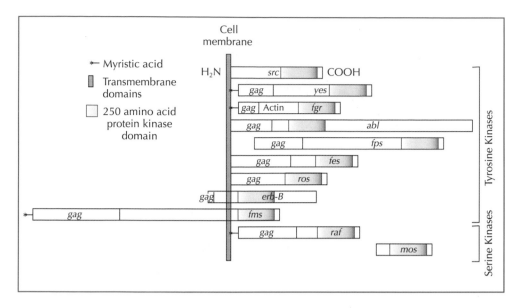

Figure 7.8 The family of retrovirus protein kinases involved in cell transformation. Many of these molecules are fusion proteins containing amino-terminal sequences derived from the viruses *gag* gene. Most of this type contain the fatty acid myristate which is added to the amino-terminus of the protein after translation and which links the protein to the inner surface of the host cell cytoplasmic membrane. In a number of cases, it has been shown that this post-translational modification is essential to the transforming action of the protein.

a distance of several kilobases from the *c-onc* gene. The best-known examples of this phenomenon occur in chickens, where insertion of *Avian leukosis virus* (ALV) activates the *myc* gene, and in mice, where *Mouse mammary tumour virus* (MMTV) insertion activates the *int* gene.

Transformation by the third class of retroviruses operates by quite a different mechanism. *Human T-cell leukaemia virus* (HTLV) and related animal viruses encode a transcriptional activator protein in the virus *tax* gene. The tax protein acts in *trans* to stimulate transcription from the virus LTR. It is believed that the protein also activates transcription of many cellular genes by interacting with transcription factors (Chapter 5). However, HTLV oncogenesis, i.e. the formation of a leukaemic tumour, has a latent period of some 20–30 years. Therefore, cell transformation (which can be mimicked *in vitro*) and tumour formation (which cannot) are not one and the same – additional events are required for the development of leukaemia. It is thought that chromosomal abnormalities which may occur in the population of HTLV-transformed cells are also required to produce a malignant tumour, although because of the difficulties of studying this lengthy process, this is not completely understood.

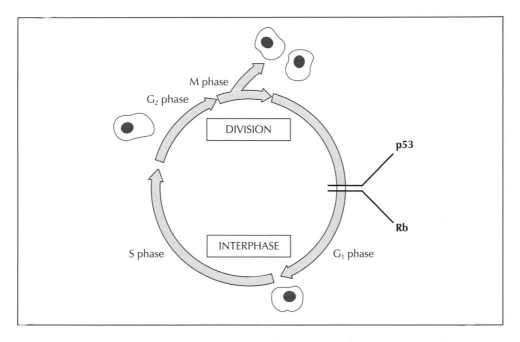

Figure 7.9 Schematic diagram showing the phases of the eukaryotic cell cycle

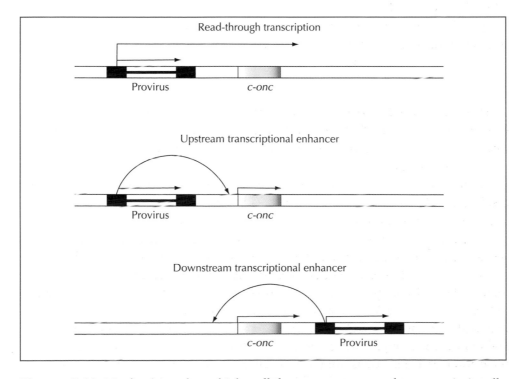

Figure 7.10 Mechanisims by which cellular oncogenes can be transcriptionally activated by retrovirus insertional mutagenesis.

Cell transformation by DNA viruses

In contrast to the **oncogenes** of retroviruses, the transforming genes of DNA tumour viruses have no cellular counterparts. Several families of DNA viruses are capable of transforming cells (Table 7.5). In general terms, the functions of their oncoproteins are much less diverse than those encoded by retroviruses. They are mostly nuclear proteins involved in the control of DNA replication which directly affect the cell cycle. They achieve their effects by interacting with cellular proteins which normally appear to have a negative regulatory role in cell proliferation. Two of the most important cellular proteins involved are known as p53 and Rb.

p53 was originally discovered by virtue of the fact that it forms complexes with SV40 T-antigen. It is now known that it also interacts with other DNA virus oncoproteins, including those of adenoviruses and papillomaviruses. The gene encoding p53 is mutated or altered in the majority of tumours, implying that loss of the normal gene product is associated with the emergence of malignantly transformed cells. Tumour cells, when injected with the native protein *in vitro* show a decreased rate of cell division and decreased tumorigenicity *in vivo*. **Transgenic** mice that do not possess an intact p53 gene are developmentally normal but are susceptible to the formation of spontaneous tumours. Therefore, it is clear that p53 plays a central role in controlling the cell cycle. p53 is believed to be a tumour suppressor or 'anti-oncogene' and has been called 'the guardian of the genome'. It is a transcription factor that activates the expression of certain cellular genes, notably *WAF1*. This gene encodes an inhibitor of G_1 cyclin-dependent kinases, causing the cell cycle to arrest at the G_1 phase (Figure 7.9). The fact that DNA viruses require ongoing cellular DNA replication for their own propagation would explain why their transforming proteins target p53.

Rb was discovered when it was noticed that the gene encoding this protein is always damaged or deleted in a tumour of the optic nerve known as retinoblastoma. Therefore, the normal function of this gene is also thought to be that of a tumour suppressor. The Rb protein forms complexes with a transcription factor called E2F. This factor is required for the transcription of adenovirus genes, but E2F is also involved in the transcription of cellular genes which drive quiescent cells into S

Table 7.5 Transforming proteins of DNA tumour viruses

Virus	Transforming protein(s)	Cellular target
Adenoviruses:	E1A + E1B	Rb, p53
Polyomaviruses (SV40)	T-antigen	p53, Rb
Papillomaviruses:		
BPV-1	E5	PDGF receptor
	E6	p53
HPV-16, HPV-18	E7	Rb

phase. The formation of inactive E2F–Rb complexes thus has the same overall effect as the action of p53 – arrest of the cell cycle at G_1. Release of E2F by replacement of E2F–Rb complexes with E1A–Rb, T-antigen–Rb or E7–Rb complexes therefore stimulates cellular and virus DNA replication.

SV40 T-antigen is one of the known virus proteins which binds p53. Chapter 5 describes the role of large T-antigen in the regulation of SV40 transcription. Infection of cells by SV40 or other polyomaviruses can result in two possible outcomes:

- Productive (**lytic**) infection
- Non-productive (**abortive**) infection.

The outcome of infection appears to be determined primarily by the cell type infected; for example, mouse polyomavirus establishes a lytic infection of mouse cells but an **abortive infection** of rat or hamster cells, while SV40 shows lytic infection of monkey cells but abortive infection of mouse cells. However, in addition to transcription, T-antigen is also involved in **genome** replication. SV40 DNA replication is initiated by binding of large T-antigen to the origin region of the genome (Figure 5.12). The function of T-antigen is controlled by phosphorylation, which decreases the ability of the protein to bind to the SV40 origin.

The SV40 **genome** is very small and does not encode all the information necessary for DNA replication. Therefore, it is essential for the host cell to enter S phase, when cell DNA and the virus genome are replicated together. Protein–protein interactions between T-antigen and DNA polymerase α directly stimulate replication of the virus genome. The precise regions of the T-antigen involved in binding to DNA, DNA polymerase α, p53 and Rb are all known (Figure 7.11). Inactivation of tumour suppressor proteins bound to T-antigen causes G_1-arrested cells to enter S phase and divide and this is the mechanism which results in transformation. However, the frequency with which abortively infected cells are transformed is low (about 1×10^{-5}).

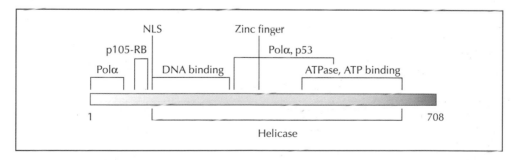

Figure 7.11 Regions of SV40 T-antigen involved in protein–protein interactions. Other functional domains of the protein involved in virus DNA replication are also shown, e.g. the helicase, ATPase and nuclear location signal (NLS) domains.

Therefore, the function of T-antigen is to alter the cellular environment to permit virus DNA replication. Transformation is a rare and accidental consequence of the sequestration of tumour suppressor proteins.

The immediate-early proteins of adenoviruses are analogous in many ways to SV40 T-antigen. E1A is a **trans-acting** transcriptional regulator of the adenovirus early genes (see Chapter 5). Like T-antigen, the E1A protein binds to Rb, inactivating the regulatory effect of this protein, permitting virus DNA replication and accidentally stimulating cellular DNA replication (see above). E1B binds p53 and reinforces the effects of E1A. The combined effect of the two proteins can be seen in the phenotype of cells transfected with DNA containing these genes (Table 7.6). However, the interaction of these transforming proteins with the cell is more complex than simple induction of DNA synthesis. Expression of E1A alone causes cells to undergo apoptosis. Expression of E1A and E1B together overcomes this response and permits transformed cells to survive and grow.

Human papillomavirus (HPV) genital infections are very common, occurring in more than 50% of young, sexually active adults, and are usually asymptomatic. Certain serotypes of HPV appear to be associated with a low risk of subsequent development of anogenital cancers such as cervical carcinoma, after an incubation period of several decades. About 500 000 new cases of cervical neoplasia are diagnosed every year, making this one of the three most common causes of cancer death in women globally. HPV is a primary cause of cervical cancer, 93% of all cervical cancers test positive for one or more high-risk type HPV. Of the 60 HPV types currently recognized, only four seem to be associated with a high risk of tumour formation (HPV-16, HPV-18, HPV-31 and HPV-45). Once again, transformation is mediated by the early gene products of the virus. However, the transforming proteins appear to vary from one type of papillomavirus to another, as shown in Table 7.5. In bovine papillomavirus, it is the E5 protein which is responsible for transformation. In HPV-16 and HPV-18, the E6 and E7 proteins are involved. The E6 protein is known to bind p53 and to target it for accelerated degradation, decreasing the intracellular level of the protein. The E7 protein has structural and functional similarities (e.g. binding to Rb) with adenovirus E1A. In general terms, it appears that two or more early proteins often cooperate to give a transformed phenotype. Although some papillomaviruses can transform cells on their own (e.g. BPV-1), others appear to require the cooperation of an activated cellular **oncogene**

Table 7.6 Role of the adenovirus E1A and E1B proteins in cell transformation

Protein	Cell phenotype
E1A	Immortalized but morphologically unaltered; not tumorigenic in animals.
E1B	Not transformed.
E1A + E1B	Immortalized and morphologically altered; tumourigenic in animals.

(e.g. HPV-16/*ras*). More confusingly, in most cases, all or part of the papillomavirus **genome**, including the putative transforming genes, is maintained in the tumour cells, whereas in some cases (e.g. BPV-4), the virus DNA may be lost after transformation, which may indicate a possible hit-and-run mechanism of transformation. Different papillomaviruses appear to use slightly different mechanisms to achieve genome replication and consequently, cell transformation may proceed via a slightly different route. It is imperative that a better understanding of these processes is obtained. There is no positive evidence that adenoviruses or polyomaviruses are involved in the formation of human tumours. In contrast, the evidence that papillomaviruses are commonly involved in the formation of malignant penile and cervical carcinomas is now very strong.

In recent years, it has emerged that p53 and Rb are major cellular sensors for **apoptosis**. Loss of these protein functions triggers apoptosis – the major anti-cancer mechanism in cells. Viruses which interfere with these proteins must thus have evolved mechanisms to counteract this effect (see discussion in Chapter 6).

VIRUSES AND CANCER

There are numerous examples of viruses which cause tumours in experimental animals. This stimulated a long search for viruses which might be the cause of cancer in humans. For many years, this search was unsuccessful, so much so that a few scientists categorically stated that viruses did not cause human tumours. Like all rash statements, this was wrong. We currently know of at least six viruses which are associated with the formation of tumours in infected humans (HHV-4/EBV, HBV, HCV, HHV-8, HPVs, HTLV). However, the relationship between virus infection and tumorigenesis is indirect and complex. The role of the HTLV tax protein in leukaemia has already been described (see Cell Transformation by Retroviruses). The evidence that papillomaviruses may be involved in human tumours is also growing. There are almost certainly many more viruses which cause human tumours, but the remainder of this chapter will describe two examples that have been intensively studied, *Epstein–Barr virus* (EBV) and *Hepatitis B virus* (HBV).

EBV was first identified in 1964 in a lymphoblastoid cell line derived from an African patient with Burkitt's lymphoma. In 1962, Dennis Burkitt described a highly malignant lymphoma whose distribution in Africa paralleled that of malaria. Burkitt recognized that this tumour was rare in India, but occurred in Indian children living in Africa, and therefore looked for an environmental cause. Initially, he thought that the tumour might be caused by a virus spread by mosquitoes (which is wrong). The association between EBV and Burkitt's lymphoma is not entirely clear cut:

- EBV is widely distributed worldwide but Burkitt's lymphoma is rare.
- EBV is found in many cell types in Burkitt's lymphoma patients, not just in the tumour cells.

■ Rare cases of EBV-negative Burkitt's lymphoma are sometimes seen in countries where malaria is not present, suggesting that there may be more than one route to this tumour.

EBV has a dual cell **tropism** for human B lymphocytes (generally a non-productive infection) and epithelial cells, in which a **productive infection** occurs. The usual outcome of EBV infection is polyclonal B-cell activation and a benign proliferation of these cells which is frequently asymptomatic but sometimes produces a relatively mild disease known as infectious mononucleosis or glandular fever. In 1968, it was shown that EBV could efficiently transform (i.e. immortalize) human B lymphocytes *in vitro*. This observation clearly strengthens the case that EBV is involved in the formation of tumours. There is now epidemiological and/or molecular evidence that EBV infection is associated with at least five human tumours:

■ Burkitt's lymphoma.
■ Nasopharyngeal carcinoma (NPC), a highly malignant tumour seen most frequently in China. There is a strong association between EBV and NPC: unlike Burkitt's lymphoma, the virus has been found in all the tumours which have been studied. Environmental factors, such as the consumption of nitrosamines in salted fish, are also believed to be involved in the formation of NPC (cf. the role of malaria in the formation of Burkitt's lymphoma).
■ B-cell lymphomas in immunosuppressed individuals, e.g. AIDS patients.
■ Some clonal forms of Hodgkin's disease.
■ X-linked lymphoproliferative syndrome (XLP), a rare condition usually seen in males where infection with EBV results in a hyperimmune response, sometimes causing a fatal form of glandular fever and sometimes cancer of the lymph nodes. XLP is an inherited defect due to a faulty gene on the X chromosome.

Cellular transformation by EBV is a complex process involving cooperative interactions between several viral proteins. There are three possible explanations to explain the link between EBV and Burkitt's lymphoma:

1 EBV immortalizes a large pool of B lymphocytes. Concurrently, malaria causes T-cell immunosuppression. There is thus a large pool of target cells in which a third event (e.g. a chromosomal translocation) results in the formation of a malignantly transformed cell. Most Burkitt's lymphoma tumours contain translocations involving chromosome 8, resulting in activation of the c-*myc* gene, which supports this hypothesis.
2 Malaria results in polyclonal B-cell activation. EBV subsequently immortalizes a cell containing a pre-existing c-*myc* translocation. This mechanism would be largely indistinguishable from the above.
3 EBV is just a passenger virus! Burkitt's lymphoma also occurs in Europe and

North America although it is very rare in these regions; however, 85% of these patients are not infected with EBV, which implies that there are other causes for Burkitt's lymphoma.

Although it has not been formally proved, it seems likely that either (1) and/or (2) are the true explanations for the origin of Burkitt's lymphoma.

Another case where a virus appears to be associated with the formation of a human tumour is that of *Hepatitis B virus* (HBV) and hepatocellular carcinoma (HCC). Hepatitis is an inflammation of the liver and as such is not a single disease. Because of the central role of the liver in metabolism, many virus infections may involve the liver. However, there are at least seven viruses which seem specifically to infect and damage hepatocytes. No two of these seven belong to the same family (see Chapter 8). HBV is the prototype member of the family *Hepadnaviridae* and causes the disease formerly known as 'serum hepatitis'. This disease was distinguished clinically from 'infectious hepatitis' (caused by other types of hepatitis virus) in the 1930s. HBV infection used to happen as a result of inoculation with human serum (e.g. blood trans-fusions, organ transplants); today it is still common among intravenous drug abusers, where it is spread by the sharing of needles and syringes. However, the virus is also transmitted sexually, by oral ingestion, and from mother to child, which accounts for familial clusters of HBV infection. All blood, organ and tissue donations in developed countries are now tested for HBV and risk of transmission is extremely low.

HBV does not replicate in tissue culture and this has seriously hindered investi-gations into its pathogenesis. Infection with the virus has three possible outcomes:

1 An acute infection followed by complete recovery and immunity from reinfection (>90% of cases).
2 Fulminant hepatitis, developing quickly and lasting a short time, causing liver fail-ure and a mortality rate of approximately 90% (<1% of cases).
3 Chronic infection, leading to the establishment of a carrier state with virus per-sistence (about 10% of cases).

There are approximately 350 million chronic HBV carriers worldwide. The total population of the world is approximately 6 billion, therefore about 5% of the world population is persistently infected with HBV. All of these chronic carriers of the virus are at 100–200 times the risk of non-carriers of developing hepatocellular carcinoma. HCC is a rare tumour in developed countries, where it represents <2% of fatal cancers. Most cases which do occur in the West are alcohol-related and this is an important clue to the pathogenesis of the tumour. However, in South-East Asia and in China, HCC is the most common fatal cancer, causing about half a million deaths every year.

Three different pathways have been proposed as possible ways in which the virus may cause the formation of the tumour: direct activation of a cellular oncogene(s), *trans*-activation of a cellular oncogene(s), or indirectly via tissue regeneration (Figure 7.12). As with EBV and Burkitt's lymphoma, the relationship between HBV and HCC is not clear cut:

- Cirrhosis (a hardening of the liver which may be the result of infections or various toxins, e.g. alcohol) appears to be a prerequisite for the development of HCC. It would appear that chronic liver damage induces tissue regeneration and that faulty DNA repair mechanisms result eventually in malignant cell transformation. Unrelated viruses which cause chronic active hepatitis, such as the flavivirus *Hepatitis C virus* (HCV), are also associated with HCC after a long latent period.
- A number of co-factors, such as aflatoxins and nitrosamines, can induce HCC-like tumours in experimental animals without virus infection. Therefore, such substances may also be involved in human HCC (cf. nitrosamines and NPC, above)
- There is no consistent evidence for the integration of the HBV **genome** or even the persistence of particular HBV genes (e.g. the X gene, which encodes a *trans*-activator protein functionally analogous to the HTLV tax protein) in tumour cells.

It is possible that all the mechanisms shown in Figure 7.12 might operate *in vivo*. The key risk factor is the development of a chronic as opposed to an acute HBV infection. This in itself is determined by a number of other factors:

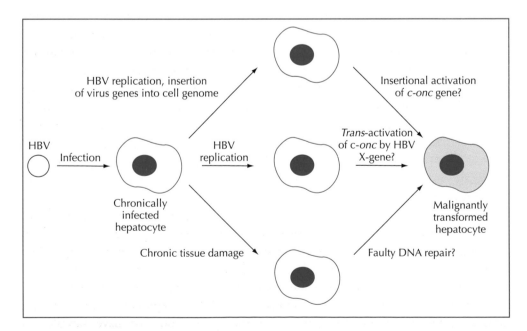

Figure 7.12 Possible mechanisms of hepatocellular carcinoma formation due to hepatitis B virus infection.

- *Age:* The frequency of chronic infections declines with increasing age at the time of infection.
- *Sex:*
  - Chronic infection: male:female ratio 1.5:1
  - Cirrhosis: male:female ratio 3:1
  - HCC: male:female ratio 6:1
- *Route of infection:* Oral or sexual infections give rise to fewer cases of chronic infection than serum infection.

Until there is a much better understanding of the pathogenesis and normal course of HBV infection it is unlikely that the reasons for these differences will be understood. There may be a happy ending to this story. A safe and effective **vaccine** which prevents HBV infection is now available and widely used in the areas of the world where HBV infection is **endemic** as part of the WHO Expanded Programme on Immunization. This will in future prevent a million deaths annually from HCC and HBV disease.

NEW AND EMERGENT VIRUSES

What constitutes a 'new' infectious agent? Are these just viruses which have never been encountered before, or are there previously known viruses which appear to have changed their behaviour? This section will describe and attempt to explain current understanding of a number of agents that meet the above criteria. Much of the information presented here is not the result of many years of study, but is derived from very recent investigations into these 'new' infectious agents. In the last few decades, there have been massive and unexpected **epidemics** caused by certain viruses. For the most part, these are not caused by completely new (i.e. previously unknown) viruses, but by viruses that were well known in the geographical areas in which they may be currently causing epidemic outbreaks of disease. Such viruses are known as **emergent viruses** (Table 7.7). There are numerous examples of such viruses which appear to have mysteriously altered their behaviour with time, with significant effects on their pathogenesis.

One of the better known examples of this phenomenon is poliovirus. It is known that poliovirus and poliomyelitis have existed in human populations for at least 4000 years. For most of this time, the pattern of disease was **endemic** rather than **epidemic**, i.e. a low, continuous level of infection in particular geographical areas. During the first half the twentieth century, the pattern of occurrence of poliomyelitis in Europe, North America and Australia changed to an epidemic one, with vast annual outbreaks of infantile paralysis. Although we do not have samples of polioviruses from earlier centuries, the clinical symptoms of the disease give no reason to believe that the virus changed substantially. Why then did the pattern of

Table 7.7 Emergent viruses		
Virus	**Family**	**Comments**
Cocoa swollen shoot	*Badnaviridae*	Has caused destruction of 200 million cocoa trees in West Africa. Deforestation increases population of mealybug vectors and disease transmission.
Hendra virus (Equine Morbillivirus)	*Paramyxoviridae*	Emerged in Brisbane, Australia, September 1994. Causes acute respiratory disease in horses with high mortality and a fatal encephalitis in humans – 2 deaths so far. The disease, normally carried by fruit bats (with no pathogenesis), re-emerged in horses in Queensland in January 1999 (no further human deaths to date).
Phocine distemper	*Paramyxoviridae*	Emerged in 1987 and caused high mortalities in seals in the Baltic and North Sea. Similar viruses subsequently recognized as responsible for cetacean (porpoise and dolphin) deaths in Irish Sea and Mediterranean. Seal numbers are steadily increasing but have not reached their pre-epizootic level. The virus was believed to have been introduced into immunologically naive seal populations by a massive migration of harp seals from the Barent Sea to northern Europe.
Rabbit haemorrhagic disease (RHD)/ rabbit calicivirus disease (RCD)/ viral haemorrhagic disease (VHD)	*Caliciviridae*	Emerged in farmed rabbits in China in 1984, spread through the UK, Europe and Mexico. Introduced to Wardang Island off the coast of South Australia to test potential for rabbit population control, the disease 'acidentally' spread to Australian mainland causing huge kill in rabbit populations. A vaccine is available to protect domestic and farmed rabbits. In August 1997 RHD was illegally introduced into the South Island of New Zealand and escaped into the USA in April 2000.

disease change so dramatically? It is believed that the reason is as follows. In rural communities with primitive sanitation facilities, poliovirus circulated freely. Serological surveys in similar contemporary situations reveal that more than 90% of children of 3 years of age have antibodies to at least one of the three serotypes of poliovirus. (Even the most virulent strains of poliovirus cause 100–200 subclinical infections for each case of paralytic poliomyelitis seen.) In such communities, infants

experience subclinical immunizing infections while still protected by maternal antibodies – a form of natural **vaccination**. The relatively few cases of paralysis and
death which do occur are likely to be overlooked, especially in view of high infant
mortality rates. During the nineteenth century, industrialization and urbanization
changed the pattern of poliovirus transmission. Dense urban populations and
increased travelling afforded opportunities for rapid transmission of the virus. In
addition, improved sanitation broke the natural pattern of virus transmission.
Children were likely to encounter the virus for the first time at a later age and without the protection of maternal antibodies. These children were at far greater risk
when they did eventually become infected and it is believed that these social changes
account for the altered pattern of disease. Fortunately, the widespread use of
poliovirus **vaccines** has since brought the situation under control in industrialized
countries (Chapter 6), and global eradication of poliovirus is anticipated by 2005.

There are many examples of the **epidemic** spread of viruses caused by movement of human populations. Measles and smallpox were not known to the Ancient
Greeks. Both of these viruses are maintained by direct person-to-person transmission
and have no known alternative hosts. Therefore, it has been suggested that it was not
until human populations in China and the Roman Empire reached a critical density that these viruses were able to propagate in an epidemic pattern and cause rec-
ognizable outbreaks of disease. Before this time, the few cases that did occur could
easily have been overlooked. Smallpox reached Europe from the Far East in AD 710
and achieved plague proportions in the eighteenth century – five reigning European
monarchs died from smallpox. However, the worst effects occurred when these
viruses were transmitted to the New World. Smallpox was (accidentally) transferred
to the Americas by Hernando Cortés in 1520. In the next two years, 3.5 million
Aztecs died from the disease and the Aztec empire was decimated by disease rather
than conquest. Although not as highly pathogenic as smallpox, epidemics of measles
subsequently finished off the Aztec and Inca civilizations. More recently, the first
contacts with isolated groups of Eskimos and tribes in New Guinea and South
America have had similarly devastating results, although on a smaller scale. These his-
torical incidents illustrate the way in which a known virus can suddenly cause illness
and death on a catastrophic scale following a change in human behaviour.

Measles and smallpox viruses are transmitted exclusively from one human host
to another. For viruses with more complex cycles of transmission, e.g. those with secondary hosts and insect vectors, control of infection becomes much more difficult
(Figure 7.13). This is particularly true of the families of viruses known collectively as
'arboviruses' (arenaviruses, bunyaviruses, flaviviruses and togaviruses). As human
territory has expanded, this has increasingly brought people into contact with the
type of environment where these viruses are found – warm, humid, vegetated areas
where insect vectors occur in high densities, such as swamps and jungles. It should
also be noted that many **emergent virus** diseases are **zoonoses,** i.e. transmitted
from animals to humans. This emphasizes the importance of the 'species barrier' in

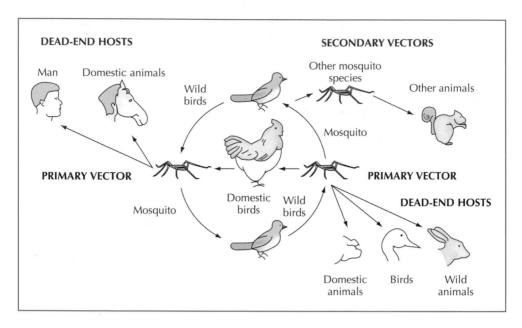

Figure 7.13 Complex transmission pattern of an 'arbovirus'.

preventing transmission of infectious diseases. A classic example from history was the mortality caused by *Yellow fever virus* during the building of the Panama Canal at the end of the nineteenth century. More recently, the increasing pace of ecological alteration in tropical areas has resulted in the resurgence of yellow fever in Central America, particularly an urban form of the disease transmitted directly from one human to another by mosquitoes.

Dengue fever is also primarily an urban disease of the tropics. It is transmitted by *Aedes aegypti*, a day-biting mosquito frequently found inside houses, which prefers to feed on humans, and some outbreaks of dengue fever have involved more than a million cases with attack rates of up to 90% of the population. There are believed to be over 40 million cases of *Dengue virus* infection worldwide each year. The disease was first described in 1780 and by 1906 it was known that the virus was transmitted by mosquitoes. The virus was isolated in 1944. Therefore, this is not a new virus, but the frequency of *Dengue virus* infection has increased dramatically in the last 20 years. F.A. Murphy (see Further Reading) suggests that this is due to factors such as:

- Population movements and the intrusion of humans and domestic animals into new arthropod habitats, particularly tropical forests.
- Deforestation, with development of new forest–farmland margins and exposure of farmers and domestic animals to new arthropods.
- Irrigation, especially primitive irrigation systems which do not take arthropod control into consideration.

- Uncontrolled urbanization, with vector populations breeding in accumulations of water (tin cans, old tyres, etc.) and sewage.
- Increased long-distance air travel, with potential for transport of arthropod vectors.
- Increased long-distance livestock transportation, with potential for carriage of viruses and arthropods (especially ticks).
- New routing of long-distance bird migration brought about by new artificial water impoundments.
- Cessation of mosquito control programmes and political upheaval resulting in degraded primary medical services.

Of more than 520 arboviruses known, at least 100 are pathogenic for humans and perhaps 20 would meet the criteria for **emergent viruses**. Attempts to control these diseases rely on twin approaches involving both the control of insect vectors responsible for transmission of the virus to humans and the development of **vaccines** to protect human populations. However, both of these approaches present considerable difficulties, the former in terms of avoiding environmental damage and the latter in terms of understanding virus pathogenesis and developing appropriate vaccines (see discussion of *Dengue virus* pathogenesis earlier).

Rift Valley fever virus was first isolated from sheep in 1930 but has caused repeated **epidemics** in sub-Saharan Africa during the last 20 years, with human infection rates in epidemic areas as high as 35%. This is an epizootic disease, transmitted from sheep to humans by a number of different mosquitoes. The construction of dams which increase mosquito populations, increasing numbers of sheep and the movement of sheep and human populations are believed to be responsible for the upsurge in this disease.

The *Hantavirus* genus (*Bunyaviridae*) is a particular cause for concern. Hantaviruses cause millions of cases of haemorrhagic fever each year in many parts of the world. Unlike arboviruses, hantaviruses are transmitted directly from rodent hosts to humans (e.g. via faeces) rather than by an invertebrate host. Hantaviruses cause two acute diseases: haemorrhagic fever with renal syndrome (HFRS) and hantavirus pulmonary syndrome (HPS). HFRS was first recognized in 1951 after an outbreak among US troops stationed in Korea. In May 1993, HPS was first recognized in the USA and a new virus, *Sin Nombre virus*, identified as the cause. It is now known that at least three different hantaviruses cause HFRS and four different viruses cause HPS. By January 1995, HPS had been recognized in 102 patients in 21 states of the USA, seven in Canada and three in Brazil with an overall mortality rate of approximately 40%. This illustrates the disease-causing potential of emerging viruses.

West Nile virus is a member of the Japanese encephalitis antigenic complex of the genus *Flavivirus*, family *Flaviviridae*. All known members of this complex are transmissible by mosquitoes and many of them can cause febrile, sometimes fatal, illnesses in humans. *West Nile virus* was first isolated in the West Nile district of Uganda in 1937 but is, in fact, the most widespread of the flaviviruses, with geographic distribution including Africa and Eurasia. Unexpectedly, an outbreak of human arboviral encephalitis attributable to a mosquito-transmitted *West Nile-like virus* (WNLV) occurred in New York, USA, and surrounding states in 1999, resulting (to January 2000) in about 50 cases and seven deaths. In this case, the virus appears to have been transmitted from wild, domestic and exotic birds by *Culex* mosquitoes (an urban mosquito that flourishes under dry conditions) – a classic pattern of arbovirus transmission. *West Nile virus* RNA has been detected in overwintering mosquitoes and in birds and the disease is now endemic in the USA.

Ebola virus has received massive attention in recent years and so will only be dealt with briefly here. The virus was first described in 1976 and since then has reappeared several times. The extreme pathogenicity of this virus has severely inhibited investigations, most of which have been carried out using molecular biological techniques. However, this predominantly molecular approach has left important questions unanswered, for example:

- *Strain variation:* Some strains of Ebola virus are highly pathogenic, whereas other strains are not. Relatively non-pathogenic strains have been isolated from monkeys imported into the USA from the Philippines. The molecular basis for these differences is unknown.
- *Natural hosts and distribution:* Most human infections appear to be associated with contact with infected primates. However, extensive ecological surveys in Central Africa have failed to show any evidence that primates (or any of the thousands of animals, plants and invertebrate species examined) are the natural reservoir for infection. Isolates from Central Africa appear to be highly pathogenic whereas those from the Philippines are apathogenic for humans.

Plant viruses can also be responsible for **emergent diseases**. Group III geminiviruses are transmitted by insect vectors (whiteflies) and their **genomes** consist of two circular, single-stranded DNA molecules (Chapter 3). These viruses cause a great deal of crop damage in plants such as tomatoes, beans, squash, cassava and cotton and their spread may be directly linked to the inadvertent worldwide dissemination of a particular biotype of the whitefly *Bemisia tabaci*. This vector is an indiscriminate feeder, encouraging rapid and efficient spread of viruses from indigenous plant species to neighbouring crops.

Occasionally, there appears an example of an emergent virus which has acquired extra genes and as a result of this new genetic capacity, becomes capable of infecting new species. A possible example of this phenomenon is seen in *Tomato spotted wilt virus* (TSWV). TSWV is a *Bunyavirus* with a very wide plant host range, infecting over 600 different species from 70 families. In recent decades, this virus has been a major agricultural pest in Asia, the Americas, Europe and Africa. Its rapid spread has been the result of dissemination of its insect vector (the thrip **Frankinellia occidentalis**) and diseased plant material. TSWV is the type species of the **Tospovirus** genus and has a similar morphology and genomic organization to the other bunyaviruses (Chapter 3). However, TSWV undergoes **propagative transmission** and it has been suggested that it may have acquired an extra gene in the M segment via **recombination**, either from a plant or from another plant virus. This new gene encodes a **movement protein** (Chapter 6), conferring the capacity to infect plants and cause extensive damage.

In addition to viruses whose ability to infect their host species appears to have changed, 'new' viruses are being discovered continually. In recent years, three new human herpesviruses have been discovered:

1 *Human herpesvirus 6 (HHV-6):* This was first isolated in 1986 in lymphocytes of patients with lymphoreticular disorders; **tropism** for CD4$^+$ lymphocytes. HHV-6 is now recognized as being an almost universal human infection. Discovery of the virus solved a longstanding mystery: the primary infection in childhood causes 'roseola infantum' or 'fourth disease', a common childhood rash whose cause was previously unknown. Antibody **titres** are highest in children and decline with age. The consequences of childhood infection appear to be mild. Primary infections of adults are rare but have more severe consequences, mononucleosis or hepatitis, and infections may be a severe problem in transplant patients.

2 *Human herpesvirus 7 (HHV-7):* This was first isolated from human CD4$^+$ cells in 1990. Its **genome** organization is similar to but distinct from that of HHV-6 and there is limited antigenic cross-reactivity between the two viruses. At present, there is no clear evidence for the direct involvement of HHV-7 in any human disease, but it may be a co-factor in HHV-6-related syndromes.

3 *Human herpesvirus 8 (HHV-8):* In 1995, sequences of a unique herpesvirus were identified in DNA samples from AIDS patients with Kaposi's sarcoma (KS) and in some non-KS tissue samples from AIDS patients. There is a strong correlation (>95%) with KS in both HIV-positive and HIV-negative patients. HHV-8 can be isolated from lymphocytes and from tumour tissue and appears to have a less ubiquitous world distribution than other HHVs, i.e. it may only be associated with a specific disease state (cf. HSV, EBV). However, the virus is not present in KS-derived cell lines, suggesting that **autocrine** or paracrine factors may be involved in the formation of KS. There is some evidence that HHV-8 may also cause other tumours such as B-cell lymphomas (± EBV as a 'helper').

Although many different virus infections may involve the liver, there are at least six viruses which seem specifically to infect and damage hepatocytes. No two of these belong to the same family! The identification of these viruses has been a long story:

- *Hepatitis B virus* (HBV) (*Hepadnavirus*): 1963
- *Hepatitis A virus* (HAV) (*Picornavirus*): 1973
- *Hepatitis delta virus* (HDV) (*Deltavirus*, see Chapter 8): 1977
- *Hepatitis C virus* (HCV) (*Flavivirus*): 1989
- *Hepatitis E virus* (HEV): 1990
- GBV-C/HGV: 1995
- 'Transfusion-transmitted virus' (TTV): 1998

Reports continue to circulate about the existence of other hepatitis viruses. Some of the agents are reported to be sensitive to chloroform (i.e. **enveloped**) while others are not. This may suggest the existence of multiple viruses, as yet undescribed, although this is still uncertain. Although the viral causes of the majority of cases of infectious human hepatatitis have now been identified, it is likely that further hepatitis viruses will be described in the future.

SUMMARY

Virus pathogenesis is a complex, variable and relatively rare state. Like the course of a virus infection, pathogenesis is determined by the balance between host and virus factors. Not all of the pathogenic symptoms seen in virus infections are caused directly by the virus – the immune system also plays a part in causing cell and tissue damage. Viruses can transform cells so that they continue to grow indefinitely. In some but not all cases, this can lead to the formation of tumours. There are at least a few well-established cases where certain viruses provoke human tumours and possibly many others that we do not yet understand. The relationship between the virus and the formation of the tumour is not a simple one, but the prevention of infection undoubtedly reduces the risk of tumour formation. New pathogenic viruses are being discovered all the time and changes in human activities result in the emergence of new or previously unrecognized diseases.

FURTHER READING

Arnaout, R.A., Lloyd, A.L., O'Brien, T.R., Goedert, J.J., Leonard, J.M., Nowak, M.A. (1999). A simple relationship between viral load and survival time in HIV-1 infection. *Proceedings of the National Academy of Sciences of the USA* 96: 11549–11553.

Clerici, M. and Shearer, G. (1993). A T_H1-T_H2 switch is a critical step in the aetiology of HIV infection. *Immunology Today* 14: 107–111.

Haase, A.T. (1999). Population biology of HIV-1 infection: viral and $CD4^+$ T cell demographics and dynamics in lymphatic tissues. *Annual Review of Immunology* 17: 625–656.

McMichael, A.J. and Phillips, R.E. (1997). Escape of human immunodeficiency virus from immune control. *Annual Review of Immunology* 15: 271–296.

Mims, C.A., Dimmock, N., Nash, A. and Stephen, A. (1995). *Mims' Pathogenesis of Infectious Disease* (4th edn). Academic Press, London. ISBN 0124982638.

Murphy, F.A. (1994). New, emerging, and reemerging infectious diseases. *Advances in Virus Research* 43: 1–52.

Morse, S.S. (Ed.). (1996). *Emerging Viruses*. Oxford University Press, New York. ISBN 0195104846.

Roulston, A., Marcellus, R.C. and Branton, P.E. (1999). Viruses and apoptosis. *Annual Review of Microbiology* 53: 577–628.

Tiollais, P. and Buendia, M. (1991). Hepatitis B virus. *Scientific American* April, 48–54.

SELF-ASSESSMENT QUESTIONS

(7.1) Are the following statements true or false?

(a) Most diseases are multi-factorial.

(b) Inflammation, fever, headaches and skin rashes are frequently not caused by virus replication, but the immune response to virus infection.

(c) The vast majority of virus infections do not result in disease.

(d) Eukaryotic cells must constantly synthesize a variety of macromolecules which require continual replacement.

(e) Virus nucleic acids act as toxins and poison cells.

(7.2) The cytopathic effects of virus infection include (true or false?):

(a) Altered shape.

(b) Detachment from the substrate.

(c) Lysis.

(d) Membrane fusion and altered permeability.

(e) Apoptosis.

(7.3) Are the following statements true or false?

(a) Shutoff is the sudden and dramatic cessation of virus macromolecular synthesis.

(b) Shutoff in poliovirus-infected cells occurs due to protease degradation of ribosomes.

(c) Lysis of adenovirus-infected cells is caused by virus-encoded molecules with a toxin-like action.

(d) Virus-induced membrane fusion causes cell transformation.

(e) The HIV gag protein is responsible for syncytium formation.

(7.4) Are the following statements true or false?
(a)   All human herpesviruses are highly cytopathic.
(b)   Retroviruses cause a variety pathogenic conditions including paraly-
        sis, arthritis and anaemia in addition to cell transformation.
(c)   Lentiviruses are the group of retroviruses most frequently associated
        with cell transformation.
(d)   HIV and other lentiviruses escape immune recognition by infecting
        monocytes.
(e)   All isolates of HIV are highly cytopathic in $CD4^+$ cells.

**(7.5) The following mechanisms may be involved in the pathogen-
esis of AIDS (true or false?):**
(a)   Antigenic variation.
(b)   T-cell anergy.
(c)   Apoptosis.
(d)   Superantigens.
(e)   Insertional activation of oncogenes.

(7.6) Are the following statements true or false?
(a)   Subacute sclerosing panencephalitis (SSPE) occurs in 10% of measles
        virus infections of adults.
(b)   Dengue haemorrhagic fever is largely due to immune-mediated dam-
        age of virus-infected cells.
(c)   Reye's syndrome can be cured by administration of aspirin during
        the initial illness.
(d)   Kawasaki disease is a rare post-infection complication of a number of
        different viruses, but most commonly influenza virus and VZV
        (chicken pox).
(e)   Guillain–Barré syndrome is a rare demyelinating disease.

(7.7) Transformed cells may display (true or false?):
(a)   loss of anchorage dependence.
(b)   loss of contact inhibition.
(c)   colony formation in semi-solid media.
(d)   decreased requirements for growth factors.
(e)   increased expression of p53.

(7.8) Are the following statements true or false?
(a)   Carcinogenesis = oncogenesis = transformation.
(b)   All acutely transforming retroviruses are replication defective.
(c)   p53 causes the cell cycle to arrest at the G_1 phase.
(d)   Rb causes the cell cycle to arrest at the G_2 phase.
(e)   Adenovirus E1A, SV40 T-antigen and HPV E7 protein all bind to p53.

(7.9) The normal functions of oncogenes may be (true or false?):
(a) Cytoplasmic protein kinases.
(b) Extracellular growth factors.
(c) G proteins involved in signal transduction.
(d) Transcription factors.
(e) Tyrosine kinases.

(7.10) Are the following statements true or false?
(a) At least six viruses are associated with the formation of human tumours.
(b) EBV has a dual cell tropism for human B lymphocytes (productive infection) and epithelial cells, in which a non-productive infection occurs.
(c) EBV infection is associated with at least four human tumours: Burkitt's lymphoma, nasopharyngeal carcinoma, B-cell lymphomas and hepatocellular carcinoma.
(d) Chronic HBV carriers are at 100–200 times the risk of non-carriers of developing hepatocellular carcinoma.
(e) Chronic active hepatitis caused by *Hepatitis C virus* (HCV) infection is associated with hepatocellular carcinoma.

Answers to Self-Assessment Questions are given in Appendix 4.

SUBVIRAL AGENTS: GENOMES WITHOUT VIRUSES, VIRUSES WITHOUT GENOMES

Learning Objectives

- On completing this chapter, you should be able to:
- Understand the concept of subviral agents
- Explain the differences between satellites and viroids
- Summarize the present state of knowledge about transmissible spongiform encephalopathies.

What is the minimum **genome** size necessary to sustain an infectious agent? Could a virus with a genome of 1700 nucleotides exist? Could an agent with a genome of 240 nucleotides exist? Could an infectious agent without any genome at all exist? Perhaps the first two alternatives might be possible, but the idea of an infectious agent without a genome seems bizarre and ridiculous. Strange as it may seem, such agents as these do exist and cause disease in animals (including humans) and plants.

SATELLITES AND VIROIDS

Satellites are small RNA molecules that are absolutely dependent on the presence of another virus for multiplication. Even viruses have their own parasites! Most satellites are associated with plant viruses, but a few are associated with **bacteriophages** or animal viruses, e.g. the *Dependovirus* genus, which are satellites of adenoviruses. Two classes of satellites can be distinguished: satellite viruses, which encode their own coat proteins, and satellite RNAs (or 'virusoids'), which use the coat protein of the helper virus (Appendix 2 ✐). The typical properties of satellites can be summarized:

- They have a genome of approximately 500–2000 nucleotides of single-stranded RNA.
- Unlike defective virus genomes, there is little or no nucleotide sequence similarity between the satellite and the helper virus genome.
- They cause distinct disease symptoms in plants which are not seen with the helper virus alone.
- Replication of satellites usually interferes with the replication of the helper virus (unlike most defective virus genomes).

Some examples of satellites are:

- Barley yellow dwarf virus satellite RNA (helper: *Luteovirus*)
- Tobacco ringspot virus satellite RNA (helper: *Nepovirus*)
- Subterranean clover mottle virus satellite RNA (helper: *Sobemovirus*).

Satellites replicate in the cytoplasm using an RNA-dependent RNA polymerase, an enzymatic activity found in plant but not animal cells.

Viroids are very small (200–400 nt), rod-like RNA molecules with a high degree of secondary structure (Figure 8.1). They have no **capsid** or **envelope** and consist only of a single nucleic acid molecule. Viroids are associated with plant diseases and are distinct from **satellites** in a number of ways (Table 8.1). The first viroid to be discovered and the best studied is potato spindle tuber viroid (PSTVd – viroid names are abbreviated 'Vd' to distinguish them from viruses). Viroids do not encode any proteins and are replicated by host cell RNA polymerase II, or possibly by the

Figure 8.1 Structure of a viroid RNA.

Table 8.1 Satellites and viroids		
Characteristic	**Satellites**	**Viroids**
Helper virus required for replication:	Yes	No
Protein(s) encoded:	Yes	No
Genome replicated by:	Helper virus enzymes	Host cell RNA polymerase II
Site of replication:	Same as helper virus (nucleus or cytoplasm)	Nucleus

product of an RNA-dependent RNA polymerase gene in some eukaryotic cells. The details of replication are not understood, but it is likely to occur by a rolling circle mechanism followed by autocatalytic cleavage and self-ligation to produce the mature viroid.

There is considerable sequence variation between different viroids and this is used as an arbitrary classification to divide viroids into genera and species (Appendix 2). However, all viroids share a common feature, a conserved central region believed to be involved in their replication (Figure 8.2). One group of viroids is capable of forming a hammerhead structure, giving them the enzymatic properties of a ribozyme (an autocatalytic, self-cleaving RNA molecule). This activity is used to cleave the multimeric structures produced during the course of replication. Other viroids use unknown host nuclear enzymes to achieve this objective. Some viroids (e.g. cadang-cadang coconut viroid, CCCVd) cause severe and lethal disease in their host plants. Others range from no apparent pathogenic effects (e.g. hop latent viroid, HLVd) to mild disease symptoms (e.g. apple scar skin viroid, ASSVd). It is not clear how viroids cause pathogenic symptoms, but obviously these must result from some perturbation of the normal host cell metabolism. They show some similarities with certain **eukaryotic** host cell sequences, in particular with an **intron** found between the 5.8S and 25S ribosomal RNAs and with the U3 snRNA which is involved in **splicing**. Therefore, it has been suggested that viroids may interfere with post-transcriptional RNA processing in infected cells. *In vitro* experiments with purified mammalian protein kinase PKR (Chapter 6) have shown that the kinase is strongly activated (phosphorylated) by viroid strains that cause severe symptoms, but far less by mild strains. Activation of a plant homologue of PKR could be the triggering event in viroid pathogenesis (see discussion of the hypersensitive response in Chapter 6).

Most viroids are transmitted by vegetative propagation, i.e. division of infected plants, although a few can be transmitted by insect vectors (**non-propagative**) or mechanically. Because viroids do not have the benefit of a protective **capsid**, viroid RNAs would be expected to be at extreme risk of degradation in the environment. However, their small size and high degree of secondary structure protects them to a

Figure 8.2 Functional regions of viroid RNA molecules.

large extent and they are able to persist in the environment for a sufficiently long period to be transferred to another host. The origins of viroids are obscure. One theory is that they may be the most primitive type of RNA **genome** – possibly left-overs from the 'RNA world' believed to have existed during the era of prebiotic evolution (see Chapter 3). Alternatively, they may have evolved at a much more recent time as the most extreme type of parasite. We may never know which of these alternatives is true, but viroids exist and cause disease in plants and in humans.

Hepatitis delta virus (HDV) is a unique chimeric molecule with some of the properties of a **satellite** virus and some of a **viroid** (Table 8.2) which causes disease in humans. HDV requires *Hepatitis B virus* (HBV) as a 'helper virus' for replication and is transmitted by the same means as HBV, benefiting from the presence of a protective coat composed of lipid plus HBV proteins. Virus preparations from HBV/HDV-infected animals contain heterologous particles distinct from those of HBV but with an irregular, ill-defined structure. These particles are composed of HBV antigens and contain the covalently closed circular HDV RNA molecule in a branched or rod-like configuration similar to that of other viroids (Figure 8.3). Unlike all other viroids, HDV encodes a protein, the δ antigen, which is a nuclear phosphoprotein. Post-transcriptional RNA editing results in the production of two slightly different forms of the protein, δAg-S (195 amino acids) which is necessary for HDV replication and δAg-L (214 amino acids) which is necessary for the assembly and release of HDV-containing particles. The HDV genome is thought to be replicated by host cell RNA polymerase II using a 'rolling circle' mechanism which produces linear concatemers that must be cleaved for infectivity. The cleavage is carried out by a ribozyme domain present in the HDV RNA, the only known example of a ribozyme in an animal virus genome.

HDV is found worldwide wherever HBV infection occurs. The interactions between HBV and HDV are difficult to study, but HDV seems to potentiate the pathogenic effects of HBV infection. Fulminant hepatitis (with a mortality rate of about 80%) is 10 times more common in co-infections than with HBV infection

Table 8.2 Properties of Hepatitis delta virus (HDV)	
Satellite-like properties	**Viroid-like properties**
Size and composition of genome – 1640 nt (about four times the size of plant viroids)	Sequence homology to the conserved central region involved in viroid replication
Single-stranded circular RNA molecule ·	
Dependent on HBV for replication – HDV RNA is packaged into coats consisting of lipids plus HBV encoded proteins	
Encodes a single polypeptide, the δ antigen	

Figure 8.3 Structure of hepatitis delta virus RNA. A region at the left end of the genome strongly resembles the RNA of plant viroids such as potato spindle tuber viroid (PSTVd), which is shown for comparison.

alone. Because HDV requires HBV for replication, it is being controlled by HBV **vaccination** (Chapter 6).

PRIONS

There are a group of transmissible, chronic, progressive infections of the nervous system which show common pathological effects and are invariably fatal. Their pathology is reminiscent of amyloid diseases such as Alzheimer's syndrome and to distinguish them from such conditions, they are known as transmissible spongiform encephalopathies (TSEs). The earliest record of any TSE dates from several centuries ago, when a disease called scrapie was first observed in sheep (see TSE in Animals). Long considered to be caused by viruses, the first doubts about the nature of the infectious agent involved in TSEs arose in the 1960s. In 1967, Tikvah Alper was the first to suggest that the agent of scrapie might replicate without nucleic acid, and in 1982, Stanley Prusiner coined the term **prion** (proteinaceous infectious particle), which, according to Prusiner, is pronounced 'pree-on'. The molecular nature of prions has not been unequivocally proved (see Molecular Biology of Prions), but the evidence that they represent a new phenomenon outside the framework of conventional scientific understanding is growing steadily stronger.

Pathology of prion diseases

All prion diseases share a similar underlying pathology, although there are significant differences between various conditions. A number of different diseases are characterized by the deposition of abnormal protein deposits in various organs, e.g. kidney, spleen, liver or brain. These 'amyloid' deposits consist of accumulations of various proteins in the form of plaques or fibrils depending on their origin. For example, Alzheimer's disease is characterized by the deposition of plaques and 'tangles' composed of β-amyloid protein. None of the 'conventional' amyloidoses are infectious diseases and extensive research has shown that they cannot be transmitted to experimental animals; they result from endogenous errors in metabolism caused by a variety of largely unknown factors. Amyloid deposits appear to be inherently cytotoxic. Although the molecular mechanisms involved in cell death are unclear, it is this effect which gives the 'spongiform encephalopathies' their name, owing to the characteristic holes in thin sections of affected brain tissue viewed under the microscope; these holes are caused by neuronal loss and gliosis. Thus deposition of amyloid is the end stage that links conventional amyloidoses and TSEs and explains the tissue damage seen in both types of disease, but does not reveal anything about their underlying causes. Definitive diagnosis of TSE cannot be made on clinical grounds alone and requires demonstration of prion protein (PrP) deposition by immunohistochemical staining of post-mortem brain tissue, molecular genetic studies or experimental transmission to animals, as discussed in the following sections.

TSEs in animals

A number of TSEs have been observed and intensively investigated in animals. In particular, scrapie is the paradigm for understanding of human TSEs. Some of these diseases are naturally occurring and have been known about for centuries, whereas others have only been observed more recently and are almost certainly causally related to one another.

Scrapie

Scrapie is a naturally occurring disease of sheep found in many parts of the world, although not universally distributed, which was first described more than 200 years ago. Scrapie appears to have originated in Spain and subsequently spread throughout Western Europe. The export of sheep from Britain in the nineteenth century is thought to have helped scrapie spread around the world. Scrapie is primarily a disease of sheep although it can also affect goats. The scrapie agent has been intensively studied and has been experimentally transmitted to laboratory animals many times (see Molecular Biology of Prions). Infected sheep show severe and progressive neurological symptoms such as abnormal gait, often repeatedly scraping against fences or posts, from which behaviour the disease takes its name. The incidence of the disease increases with the age of the animals. Some countries, such as Australia and New Zealand, have eliminated scrapie by slaughtering infected sheep and the imposition of rigorous import controls. Work in Iceland has shown that the land on which infected sheep graze may retain the condition and infect sheep up to three years later.

The incidence of scrapie in a flock is related to the breed of sheep. Some breeds are relatively resistant to the disease while others are prone to it, indicating genetic control of susceptibility. In recent years the occurrence of TSE in sheep in the UK closely parallels the incidence of BSE in cattle (Figure 8.4). This is probably due to infection with the BSE agent (to which sheep are known to be sensitive) via infected feed (see below). The natural mode of transmission between sheep is unclear. Lambs of scrapie-infected sheep are more likely to develop the disease, but the reason for this is unclear. Symptoms of scrapie are not seen in sheep of less than one and a half years old, which indicates that the incubation period of scrapie is at least this long. The first traces of infectivity can be detected in the tonsils, mesenteric lymph nodes and intestines of sheep 10–14 months old, which suggests an oral route of infection. The infective agent is present in the membranes of the embryo but it has not been demonstrated in colostrum or milk or in the tissues of the newborn lambs.

Transmissible mink encephalopathy (TME)

TME is a rare disease of farmed mink caused by exposure to a scrapie-like agent in feed. The disease was first identified in Wisconsin, USA, in 1947 and has also been recorded in Canada, Finland, Germany and Russia. Like other TSEs, TME is a slow progressive neurological disease. Early symptoms include changes in habits and clean-

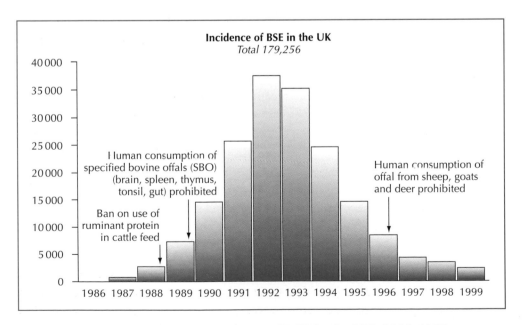

Figure 8.4 Reported incidence of BSE in the UK, 1986–1999.

liness as well as difficulty in eating or swallowing. TME-infected mink become hyperexcitable and begin arching their tails over their backs, ultimately losing loco-motor coordination. Natural TME has a minimum incubation period of 7–12 months and although exposure is generally through oral routes, horizontal mink-to-mink transmission cannot be ruled out. The origin of the transmissible agent in TME appears to be contaminated foodstuffs but this is discussed further below (see BSE).

Feline spongiform encephalopathy (FSE)

FSE was recognized in the UK in May 1990 as a scrapie-like syndrome in domestic cats resulting in ataxia (irregular and jerky movements) and other symptoms typical of spongiform encephalopathies. By December 1997, a total of 81 cases had been reported in the UK. In addition, FSE has been recorded in a domestic cat in Norway and in three species of captive wild cats (cheetahs, puma and ocelot). Inclusion of cattle offal in commercial pet foods was banned in the UK in 1990, so the incidence of this disease is expected to decline rapidly (see BSE).

Chronic wasting disease (CWD)

A disease similar to scrapie which affects deer and captive exotic ungulates (e.g. nyala, oryx, kudu, etc.), CWD was first recognized in captive deer and elk in the western United States in 1967 and appears to be **endemic** in origin. The incidence in wild deer and elk is up to 15% in Colorado. This is worrying, since prions taken from the brains of infected deer and elk are able to convert normal human prion to a protease-resistant form, a well-studied test for the ability to cause human disease (see below).

Bovine spongiform encephalopathy (BSE)

BSE was first recognized in dairy cattle in the UK in 1986 as a typical spongiform encephalopathy. Affected cattle showed altered behaviour and a staggering gait, giv-ing the disease its name in the press of 'mad cow disease'. On microscopic examina-tion, the brains of affected cattle showed extensive spongiform degeneration. It was concluded that BSE resulted from the use of contaminated foodstuffs. To obtain higher milk yields and growth rates, the nutritional value of feed for farmed animals was routinely boosted by the addition of protein derived from waste meat products and bonemeal (MBM) prepared from animal carcasses, including sheep and cows. This practice was not unique to the UK but was widely followed in most developed countries. By January 2000, a total of 179 256 cases of BSE had been reported in the UK and 1392 cases elsewhere (including Switzerland, Ireland, Portugal, France, Germany, Italy, Oman, Canada, Denmark and the Falklands) (Figure 8.4).

The initial explanation for the emergence of BSE in the UK was as follows. Because scrapie is **endemic** in Britain, it was assumed that this was the source of the infectious agent in the feed. Traditionally, MBM was prepared by a rendering process involving steam treatment and hydrocarbon extraction, resulting in two products, a protein-rich fraction called 'greaves' containing about 1% fat from which MBM was

produced and a fat-rich fraction called 'tallow' which was put to a variety of indus-
trial uses. In the late 1970s, the price of tallow fell and the use of expensive hydro-
carbons in the rendering process was discontinued, producing an MBM product
containing about 14% fat in which the infectious material may not have been inactivated. As a result, a ban on the use of ruminant protein in cattle feed was introduced
in July 1988 (Figure 8.4). In November 1989, human consumption of specified
bovine offals thought most likely to transmit the infection (brain, spleen, thymus,
tonsil and gut) was prohibited. A similar ban on consumption of offals from sheep,
goats and deer was finally announced in July 1996 to counter concerns about transmission of BSE to sheep. The available evidence suggests that milk and dairy products do not contain detectable amounts of the infectious agent. The total number of
BSE cases continued to rise, as would be expected from the long incubation period
of the disease, and the peak incidence was reached in the last quarter of 1992, since
when the number of new cases has started to fall.

   Unfortunately, there are a number of false assumptions in the above reasoning:

- It is now known that none of the rendering processes used before or after the
  1980s completely inactivates the infectivity of prions. Therefore cattle would have
  been exposed to scrapie prions in all countries worldwide where scrapie was present and MBM was used, not just in the UK in the 1980s. For example, the incidence of scrapie in the USA is hard to determine but in the eight years after the
  level of compensation for slaughter of infected sheep was raised to $300 in 1977,
  the reported number of cases went up tenfold to a peak of about 50 affected flocks
  a year.
- BSE is not scrapie. The biological properties of the scrapie and BSE agents are distinct, e.g. transmissibility to different animal species and pattern of lesions produced in infected animals (see Molecular Biology of Prions). There is no evidence
  to support the assumption that BSE is scrapie in cows. The only feasible interpretation based on present knowledge is that BSE originated as an endogenous
  bovine (cow) prion which was amplified by the feeding of cattle-derived protein
  in MBM back to cows. Thus the emergence of BSE in the UK appears to have
  been due to a chance event compounded by poor husbandry practices, i.e. use of
  MBM in ruminant feed.
- The reported international distribution of BSE is at odds with established facts.
  Germany, Spain and Italy each imported approximately 13 000 British cattle plus
  1200 tonnes of British MBM at the height of the epidemic, while the USA
  imported 126 cattle and 44 tonnes of MBM from the UK. Approximately 40 000
  tonnes of MBM were exported from the UK between 1985 and 1988; France
  alone imported at least 17 000 tonnes during this period and yet has only reported
  20 cases of BSE compared with nearly 100 000 in the UK during the same
  period. During 1985–1990 the UK exported 57 900 cattle. These animals would
  have resulted in 1668 cases of BSE had they remained in the UK, but only a small

fraction of these cases have been reported by the recipient countries. The United States Department of Agriculture (USDA) maintains that no cases of BSE have been confirmed in the USA, but TME in the USA has been found in mink fed on 'downer cows' and never fed on sheep which therefore could not have been exposed to scrapie (see Further Reading).

Important unanswered questions remain concerning BSE. Many of these are raised by the large number of infected cattle (>41 000) born after the 1988 feed ban. It is now generally acknowledged that the feed ban was initially improperly enforced and moreover, only applied to cattle feed. The same mills that were producing cattle feed were also producing sheep, pig and poultry food containing MBM, allowing many opportunities for contamination. As a result, in March 1996 the use of all mammalian MBM in animal feed was prohibited in the UK. It is now known that vertical transmission of BSE in herds can occur at a frequency of 1–10%. Similarly, there is a possibility of environmental transmission similar to that known to occur with scrapie (above). Apart from the economic damage done by BSE, the main concern at present is the possible risk to human health (discussed below).

Human TSEs

There are four recognized human TSEs (summarized in Table 8.3). Understanding of human TSEs is derived largely from studies of the animal TSEs already described. There are believed to be three sources from which human TSEs originate:

- *Sporadic*: Creutzfeldt-Jakob disease (CJD) arises spontaneously at a frequency of about one in a million people per year with little variation worldwide. The average age at onset of disease is about 65 and the average duration of illness about three months. This category accounts for 90% of all human TSE, but only about 1% of sporadic CJD cases are transmissible to mice.
- *Iatrogenic/acquired TSE*: This occurs due to recognized risks, e.g. neurosurgery, transplantation, etc. About 50 cases of TSE were caused in young people who received injections of human growth hormone or gonadotrophin derived from pooled cadaver pituitary gland extracts, a practice which has now been discontinued in favour of recombinant DNA-derived hormone.
- *Familial*: Approximately 10% of human TSEs are familial, i.e. inherited. There are a number of mutations in the human *PrP* gene which are known to give rise to TSE as an autosomal dominant trait acquired by hereditary mendelian transmission (Figure 8.5).

Kuru was the first human spongiform encephalopathy to be investigated in detail and is possibly one of the most fascinating stories to have emerged from any epidemiological investigation. The disease occurred primarily in 169 villages occupied by the

Table 8.3 Transmissible spongiform encephalopathies (TSEs) in humans

Disease	Description	Comments
Creutzfeldt-Jakob disease (CJD)	Spongiform encephalopathy in cerebral and/or cerebellar cortex and/or subcortical grey matter, or encephalopathy with prion protein (PrP) immunoreactivity (plaque and/or diffuse synaptic and/or patchy/perivacuolar types).	Three forms: sporadic, iatrogenic (recognized risk, e.g. neurosurgery), familial (same disease in first-degree relative).
Fatal familial insomnia (FFI)	Thalamic degeneration, variable spongiform change in cerebrum.	Occurs in families with PrP_{178} Asp-Asn mutation.
Gerstmann-Straussler-Scheinker disease (GSS)	Encephalo(myelo)pathy with multicentric PrP plaques.	Occurs in families with dominantly inherited progressive ataxia and/or dementia.
Kuru	Characterized by large amyloid plaques.	Occurs in the Fore population of New Guinea due to ritual cannibalism, now eliminated.

Fore tribes in the highlands of New Guinea. The first cases were recorded in the 1950s and involved progressive loss of voluntary neuronal control, followed by death less than a year after the onset of symptoms. The key to the origin of the disease was provided by the profile of its victims – it was never seen in young children, rarely in adult men and was most common in both male and female adolescents and in adult

Figure 8.5 Mutations in the human *PrP* gene.

women. The Fore people practised ritual cannibalism as a rite of mourning for their dead. Women and children participated in these ceremonies but adult men did not take part, explaining the age/sex distribution of the disease. The incubation period for kuru can be in excess of 30 years, but in most cases is somewhat shorter. The practice of ritual cannibalism was discouraged in the late 1950s and the incidence of kuru declined dramatically. Kuru has now disappeared.

The above description covers the known picture of human TSEs which has been painstakingly built up over several decades. There is no evidence that any human TSE is traditionally acquired by an oral route, e.g. eating scrapie-infected sheep. There are good reasons why this should be (see Molecular Biology of Prions). However, in April 1996, a new variant of CJD (vCJD) was described in the UK. These vCJD cases share unusual features which distinguish them from other forms of CJD:

- An early age of onset or death (average 27 years, cf. 65 for CJD).
- A prolonged duration of illness (average 13 months, cf. 3 months for CJD).
- A predominantly psychiatric presentation including anxiety, depression, withdrawal and behavioural changes rather than neurological symptoms.
- The subsequent development of a cerebellar syndrome with ataxia.
- Forgetfulness and memory disturbance develop and progress to severe cognitive impairment.
- Myoclonus (involuntary muscular contractions) developing in the majority of patients.
- Absence of the typical EEG appearances of CJD.
- Neuropathologic spongiform change, neuronal loss and astrocytic gliosis most evident in the basal ganglia and thalamus. The most striking and consistent neuropathological feature is amyloid plaque formation reminiscent of that seen in kuru extensively distributed throughout the cerebrum and cerebellum.

The official UK Spongiform Encephalopathy Advisory Committee concluded that vCJD is 'a previously unrecognized and consistent disease pattern' and that 'although there is no direct evidence of a link, on current data and in the absence of any credible alternative the most likely explanation at present is that these cases are linked to exposure to BSE'. By August 2000, 82 people had died of vCJD in the UK and several more in other countries. Current investigations and modelling of the epidemic suggest that the maximum number of deaths from vCJD in the UK is likely to be 14 000 or less – hardly a comforting thought.

Molecular biology of prions

The evidence that prions are not conventional viruses is based on the fact that nucleic acid is not necessary for infectivity since they show:

- *Resistance to heat inactivation*: Infectivity is reduced but not eliminated by high-temperature autoclaving (135°C for 18 min). Some infectious activity is even retained after treatment at 600°C, suggesting that an inorganic molecular template is capable of nucleating the biological replication of the agent.
- *Resistance to radiation damage*: Infectivity was found to be resistant to short-wave ultraviolet radiation and to ionizing radiation. These treatments inactivate infectious organisms by causing damage to the **genome**. There is an inverse relationship between the size of target nucleic acid molecule and the dose of radioactivity or ultraviolet light needed to inactivate them, i.e. large molecules are sensitive to much lower doses than are smaller molecules (Figure 8.6). The scrapie agent was found to be highly resistant to both ultraviolet light and ionizing radiation, indicating that any nucleic acid present must be less than 80 nucleotides.
- *Resistance to DNAse and RNAse treatment, to psoralens and to Zn^{2+} catalysed hydrolysis*: All of these treatments inactivate nucleic acids.
- *Sensitivity to urea, SDS, phenol and other protein-denaturing chemicals.*

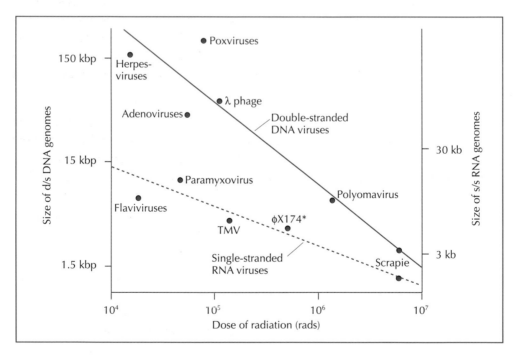

Figure 8.6 Radiation sensitivity of infectious agents. The dose of ionizing radiation required to destroy the infectivity of an infectious agent is dependent on the size of its genome. Larger genomes (e.g. double-stranded DNA viruses – upper line) present a larger 'target' and therefore are more sensitive than smaller genomes (e.g. single-stranded RNA viruses – lower line; N.B. φX174 has a single-stranded DNA genome). The scrapie agent is considerably more resistant to radiation than any known virus (note log scale on vertical axis).

All these characteristics indicate an agent with the properties of a protein rather than a virus. A protein of 254 amino acids, PrP^{Sc}, is associated with scrapie infectivity. Biochemical purification of scrapie infectivity results in preparations highly enriched in PrP^{Sc} and purification of PrP^{Sc} results in enrichment of scrapie activity. In 1984, Prusiner determined the sequence of 15 amino acids at the end of purified PrP^{Sc}. This led to the discovery that all mammalian cells contain a gene (*Prnp*) which encodes a protein identical to PrP^{Sc}, termed PrP^{C}. No biochemical differences between PrP^{C} and PrP^{Sc} have been determined, although unlike PrP^{C}, PrP^{Sc} is partly resistant to protease digestion, resulting in the formation of a 141 amino acid protease-resistant fragment which accumulates as fibrils in infected cells (Figure 8.7). Only a proportion of the total PrP in diseased tissue is present as PrP^{Sc}, but this has been shown to be the infectious form of the PrP protein, since highly purified PrP^{Sc} is infectious when used to inoculate experimental animals. Like other infectious agents, there is a dosage effect which gives a strong correlation between the amount of PrP^{Sc} in an inoculum and the incubation time until the development of disease.

Thus TSEs, which behave like infectious agents, appear to be caused by an endogenous gene/protein (Figure 8.8). Susceptibility of a host species to prion infection is co-determined by the prion inoculum and the *Prnp* gene. Disease incubation times for individual prion isolates vary in different strains of inbred mice but for a given isolate in a particular strain are remarkably consistent. These observations have resulted in two important concepts:

1 *Prion strain variation*: At least 15 different strains of PrP^{Sc} have been recognized. These can be distinguished by the incubation time to the onset of disease and the type and distribution of lesions within the CNS in inbred strains of mice. Thus prions can be 'fingerprinted' and BSE can be distinguished from scrapie or CJD.
2 *The species barrier*: When prions are initially transmitted from one species to another, disease develops only after a very long incubation period, if at all. On serial passage in the new species, the incubation time often decreases dramatically and then

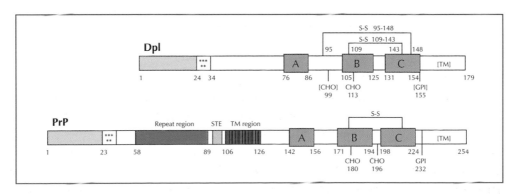

Figure 8.7 Structure of the prion (PrP) and doppel (Dpl) proteins.

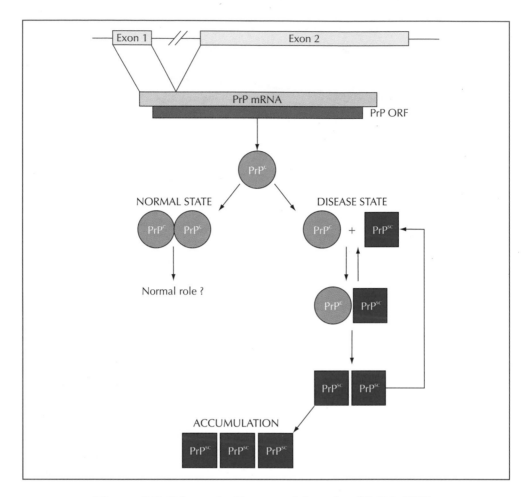

Figure 8.8 Schematic diagram of the role of PrP in TSEs.

stabilizes. This species barrier can be overcome by introducing a PrP transgene from the prion donor, e.g. hamster, into the recipient mice (Figure 8.9).

However, PrP^C and PrP^{Sc} are not post-translationally modified and the genes which encode them are not mutated, i.e. this is distinct from mendelian inheritance of familial forms of CJD. How such apparently complex behaviour can be 'encoded' by a 254 amino acid protein has not been firmly established, but there is evidence that the fundamental difference between the infectious, pathogenic form (PrP^{Sc}) and the endogenous form (PrP^C) results from a change in the conformation of the folded protein, which adopts a conformation rich in β-sheet (Figure 8.10).

Transgenic 'knockout' $Prnp^{0/0}$ mice, which do not possess an endogenous prion gene, are completely immune to the effects of PrP^{Sc} and do not propagate infectivity to normal mice, indicating that production of endogenous PrP^C is an essential part of the disease process in TSEs and that the infectious inoculum of PrP^{Sc} does not repli-

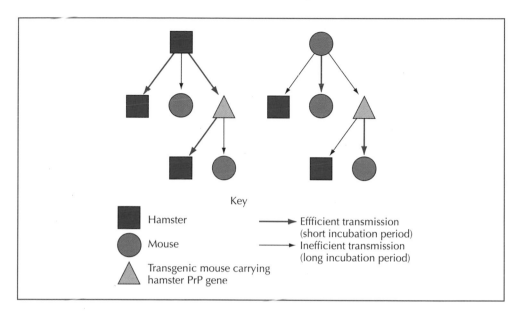

Key

■ Hamster

● Mouse

▲ Transgenic mouse carrying
hamster PrP gene

⟶ Effficient transmission
(short incubation period)

⟶ Inefficient transmission
(long incubation period)

Figure 8.9 Experimental transmission of scrapie to animals demonstrates an apparent species barrier. Hamster-to-hamster and mouse-to-mouse transmission results in the onset of disease after a relatively short incubation period (75 days and 175 days, respectively). Transmission from one host species to another is much less efficient and disease occurs only after a much longer incubation period. Transmission of hamster-derived PrP to transgenic mice carrying several copies of the hamster PrP gene (the darker mice in this figure) is much more efficient, whereas transmission of mouse-derived PrP to the transgenic mice is less efficient. Subsequent transmission from the transgenic mice implies that some modification of the properties of the agent seems to have occurred.

cate *per se*. Unfortunately, these experiments have given few clues to the normal role of PrP^C. Most *Prnp*$^{0/0}$ mice are developmentally normal and do not have CNS abnormalities, suggesting that loss of normal PrP^C function is not the cause of TSE and that the accumulation of PrP^{Sc} is responsible for disease symptoms. However, one strain of *Prnp*$^{0/0}$ mouse was found to develop late-onset ataxia and neurological degeneration. This observation led to the discovery of another gene called *Prnd* close to the *Prnp* gene which encodes a 179 amino acid PrP-like protein designated doppel (Dpl), overexpression of which appears to cause neurodegeneration (Figure 8.7). Like *Prnp*, this gene is conserved in vertebrates including humans and may have arisen from *Prnp* by gene duplication. It is suspected that there may be other members of the *Prn* gene family.

The URE3 protein of the yeast *Saccharomyces cerevisiae* has properties very reminiscent of PrP. Other PrP-like proteins are also known, e.g. PSI in yeast and Het-s* in the fungus *Podospora*. URE3 modifies a cellular protein Ure2p causing altered nitrogen metabolism; similarly, the PSI phenotype involves a self-propagating aggregation

Figure 8.10 Conformatioal changes in PrP.

of Ure2p and the cellular protein Sup35p. Cells 'infected' with URE3 can be 'cured' by treatment with protein-denaturing agents such as guanidium, which is believed to cause refolding of URE3 to the Ure2p conformation. The explanation for the inherited familial forms of prion disease is therefore presumably that inherited mutations enhance the rate of spontaneous conversion of PrP^C into PrP^{Sc}, permitting disease manifestation within the lifetime of an affected individual. This concept also suggests that the sporadic incidence of CJD can be accounted for by somatic mutation of the *PrP* gene and offers a possible explanation for the emergence of BSE, i.e. spontaneous mutation of a bovine PrP gene resulted in infectious prions which were then amplified through the food chain. In recent years, the construction of **transgenic** animals has cast further light on the above ideas.

The prion hypothesis is revolutionary and has justifiably met with a somewhat sceptical reception. As Stanley Prusiner wrote in his 1997 Nobel Prize acceptance speech:

> While the scepticism about prions was once well justified and formed the basis for a vigorous scientific debate, the wealth of available data now renders such arguments moot. In summary, no single hypothesis involving a virus can

explain the findings . . . While no single experiment can refute the existence of the 'scrapie virus,' all of the data taken together from numerous experimental studies present an impressive edifice which argues that the 50–year quest for a virus has failed because it does not exist!

Certainly, the prion story is not complete. It is still possible to construct numerous alternative theories of varying degrees of complexity (and plausibility!) to fit the experimental data. Science progresses by the construction of experimentally verifiable hypotheses. For many years, research into spongiform encephalopathies has been agonizingly slow because each individual experiment has taken at least one and in some cases many years to complete. With the advent of molecular biology, this has now become a fast-moving and dynamic field. The next few years will undoubtedly reveal more information about the cause of these diseases and will probably provide much food for thought about the interaction between infectious agents and the host in the pathogenesis of infectious diseases.

SUMMARY

A variety of novel infectious agents cause disease in plants, in animals and in humans. Several types of non-viral subcellular pathogens have disease-causing potential. These include **satellites**, **viroids** and **prions**. Conventional strategies to combat virus infections, such as drugs and **vaccines**, have no effect on these unconventional agents. A full understanding of the biology of these novel infectious entities will be necessary before means of treatment for the diseases they cause will become available.

FURTHER READING

Belay, E.D. (1999). Transmissible spongiform encephalopathies in humans. *Annual Review of Microbiology* 53: 283–314.

Collinge, J. and Palmer, M.S. (Eds) (1997). *Prion Diseases*. Oxford University Press, Oxford. ISBN 0198547897.

Diener, T.O. (Ed.) (1987). *The Viroids*. Plenum Press, New York.

Dodds, J.A. (1998). Satellite tobacco mosaic virus. *Annual Review of Phytopathology* 36: 295–310.

Klitzman, R. (1998). *The Trembling Mountain: A Personal Account of Kuru, Cannibals, and Mad Cow Disease*. Plenum Press, New York. ISBN 030645792X.

Lai, M.M.C. (1995). The molecular biology of hepatitis delta virus. *Annual Review of Biochemistry* 64: 259–286.

McKenzie, D., Bartz, J.C. and Marsh, R.F. (1996). Transmissible mink encephalopathy. *Seminars in Virology* 7: 201–206.

Moore, R.C., Lee, I.Y., Silverman, G.L. *et al.* (1999). Ataxia in prion protein (PrP)-

deficient mice is associated with upregulation of the novel PrP-like protein doppel. *Journal of Molecular Biology* 292: 797–817.

Prusiner, S.B. (1998). Prions. *Proceedings of the National Academy of Sciences of the USA* 95: 13363–13383.

Wickner, R.B. (1997). *Prion Diseases of Mammals and Yeast.* Springer-Verlag, Berlin. ISBN 3540624538.

SELF-ASSESSMENT QUESTIONS

(8.1) Are the following statements true or false?
(a)   Satellites encode their own coat proteins.
(b)   Viroids use the coat protein of their helper virus.
(c)   The nucleotide sequence of satellites is related to the helper virus genome.
(d)   Viroids are 200–400 nucleotides long.
(e)   All viroids have a conserved region involved in their replication.

(8.2) Are the following statements true or false?
(a)   Viroids cause disease by interfering with cellular DNA replication.
(b)   *Hepatitis delta virus* (HDV) δAg-S is necessary for the assembly and release of HDV-containing particles.
(c)   HDV δAg-L is necessary for HDV replication.
(d)   HDV has some of the properties of a satellite virus and some of a viroid.
(e)   HDV infection without HBV coinfection is associated with fulminant hepatitis.

(8.3) The following diseases are caused by prions (true or false?):
(a)   Alzheimer's syndrome.
(b)   Coconut cadang-cadang disease.
(c)   Chronic wasting disease (CWD).
(d)   Creutzfeldt-Jakob disease (CJD).
(e)   Fatal familial insomnia (FFI).

(8.4) Are the following statements true or false?
(a)   Scrapie was first described in 1982.
(b)   Scrapie is endemic in the UK and USA.
(c)   Transmissible mink encephalopathy (TME) occurs only in the USA.
(d)   More than 179 000 cases of BSE have been reported in the UK and at least 70 people have died of vCJD.
(e)   BSE is caused by scrapie-infected feed.

(8.5) Are the following statements true or false?

(a)   There are three sources of human TSEs: sporadic, iatrogenic/acquired and familial/inherited.

(b)   Sporadic Creutzfeldt–Jakob disease (CJD) accounts for about 90% of human TSE.

(c)   Kuru is an inherited form of TSE.

(d)   The incidence of CJD is similar worldwide.

(e)   Only about 1% of sporadic CJD cases are transmissible to mice.

(8.6) Prion infectivity is inactivated by the following treatments (true or false?):

(a)   Heating to 135°C for 30 min.

(b)   Heating to 600°C for 15 min.

(c)   DNAse treatment.

(d)   RNAse treatment.

(e)   Phenol.

(8.7) PrP^C (true or false?):

(a)   is a 254 amino acid protein.

(b)   is encoded by a cellular gene.

(c)   is converted by PrP^{Sc} to a protease-resistant form.

(d)   consists of 30% α–helix and 43% β–sheet.

(e)   is resistant to short-wave ultraviolet radiation and to ionizing radiation.

(8.8) Are the following statements true or false?

(a)   Transgenic animals which do not possess an endogenous prion gene are immune to the effects of PrP^{Sc}.

(b)   Transgenic animals which do not possess an endogenous prion gene develop a variety of tumours.

(c)   Human PrP differs from mouse PrP at 28 of 254 amino acids.

(d)   The BSE agent is indistinguishable from that of scrapie.

(e)   The 'species barrier' prevents the efficient transfer of infectious prions from one species to another.

(8.9) Are the following statements true or false?

(a)   The URE3 protein of yeast has the properties of a prion.

(b)   The URE3 phenotype of yeast can be 'cured' by treatment with guanidium.

(c)   Prion-like proteins have also been found in fungi.

(d)   Prions cause disease in plants.

(e)   The prion hypothesis is the only possible interpretation for TSEs.

Answers to Self-Assessment Questions are given in Appendix 4.

GLOSSARY AND ABBREVIATIONS

Terms shown in the text in **bold blue** are defined in this glossary.

Guide to pronunciation is shown in parentheses: this information is only intended as a guide – there are alternative pronunciations and regional differences in the way many words are pronounced.

abortive infection
('a–bore–tiv in–fec–shon')

The initiation of infection without completion of the infectious cycle and, therefore, without the production of infectious particles (cf. **productive infection**).

adjuvant
('aj–oo–vant')

A substance included in a medication to improve the action of the other constituents; usually, a component of vaccines which boosts their immunogenicity, e.g. aluminium sulphate.

ambisense
('ambi–sense')

A single-stranded virus genome which contains genetic information encoded in both the positive (i.e. virus-sense) and negative (i.e. complementary) orientations, e.g. *Bunyaviridae* and *Arenaviridae* (see Chapter 3).

anergy
('an–er–gee')

An immunologically unresponsive state in which lymphocytes are present but not functionally active.

apoptosis
('ap–a–tow–sis')

The genetically programmed death of certain cells which occurs during various stages in the development of multicellular organisms and may also be involved in control of the immune response.

assembly
('ass-embly')
A late phase of viral replication during which all the components necessary for the formation of a mature virion collect at a particular site in the cell and the basic structure of the virus particle is formed (see Chapter 4).

attachment
('a-tatch-ment')
The initial interaction between a virus particle and a cellular receptor molecule; the phase of viral replication during which this occurs (see Chapter 4).

attenuated
('at-ten-u-ated')
A pathogenic agent which has been genetically altered and displays decreased virulence. Attenuated viruses are the basis of live virus vaccines (see Chapter 6).

autocrine
('auto-krine')
The production by a cell of a growth factor which is required for its own growth. Such positive feedback mechanisms may result in cellular transformation (see Chapter 7).

avirulent
('a-vir-u-lent')
An infectious agent which has *no* disease-causing potential. It is doubtful if such agents really exist – even the most innocuous organisms may cause disease in certain circumstances, e.g. in immuno-compromised hosts.

bacteriophage
('bac-teer-ee-o-fage')
A virus which replicates in a bacterial host cell.

bp
('base pair')
Base pair – a single pair of nucleotide residues in a double-stranded nucleic acid molecule held together by Watson–Crick hydrogen bonds (see **kbp**).

budding
('bud-ding')
A mechanism involving release of virus particle from an infected cell by extrusion through a membrane. The site of budding may be at the surface of the cell or may involve the cytoplasmic or nuclear membranes depending on the site of assembly. Virus **envelopes** are acquired during budding

capsid
('cap-sid')
The protective protein coat of a virus particle (see Chapter 2).

chromatin
('cro-mat-in')
The ordered complex of DNA plus proteins (histones and non-histone chromosomal proteins) found in the nucleus of **eukaryotic** cells.

cis-**acting**
('sis-acting')
A genetic element which affects the activity of contiguous (i.e. on the same nucleic acid molecule) genetic regions; e.g. transcriptional promoters and enhancers are *cis*-acting sequences adjacent to the genes whose transcription they control.

complementation
('comp-lee-men-tay-shon')
The interaction of virus gene products in infected cells that results in the yield of one or both of the parental mutants being enhanced while their genotypes remain unchanged.

conditional mutant
('con-dish-on-al mu-tant')
A mutant phenotype which is replication competent under 'permissive' conditions but not under 'restrictive' or 'non-permissive' conditions; e.g. a virus with a temperature sensitive (t.s.) mutation may be able to replicate at the permissive temperature of 33°C but unable to replicate or severely inhibited at the non-permissive temperature of 38°C.

conditional lethal mutant
('con-dish-on-al lee-thal mu-tant')
A conditional mutation whose phenotype is (relatively) unaffected under permissive conditions but which is severely inhibitory under non-permissive conditions.

cytopathic effect (c.p.e.)
('sy-toe-path-ik ee-fect')
Cellular injury caused by virus infection; the effects of virus infection on cultured cells, visible by microscopic or direct visual examination (see Chapter 7).

defective interfering (D.I.) particles
('dee-fect-ive inter-feer-ing part-ik-els')
Particles encoded by genetically deleted virus genomes which lack one or more essential functions for replication.

ds
('double stranded')
Double-stranded (nucleic acid).

eclipse period
('ee-clips peer-ee-od')
An early phase of infection when virus particles have broken down after penetrating cells, releasing their genomes within the host cell as a prerequisite to replication. Often used to refer specifically to bacteriophages (see Chapter 4).

emergent virus
('ee-merge-ent vy-rus')
A virus identified as the cause of an increasing incidence of disease, possibly as a result of changed environmental or social factors (see Chapter 7).

endemic
('en-dem-ik')
A pattern of disease which recurs or is commonly found in a particular geographic area (cf. **epidemic**).

enhancer
('en-han-ser')
Cis-acting genetic elements which potentiate the transcription of genes or translation of mRNAs.

envelope
('en-vel-ope')
An outer (bounding) lipoprotein bilayer membrane possessed by many viruses. (N.B. Some viruses contain lipid as part of a complex outer layer, but

these are not usually regarded as enveloped unless a bilayer unit membrane structure is clearly demonstrable).

epidemic
('epy-dem-ik')
A pattern of disease characterized by a rapid increase in the number of cases occurring and widespread geographical distribution (cf. **endemic**). An epidemic which encompasses the entire world is known as a **pandemic**.

eukaryote/eukaryotic
('u-kary-ote')
An organism whose genetic material is separated from the cytoplasm by a nuclear membrane and divided into discrete chromosomes.

exon
('x-on')
A region of a gene expressed as protein after the removal of **introns** by post-transcriptional splicing.

fusion protein
('few-shon pro-teen')
A virus protein required and responsible for fusion of the virus **envelope** (or sometimes, the **capsid**) with a cellular membrane and consequently, for entry into the cell (see Chapter 4).

genome
('gee-nome *or* gen-ome')
The nucleic acid comprising the entire genetic information of an organism.

helix
('hee-licks')
A cylindrical solid formed by stacking repeated subunits in a constant relationship with respect to their amplitude and pitch (see Chapter 2). **Helical**: like a helix.

haemagglutination
('hay-ma-glut-in-nation')
The (specific) agglutination of red blood cells by a virus or other protein.

heterozygosis
('het-er-o-zy-go-sis')
Aberrant packaging of multiple genomes may on occasion result in multiploid particles (i.e. containing more than a single genome) which are therefore heterozygous.

hnRNA
('heavy nuclear RNA')
'Heterogeneous nuclear RNA' or 'heavy nuclear RNA' – the primary, unspliced transcripts found in the nucleus of eukaryotic cells.

hyperplasia
('hyper-play-see-a')
Excessive cell division or the growth of abnormally large cells. In plants, results in the production of swollen or distorted areas due to the effects of plant viruses.

hypoplasia
('high-po-play-see-a')
Localized retardation of cell growth. Numerous plant viruses cause this effect, frequently leading to **mosaicism** (the appearance of thinner, yellow areas on the leaves).

icosahedron
('eye-cos-a-heed-ron')
A solid shape consisting of 20 triangular faces arranged around the surface of a sphere – the basic

	symmetry of many virus particles (see Chapter 2). **Icosahedral**: like an icosahedron.
immortalized cell ('im-mort-al-ized sell')	A cell capable of indefinite growth (i.e. number of cell divisions) in culture. On rare occasions, immortalized cells arise spontaneously but are more commonly caused by mutagenesis as a result of virus **transformation** (see Chapter 7).
inclusion bodies ('in-klusion bod-ees')	Subcellular structures formed as a result of virus infection. Often a site of virus assembly (see Chapter 4).
IRES (Internal Ribosome Entry Site) ('eye-res')	An RNA secondary structure found in the 5′ untranslated region (UTR) of (+)sense RNA viruses such as picornaviruses and flaviviruses, which functions as a 'ribosome landing pad', allowing internal initiation of translation on the vRNA.
intron ('in-tron')	A region of a gene removed after transcription by splicing and consequently not expressed as protein (cf. **exon**).
isometric ('eye-so-met-rik')	A solid displaying **cubic** symmetry, of which the icosahedron is one form.
kb ('kilobase')	1000 nucleotide residues – a unit of measurement of single-stranded nucleic acid molecules. Sometimes (wrongly) used to mean **kbp** (below).
kbp ('kilobase pair')	1000 base pairs (see above) – a unit of measurement of double-stranded nucleic acid molecules.
latent period ('lay-tent peer-ee-od')	The time after infection before the first new extracellular virus particles appear (see Chapter 4).
lysogeny ('lie-soj-en-ee')	Persistent, latent infection of bacteria by **temperate bacteriophages** such as phage λ.
lytic virus ('lit-ik-vy-rus')	Any virus (or virus infection) which results in the death of infected cells and their physical breakdown.
maturation ('mat-yoor-ay-shon')	A late phase of virus infection during which newly formed virus particles become infectious. Usually involves structural changes in the particle resulting from specific cleavages of capsid proteins to form the mature products, or conformational changes in proteins during assembly (see Chapter 4).
monocistronic ('mono-sis-tron-ik')	A messenger RNA that consists of the transcript of a single gene and which therefore encodes a single polypeptide; a virus genome which produces such an mRNA (cf. **polycistronic**).

monolayer ('mono-layer')	A flat, contiguous sheet of adherent cells attached to the solid surface of a culture vessel.
mosaicism ('mo-say-iss-cis-em')	The appearance of thinner, yellow areas on the leaves of plants caused by the cytopathic effects of plant viruses.
movement proteins ('move-ment pro-teen')	Specialized proteins encoded by plant viruses which modify plasmodesmata (channels which pass through cell walls connecting the cytoplasm of adjacent cells) and cause virus nucleic acids to be transported from one cell to the next, permitting the spread of a virus infection.
mRNA ('messenger RNA')	Messenger RNA.
multiplicity of infection (m.o.i.) ('multi-pliss-itty of in-fec-shon')	The (average) number of virus particles which infect each cell in an experiment.
necrosis ('neck-ro-sis')	Cell death, particularly that caused by an external influence (cf. **apoptosis**).
negative-sense ('neg-at-iv sense')	The nucleic acid strand with a base sequence complementary to the strand which contains the protein-coding sequence of nucleotide triplets *or* a virus whose genome consists of a negative-sense strand. (Also 'minus-sense' or '(-)sense'.)
non-propagative ('non prop-a-gate-iv')	A term describing the transmission via secondary hosts (such as arthropods) of viruses which do not replicate in the vector organism, e.g. gemini-viruses. Also known as 'non-circulative transmission', i.e. the virus does not circulate in the vector population.
nt ('nucleotide')	A single nucleotide residue in a nucleic acid molecule.
nucleocapsid ('new-clio-cap-sid')	An ordered complex of proteins plus the nucleic acid genome of a virus.
oncogene ('on-co-gene')	A gene which encodes a protein capable of inducing cellular **transformation**.
ORF ('open reading frame')	Open reading frame – a region of a gene or mRNA which encodes a polypeptide, bounded by an AUG translation start codon at the 5′ end and a termination codon at the 3′ end. Not to be confused with the poxvirus called orf.

packaging signal ('pack–a–jing sig–nal')	A region of a virus genome with a particular nucleotide sequence or structure which specifically interacts with a virus protein(s) resulting in the incorporation of the genome into a virus particle.
pandemic ('pan–dem–ik')	An **epidemic** which encompasses the entire world.
penetration ('pen–ee–tray–shon')	The phase of virus replication at which the virus particle or genome enters the host cell (see Chapter 4).
phage ('fage')	See **bacteriophage**
phenotypic mixing ('fee–no–tip–ik mix–ing')	Individual progeny viruses from a mixed infection which contain structural proteins derived from both parental viruses.
plaque ('plak')	A localized region in a cell sheet or overlay in which cells have been destroyed or their growth retarded by virus infection.
plaque-forming units (p.f.u.) ('plak forming units')	A measure of the amount of viable virus present in a virus preparation. Includes both free virus particles and infected cells containing infectious particles ('infectious centres').
plasmid ('plas-mid')	An extrachromosomal genetic element capable of autonomous replication.
polycistronic ('poly-sis-tron-ik')	A messenger RNA which encodes more than one polypeptide (cf. **monocistronic**).
polyprotein ('poly-pro-teen')	A large protein which is post-transcriptionally cleaved by proteases to form a series of smaller proteins with differing functions.
positive-sense ('pos-it-iv sense')	The nucleic acid strand with a base sequence which contains the protein-coding sequence of nucleotide triplets *or* a virus whose genome consists of a positive-sense strand. (Also 'plus-sense' or '(+)sense'.)
primary cell ('pri-mary sell')	A cultured cell explanted from an organism which is capable of only a limited number of divisions (cf. **immortalized cell**).
prion ('pree-on')	A proteinaceous infectious particle, believed to be responsible for transmissible spongiform encephalopathies such as Creutzfeldt–Jakob disease (CJD) or bovine spongiform encephalopathy (BSE) (see Chapter 8).

productive infection ('pro–duct–iv in–fect–shon')	(A 'complete' virus infection in which further infectious particles are produced (cf. **abortive infection**).
prokaryote ('pro–kary–ote')	An organism whose genetic material is not separated from the cytoplasm of the cell by a nuclear membrane
promoter ('pro–mote–er')	A *cis*-**acting** regulatory region upstream of the coding region of a gene which promotes transcription by facilitating the assembly of proteins in transcriptional complexes.
propagative transmission ('prop–a–gate–ive tran–mish–on')	A term describing the transmission via secondary hosts (such as arthropods) of viruses which are able to replicate in both the primary host and the vector responsible for their transmission, e.g. plant reoviruses. Also known as 'circulative transmission', i.e. the virus circulates in the vector population.
prophage ('pro–fage')	The lysogenic form of a temperate bacteriophage genome integrated into the genome of the host bacterium.
provirus ('pro–vy–rus')	The double-stranded DNA form of a retrovirus genome integrated into the **chromatin** of the host cell.
pseudoknot ('s'yoo–doh–not')	An RNA secondary structure which causes 'frameshifting' during translation, producing a hybrid peptide containing information from an alternative reading frame.
pseudorevertant ('s'yoo–doh–re–vert–ant')	A virus with an apparently wild-type phenotype but which still contains a mutant genome – may be the result of genetic **suppression**
pseudotyping ('s'yoo–doh–type–ing')	Where the genome of one virus is completely enclosed within the capsid, or more usually the envelope, of another virus. An extreme form of **phenotypic mixing**
quasi-equivalence ('kwayz–eye–ee–kwiv–al–ense')	A principle describing a means of forming a regular solid from irregularly shaped subunits in which sub-units in *nearly* the same local environment form *nearly* equivalent bonds with their neighbours (see Chapter 2).
quasi-species ('kwayz–eye–spee–sees')	A complex mixture of rapidly evolving and competing molecular variants of RNA virus genomes which occurs in most populations of RNA viruses.

receptor ('ree–sep–tor')	A specific molecule on the surface of a cell to which a virus attaches as a preliminary to entering the cell. May consist of proteins or the sugar residues present on glycoproteins or glycolipids in the cell membrane (see Chapter 4).
recombination ('ree–com–bin–nation')	The physical interaction of virus genomes in a **superinfected** cell resulting in progeny genomes which contain information in non-parental combinations.
release ('ree–lease')	A late phase of virus infection during which newly formed virus particles leave the cell (see Chapter 4).
replicase ('rep–lick–aze')	An enzyme responsible for replication of RNA virus genomes (see **transcriptase**).
replicon ('rep–lick–on')	A nucleic acid molecule containing the information necessary for its own replication; includes both **genomes** and other molecules such as **plasmids** and **satellites**.
retrotransposon ('ret–tro–trans–pose–on')	A transposable genetic element closely resembling a retrovirus genome, bounded by long terminal repeats (see Chapter 3).
satellites ('sat–el–ites')	Small RNA molecules (500–2000 nt) which are dependent on the presence of a helper virus for replication but unlike defective viruses, show no sequence homology to the helper virus genome. Larger satellite RNAs may encode a protein (cf. **viroids**, **virusoids**).
shutoff ('shut–off')	A sudden and dramatic cessation of most host cell macromolecular synthesis which occurs during some virus infections, resulting in cell damage and/or death (see Chapter 7).
splicing ('sp–lice–ing')	Post-transcriptional modification of primary RNA transcripts which occurs in the nucleus of **eukaryotic** cells during which **introns** are removed and **exons** are joined together to produce cytoplasmic **mRNAs**
superantigens ('super–anti–gens')	Molecules which short-circuit the immune system, resulting in massive activation of T cells by binding to both the variable region of the β chain of the T-cell receptor (Vβ) and to MHC class II molecules, cross-linking them in a non-specific way (Figure 7.3).

superinfection
('super-infect-shon')

Infection of a single cell by more than one virus particle, especially two viruses of distinct types, *or* deliberate infection of a cell designed to rescue a mutant virus.

suppression
('sup-press-shon')

The inhibition of a mutant phenotype by a second suppressor mutation, which may be either in the virus genome or in that of the host cell (see Chapter 3).

syncytium
('sin-sit-ee-um')

A mass of cytoplasm containing several separate nuclei enclosed in a continuous membrane resulting from the fusion of individual cells. Plural **syncytia**.

systemic infection
('sis-tem-ik infect-shon')

An infection involving multiple parts of a multi-cellular organism.

temperate bacteriophage
('temper-ate bac-teer-ee-o-fage')

A bacteriophage capable of establishing a **lysogenic** infection (cf. virulent bacteriophage, a bacteriophage which is not capable of establishing a lysogenic infection and always kills the bacteria in which it replicates).

terminal redundancy
('ter-minal ree-dun-dance-ee')

Repeated sequences present at the ends of a nucleic acid molecule.

titre
('tight-er' *or* 'teet-er')

A relative measure of the amount of a substance (e.g. virus or antibody) present in a preparation.

trans-**acting**
('trans-acting')

A genetic element encoding a diffusible product which acts on regulatory sites whether or not these are contiguous with the site from which they are produced, e.g. proteins which bind to specific sequences present on any stretch of nucleic acid present in a cell, such as transcription factors (cf. *cis*-**acting**).

transcriptase
('trans-crypt-aze')

An enzyme, usually packaged into virus particles, responsible for the transcription of RNA virus genomes (see **replicase**).

transfection
('trans-fect-shon')

Infection of cells mediated by the introduction of nucleic acid rather than by virus particles.

transformation
('trans-form-ay-shon')

Any change in the morphological, biochemical or growth parameters of a cell.

transgenic
('trans-gene-ik' *or* 'trans-gen-ik')

A genetically manipulated eukaryotic organism (animal or plant) which contains additional genetic information from another species. The additional genes may be carried and/or expressed only in the somatic cells of the transgenic organism, or in the cells of the germline, in which case they may be inheritable by any offspring.

transposons ('trans–pose–ons')	Specific DNA sequences which are able to move from one position in the genome of an organism to another (see Chapter 3).
triangulation number ('tri-ang-u-lay-shon num-ber')	A numerical factor which defines the symmetry of an icosahedral solid (see Chapter 2).
tropism ('trope-ism')	The types of tissues or host cells in which a virus is able to replicate.
uncoating ('un–coat–ing')	A general term for the events which occur after the penetration of a host cell by a virus particle, in which the virus capsid is completely or partially removed and the genome exposed, usually in the form of a nucleoprotein complex (see Chapter 4).
vaccine ('vax-seen')	A preparation containing an antigenic molecule or mixture of such molecules designed to elicit an immune response. Virus vaccines can be divided into three basic types: subunit, inactivated and live vaccines (see Chapter 6).
vaccination ('vax-sin-ay-shon')	The administration of a **vaccine**
variolation ('var-ee-o-lay-shon')	The ancient practice of inoculating immunologically naive individuals with material obtained from small-pox patients – a primitive form of vaccination (see Chapter 1).
virion ('vir-ee-on')	Morphologically complete (mature) infectious virus particle.
viroid ('vy-royd')	Autonomously replicating plant pathogens consisting solely of unencapsidated, single-stranded, circular (rod-like) RNAs of 200–400 nucleotides. Viroids do not encode any protein products. Some viroid RNAs have ribozyme activity (self-cleavage) (cf. **satellites, virusoids**).
virusoids ('vy-rus-oyds')	Small satellite RNAs with a circular, highly base-paired structure similar to viroid. Depend on a host virus for replication and encapsidation but do encode any proteins. All virusoid RNAs studied so far have ribozyme activity (cf. **satellites, viroids**).
virus-attachment protein ('vyr-us at-tatch-ment pro-teen')	A virus protein responsible for the interaction of a virus particle with a specific cellular receptor molecule.
zoonosis ('zoo-no-sis')	Infection transmitted from an animal to a human. Plural: **zoonoses**

CLASSIFICATION OF SUBCELLULAR INFECTIOUS AGENTS

Classifying subcellular infectious agents is more complex than it may appear at first sight and it is appropriate to start with a few definitions:

- *Systematics* is the science of organizing the history of the evolutionary relationships of organisms.
- *Classification* is determining the evolutionary relationships between organisms.
- *Identification* is recognizing the place of an organism in an existing classification scheme, often using dichotomous keys to identify the organism.
- *Taxonomy* (nomenclature) is assigning scientific names according to agreed international scientific rules. The official taxonomic groups (from the largest to the smallest are):

  - Kingdom (e.g. animals, plants, bacteria – does not apply to viruses)
  - Phylum (e.g. vertebrates – does not apply to viruses)
  - Class (group of related orders – does not apply to viruses)
  - Order (group of related families)
  - Family (group of related genera)
  - Genus (group of related species)
  - Species – the smallest taxonomic group.

The importance of virus identification has been discussed in Chapter 4. Subcellular agents present a particular problem for taxonomists. They are too small to be seen without electron microscopes but very small changes in molecular structure may give rise to agents with radically different properties. The vast majority of viruses which are known have been studied because they have pathogenic potential for humans, animals or plants. Therefore, the disease symptoms caused by infection are one criterion used to aid classification. The physical structure of a virus particle can be determined directly (by electron microscopy) or indirectly (by biochemical or sero-logical investigation) and is also used in classification. However, the structure and sequence of the virus genome continues to increase in importance as molecular biological analysis provides a rapid and sensitive way to detect and differentiate many diverse viruses.

In 1966, the International Committee on Nomenclature of Viruses was estab-lished and produced the first unified scheme for virus classification. In 1973, this committee expanded its objectives and renamed itself the International Committee on Taxonomy of Viruses (ICTV); it meets every four years. Rules for virus taxonomy have been established, some of which include:

- Latin binomial names (e.g. *Rhabdovirus carpio*) are not used. No person's name should be used in nomenclature. Names should have international meaning.
- A virus name should be meaningful and should consist of as few words as poss-ible. Serial numbers or letters are not acceptable as names.
- A virus species is a polythetic class (i.e. a group whose members always have sev-eral properties in common, although no single common attribute is present in all of its members) of viruses that constitute a replicating lineage and occupy a par-ticular ecological niche.
- A genus is a group of virus species sharing common characters. Approval of a new genus is linked to the acceptance of a type species, i.e. a species which displays the typical characteristics on which the genus is based.
- A family is a group of genera with common characters. Approval of a new family is linked to the acceptance of a type genus.

In general terms, groups of related viruses are divided into families whose names end in the suffix *-viridae* (e.g. *Poxviridae*). In most cases, a higher level of classification than the family has not been established, although three orders (groups of related families) have now been recognized (see Chapter 3). In a few cases, very large families have been subdivided into subfamilies, and end in the suffix *-virinae*. Subspecies, strains, isolates, variants, mutants and artificially created laboratory recombinants are not officially recognized by the ICTV.

- The names of virus orders, families, subfamilies, genera and species should be written in italics with the first letter capitalized.
- Other words are not capitalized unless they are proper nouns, e.g. *Tobacco mosaic virus*, *Poliovirus*, *Murray River encephalitis virus*.
- This format should only be used when official taxonomic entities are referred to – it is not possible to centrifuge the species *Poliovirus* for example, but it is poss-ible to centrifuge poliovirus. Italics and capitalization are not used for vernacular usage (e.g. rhinoviruses, cf. the genus *Rhinovirus*), for acronyms (e.g. HIV-1), nor for adjectival forms (e.g. poliovirus polymerase).

■ See M.H.V.Van Regenmortel (1999) How to write the names of virus species. *Archives of Virology* 144(5): 1041–1042.

The seventh report of the ICTV was published in 2000 (H.V. Van Regenmortel, D.H.L. Bishop, M.H.Van Regenmortel and Claude M. Fauquet (Eds) (2000). *Virus Taxonomy: Seventh Report of the International Committee on Taxonomy of Viruses.* Academic Press, London. ISBN 0123702003) and the information in this appendix is drawn from that report. More than 1550 virus species belonging to 3 orders, 56 families, 9 subfamilies and 233 genera are recognized in the report. These well-characterized viruses are an unknown proportion of the total number of viruses that exist. By the time of the next ICTV meeting, undoubtedly many more viruses will have been added to the list.

GROUP I: dsDNA VIRUSES

Order *Caudovirales* – Tailed bacteriophages

Family (Subfamily)	Genus	Type species	Hosts
Myoviridae	T4-like phages	Enterobacteria phage T4	Bacteria
	P1-like phages	Enterobacteria phage P1	Bacteria
	P2-like phages	Enterobacteria phage P2	Bacteria
	Mu-like phages	Enterobacteria phage Mu	Bacteria
	SP01-like phages	Bacillus phage SP01	Bacteria
	φH-like phages	Halobacterium virus φH	Bacteria
Podoviridae	T7-like phages	Enterobacteria phage T7	Bacteria
	P22-like phages	Enterobacteria phage P22	Bacteria
	φ29-like phages	Bacillus phage φ29	Bacteria
Siphoviridae	λ-like phages	Enterobacteria phage λ	Bacteria
	T1-like phages	Enterobacteria phage T1	Bacteria
	T5-like phages	Enterobacteria phage T5	Bacteria
	L5-like phages	Mycobacterium phage L5	Bacteria
	c2-like phages	Lactococcus phage c2	Bacteria
	ψM1-like phages	Methanobacterium virus ψM1	Bacteria
Ascoviridae	Ascovirus	Spodoptera frugiperda ascovirus	Invertebrates
Adenoviridae	Mastadenovirus	Human adenovirus C	Vertebrates
	Aviadenovirus	Fowl adenovirus A	Vertebrates
Asfarviridae	Asfivirus	African swine fever virus	Vertebrates
Baculoviridae	Nucleopolyhedrovirus	Autographa californica nucleopolyhedrovirus	Invertebrates
	Granulovirus	Cydia pomonella granulovirus	Invertebrates

continued

Order *Caudovirales* – Tailed bacteriophages

Family (Subfamily)	Genus	Type species	Hosts
Corticoviridae	*Corticovirus*	*Alteromonas phage PM2*	Bacteria
Fuselloviridae	*Fusellovirus*	*Sulfolobus virus SSV1*	Archaea
Herpesviridae:	*Simplexvirus*	*Human herpesvirus 1*	Vertebrates
Alphaherpesvirinae	*Varicellovirus*	*Human herpesvirus 3*	Vertebrates
Betaherpesvirinae	*Cytomegalovirus*	*Human herpesvirus 5*	Vertebrates
	Muromegalovirus	*Murine herpesvirus 1*	Vertebrates
	Roseolovirus	*Human herpesvirus 6*	Vertebrates
Gammaherpesvirinae	*Lymphocryptovirus*	*Human herpesvirus 4*	Vertebrates
	Rhadinovirus	*Simian herpesvirus 2*	Vertebrates
Iridoviridae	*Iridovirus*	*Invertebrate iridescent virus 6*	Invertebrates
	Chloriridovirus	*Invertebrate iridescent virus 3*	Invertebrates
	Ranavirus	*Frog virus 3*	Vertebrates
	Lymphocystivirus	*Lymphocystis disease virus 1*	Vertebrates
Lipothrixviridae	*Lipothrixvirus*	*Thermoproteus virus 1*	Archaea
Polyomaviridae	*Polyomavirus*	*Simian virus 40*	Vertebrates
Papillomaviridae	*Papillomavirus*	*Cottontail rabbit papillomavirus*	Vertebrates
Phycodnaviridae	*Chlorovirus*	*Paramecium bursaria Chlorella virus 1*	Algae
	Prasinovirus	*Micromonas pusilla virus SP1*	Algae
	Prymnesiovirus	*Chryosochromomulina brevifilium virus PW1*	Algae
	Phaeovirus	*Extocarpus siliculosus virus 1*	Algae
Plasmaviridae	*Plasmavirus*	*Acholeplasma phage L2*	Mycoplasma
Polydnaviridae	*Ichnovirus*	*Campoletis sonorensis ichnovirus*	Invertebrates
	Bracovirus	*Cotesia melanoscela brachovirus*	Invertebrates
Poxviridae:	*Orthopoxvirus*	*Vaccinia virus*	Vertebrates
Chordopoxvirinae	*Parapoxvirus*	*Orf virus*	Vertebrates
	Avipoxvirus	*Fowlpox virus*	Vertebrates
	Capripoxvirus	*Sheeppox virus*	Vertebrates
	Leporipoxvirus	*Myxoma virus*	Vertebrates
	Suipoxvirus	*Swinepox virus*	Vertebrates
	Molluscipoxvirus	*Molluscum contagiosum virus*	Vertebrates
	Yatapoxvirus	*Yaba monkey tumour virus*	Vertebrates
Entomopoxvirinae	*Entomopoxvirus A*	*Melolontha melolontha entomopoxvirus*	Invertebrates
	Entomopoxvirus B	*Amsacta moorei entomopoxvirus*	Invertebrates
	Entomopoxvirus C	*Chironomus luridus entomopoxvirus*	Invertebrates
	Rhizidovirus	*Rhizidomyces virus*	Fungi
Rudiviridae	*Rudivirus*	*Sulfolobus virus SIRV1*	Archaea
Tectiviridae	*Tectivirus*	*Enterobacteria phage PRD1*	Bacteria

GROUP II: ssDNA VIRUSES

Family (Subfamily)	Genus	Type species	Hosts
Circoviridae	Circovirus	Porcine circovirus	Vertebrates
	Gyrovirus	Chicken anaemia virus	Vertebrates
Geminiviridae	Mastrevirus	Maize streak virus	Plants
	Curtovirus	Beet curly top virus	Plants
	Topocuvirus	Tomato pseudo-curly top virus	Plants
	Begomovirus	Bean golden mosaic virus	Plants
Inoviridae	Inovirus	Enterobacteria phage M13	Bacteria
	Plectrovirus	Acholeplasma phage MV-L51	Bacteria
Microviridae	Microvirus	Enterobacteria φX174	Bacteria
	Spiromicrovirus	Spiroplasma phage 4	Spiroplasma
	Bdellomicrovirus	Bdellovibrio phage MAC1	Bacteria
	Chlamydiamicrovirus	Chlamydia phage 1	Bacteria
	Nanovirus	Subterranean clover stunt virus	Plants
Parvoviridae:	Parvovirus	Mice minute virus	Vertebrates
Parvovirinae	Erythrovirus	B19 virus	Vertebrates
	Dependovirus	Adeno-associated virus 2	Vertebrates
Densovirinae	Densovirus	Junonia coenia densovirus	Invertebrates
	Iteravirus	Bombyx mori densovirus	Invertebrates
	Brevidensovirus	Aedes aegypti densovirus	Invertebrates

GROUP III: dsRNA VIRUSES

Family (Subfamily)	Genus	Type species	Hosts
Birnaviridae	Aquabirnavirus	Infectious pancreatic necrosis virus	Vertebrates
	Avibirnavirus	Infectious bursal disease virus	Vertebrates
	Entomobirnavirus	Drosophila X virus	Invertebrates
Cystoviridae	Cystovirus	Pseudomonas phage φ6	Bacteria
Hypoviridae	Hypovirus	Cryphonectria hypovirus 1–EP713	Fungi
Partitiviridae	Partitivirus	Gaeumarmomyces graminis virus 019/6–A	Fungi
	Chrysovirus	Penicillium chrysogenum virus	Fungi
	Alphacryptovirus	White clover cryptic virus 1	Plants
	Betacryptovirus	White clover cryptic virus 2	Plants
Reoviridae	Orthoreovirus	Mammalian orthoreovirus	Vertebrates
	Orbivirus	Bluetongue virus	Vertebrates
	Rotavirus	Rotavirus A	Vertebrates
	Coltivirus	Colorado tick fever virus	Vertebrates

continued

Family (Subfamily)	Genus	Type species	Hosts
	Aquareovirus	Golden shiner virus	Vertebrates
	Cypovirus	Cypovirus 1	Invertebrates
	Fijivirus	Fiji disease virus	Plants
	Phytoreovirus	Wound tumour virus	Plants
	Oryzavirus	Rice ragged stunt virus	Plants
Totiviridae	Totivirus	Saccharomyces cerevisiae virus L-A	Fungi
	Giardiavirus	Giardia lamblia virus	Protozoa
	Leishmaniavirus	Leishmania RNA virus 1–1	Protozoa

GROUP IV: (+)SENSE RNA VIRUSES

Order *Nidovirales* – 'Nested' viruses

Family (Subfamily)	Genus	Type species	Hosts
Arteriviridae	Arterivirus	Equine arteritis virus	Vertebrates
Coronaviridae	Coronavirus	Infectious bronchitis virus	Vertebrates
	Torovirus	Equine totovirus	Vertebrates
	Allexivirus	Shallot virus X	Plants
Astroviridae	Astrovirus	Human astrovirus 1	Vertebrates
Barnaviridae	Barnavirus	Mushroom bacilliform virus	Fungi
	Benyvirus	Beet necrotic yellow vein virus	Plants
Bromoviridae	Alfamovirus	Alfalfa mosaic virus	Plants
	Bromovirus	Brome mosaic virus	Plants
	Cucumovirus	Cucumber mosaic virus	Plants
	Ilarvirus	Tobacco streak virus	Plants
	Oleavirus	Olive latent virus 2	Plants
Caliciviridae	Lagovirus	Rabbit haemorrhagic disease virus	Vertebrates
	Norwalk-like viruses	Norwalk virus	Vertebrates
	Sapporo-like viruses	Sapporo virus	Vertebrates
	Vesivirus	Swine vesicular exanthema virus	Vertebrates
	Capillovirus	Apple stem grooving virus	Plants
	Carlavirus	Carnation latent virus	Plants
Closteroviridae	Closterovirus	Beet yellows virus	Plants
	Idaeovirus	Raspberry bushy dwarf virus	Plants
Comoviridae	Comovirus	Cowpea mosaic virus	Plants
	Fabavirus	Broad bean wilt virus 1	Plants
	Nepovirus	Tobacco ringspot virus	Plants

Family (Subfamily)	Genus	Type species	Hosts
Cricket paralysis-like viruses		Cricket paralysis virus	Invertebrates
Flaviviridae	Flavivirus	Yellow fever virus	Vertebrates
	Pestivirus	Bovine diarrhea virus 1	Vertebrates
	Hepacivirus	Hepatitis C virus	Vertebrates
Foveavirus		Apple stem pitting virus	Plants
Furovirus		Soil-borne wheat mosaic virus	Plants
Hepatitis E-like viruses		Hepatitis E virus	Vertebrates
Hordeivirus		Barley stripe mosaic virus	Plants
Leviviridae	Levivirus	Enterobacteria phage MS2	Bacteria
	Allolevivirus	Enterobacteria phage Qβ	Bacteria
Luteoviridae	Luteovirus	Cereal yellow dwarf virus-PAV	Plants
	Polerovirus	Potato leafroll virus	Plants
	Enamovirus	Pea enation mosaic virus-1	Plants
Machlomovirus		Maize chlorotic mottle virus	Plants
Marafivirus		Maize rayado fino virus	Plants
Narnaviridae	Narnavirus	Saccharomyces cerevisiae narnavirus 20S	Fungi
	Mitovirus	Cryphonectria parasitica mitovirus 1-NB631	Fungi
Nodaviridae	Alphanodoavirus	Nodamura virus	Invertebrates
	Betanodovirus	Striped jack nervous necrosis virus	Vertebrates
Pecluvirus		Peanut clump virus	Plants
Ourmiavirus		Ourmiavirus melon virus	Plants
Picornaviridae	Enterovirus	Poliovirus	Vertebrates
	Rhinovirus	Human rhinovirus A	Vertebrates
	Hepatovirus	Hepatitis A virus	Vertebrates
	Cardiovirus	Encephalomyocarditis virus	Vertebrates
	Aphtovirus	Foot-and-mouth disease virus O	Vertebrates
	Parechovirus	Human parechovirus	Vertebrates
	Erbovirus	Equine rhinitis B virus	Vertebrates
	Kobuvirus	Aichi virus	Vertebrates
	Teschovirus	Porcine teschovirus	Vertebrates
Pomovirus		Potato mop-top virus	Plants
Potexvirus		Potato virus X	Plants
Potyviridae	Potyvirus	Potato virus Y	Plants
	Ipovirus	Sweet potato mild mottle virus	Plants
	Macluravirus	Maclura mosaic virus	Plants
	Rymovirus	Ryegrass mosaic virus	Plants
	Tritimovirus	Wheat streak mosaic virus	Plants
	Bymovirus	Barley yellow mosaic virus	Plants
Sequiviridae	Sequivirus	Parsnip yellow fleck virus	Plants
	Waikavirus	Rice tungro spherical virus	Plants

continued

Order *Nidovirales* – 'Nested' viruses

Family (Subfamily)	Genus	Type species	Hosts
	Sobemovirus	Southern bean mosaic virus	Plants
Tetraviridae	Betatetravirus	Nudaurelia capensis β virus	Invertebrates
	Omegatetravirus	Nudaurelia capensis ω virus	Invertebrates
	Tobamovirus	Tobacco mosaic virus	Plants
	Tobravirus	Tobacco rattle virus	Plants
Tombusviridae	Tombusvirus	Tomato bushy stunt virus	Plants
	Avenavirus	Oat chlorotic stunt virus	Plants
	Aureusvirus	Pothos latent virus	Plants
	Carmovirus	Carnation mottle virus	Plants
	Dainthovirus	Carnation ringspot virus	Plants
	Machlomovirus	Maize chlorotic mottle virus	Plants
	Necrovirus	Tobacco necrosis virus	Plants
	Panicovirus	Panicum mosaic virus	Plants
Togaviridae	Alphavirus	Sindbis virus	Vertebrates
	Rubivirus	Rubella virus	Vertebrates
	Trichovirus	Apple chlorotic leaf spot virus	Plants
	Tymovirus	Turnip yellow mosaic virus	Plants
	Umbravirus	Carrot mottle virus	Plants
	Vitivirus	Grapevine virus A	Plants

GROUP V: (–)SENSE RNA VIRUSES

Order *Mononegavirales*

Family (Subfamily)	Genus	Type species	Hosts
Bornaviridae	Bornavirus	Borna disease virus	Vertebrates
Filoviridae	Marburg-like viruses	Marburg virus	Vertebrates
	Ebola-like viruses	Ebola virus	Vertebrates
Paramyxoviridae:	Respirovirus	Sendai virus	Vertebrates
Paramyxovirinae	Morbillivirus	Measles virus	Vertebrates
	Rubulavirus	Mumps virus	Vertebrates
Pneumovirinae	Pneumovirus	Human respiratory syncytial virus	Vertebrates
	Metapneumovirus	Turkey rhinotracheitis virus	Vertebrates
Rhabdoviridae	Vesiculovirus	Vesicular stomatitis Indiana virus	Vertebrates
	Lyssavirus	Rabies virus	Vertebrates
	Ephemerovirus	Bovine ephemeral fever virus	Vertebrates
	Novirhabdovirus	Infectious haematopoetic necrosis virus	Vertebrates

Family (Subfamily)	Genus	Type species	Hosts
	Cytorhabdovirus	Lettuce necrotic yellows virus	Plants
	Nucleorhabdovirus	Potato yellow dwarf virus	Plants
Arenaviridae	Arenavirus	Lymphocytic choriomeningitis virus	Vertebrates
Bunyaviridae	Bunyavirus	Bunyamwera virus	Vertebrates
	Hantavirus	Hantaan virus	Vertebrates
	Nairovirus	Nairobi sheep disease virus	Vertebrates
	Phlebovirus	Sandfly fever Sicilian virus	Vertebrates
	Tospovirus	Tomato spotted wilt virus	Plants
Deltavirus		Hepatitis delta virus	Vertebrates
Ophiovirus		Citrus psorosis virus	Plants
Orthomyxoviridae	Influenza A virus	Influenza A virus	Vertebrates
	Influenza B virus	Influenza B virus	Vertebrates
	Influenza C virus	Influenza C virus	Vertebrates
	Thogotovirus	Thogoto virus	Vertebrates
Tenuivirus		Rice stripe virus	Plants

GROUP VI: RNA REVERSE TRANSCRIBING VIRUSES

Family (Subfamily)	Genus	Type species	Hosts
Retroviridae	Alpharetrovirus	Avian leukosis virus	Vertebrates
	Betaretrovirus	Mouse mammary tumour virus	Vertebrates
	Gammaretrovirus	Murine leukaemia virus	Vertebrates
	Deltaretrovirus	Bovine leukaemia virus	Vertebrates
	Epsilonretrovirus	Walley dermal sarcoma virus	Vertebrates
	Lentivirus	Human immunodeficiency virus 1	Vertebrates
	Spumavirus	Human spumavirus	Vertebrates
Metaviridae	Metavirus	Saccharomyces cerevisiae Ty3 virus	Fungi
	Errantivirus	Drosophila melanogaster gypsy virus	Invertebrates
Pseudoviridae	Pseudovirus	Saccharomyces cerevisiae Ty1 virus	Invertebrates
	Hemivirus	Drosophila melanogaster copia virus	Invertebrates

GROUP VII: DNA REVERSE TRANSCRIBING VIRUSES

Family (Subfamily)	Genus	Type species	Hosts
Hepadnaviridae	Orthohepadnavirus	Hepatitis B virus	Vertebrates
	Avihepadnavirus	Duck hepatitis B virus	Vertebrates
Caulimoviridae	Caulimovirus	Cauliflower mosaic virus	Plants
	Badnavirus	Commelina yellow mottle virus	Plants

SUBVIRAL AGENTS: VIROIDS

Family (Subfamily)	Genus	Type species	Hosts
Pospiviroidae	Pospiviroid	Potato spindle tuber viroid	Plants
	Hostuviroid	Hop stunt viroid	Plants
	Cocadviroid	Coconut cadang-cadang viroid	Plants
	Apscaviroid	Apple scar skin viroid	Plants
	Coleviroid	Coleus blumei viroid 1	Plants
Avsunviroidae	Avsunviroidae	Avocado sunblotch viroid	Plants
	Pelamonviroid	Peach latent mosaic viroid	Plants

SUBVIRAL AGENTS: SATELLITES AND PRIONS

Family (Subfamily)	Genus	Type species	Hosts
Satellites			Invertebrates
			Plants
			Fungi
Prions			Vertebrates
			Fungi

THE HISTORY OF VIROLOGY

'If I have seen further it is by standing on the shoulders of Giants.'
(Isaac Newton in a letter to Robert Hooke, 5 February 1676)

1796: **Edward Jenner** (1749–1823) used cowpox to **vaccinate** against smallpox. Although Jenner is commonly given the credit for vaccination, **variolation**, the practice of deliberately infecting people with smallpox to protect them from the worst type of the disease, had been practised in China at least two thousand years previously. In 1774, a farmer named Benjamin Jesty had vaccinated his wife and two sons with cowpox taken from the udder of an infected cow and had written about his experience (see 1979). Jenner was the first person to deliberately vaccinate against any infectious disease, i.e. to use a preparation containing an antigenic molecule or mixture of such molecules designed to elicit an immune response.

1885: **Louis Pasteur** (1822–1895) experimented with rabies vaccination, using the term 'virus' (Latin, poison) to describe the agent. Although Pasteur did not discriminate between viruses and other infectious agents, he originated the terms 'virus' and 'vaccination' (in honour of Jenner) and developed the scientific basis for Jenner's experimental approach to vaccination.

1886: **John Buist** (a Scottish pathologist) stained lymph from skin lesions of a smallpox patient and saw 'elementary bodies' which he thought were the spores of micrococci. These were in fact smallpox virus particles – just large enough to see with the light microscope.

1892: **Dmiti Iwanowski** (1864–1920) described the first 'filterable' infectious agent – *Tobacco mosaic virus* (TMV) – smaller than any known bacteria. Iwanowski was the first person to discriminate between viruses and other infectious agents, although he was not fully aware of the significance of this finding.

1898: **Martinus Beijerinick** (1851–1931) extended Iwanowski's work with TMV and formed the first clear concept of the virus 'contagium vivum fluidum' – soluble living germ. Beijerinick confirmed and extended

Iwanowski's work and was the person who developed the concept of the virus as a distinct entity.

Freidrich Loeffler (1852–1915) and **Paul Frosch** (1860–1928) demonstrated that foot-and-mouth disease is caused by such 'filterable' agents. Loeffler and Frosch were the first to prove that viruses could infect animals as well as plants.

1900:   **Walter Reed** (1851–1902) demonstrated that yellow fever is spread by mosquitoes. Although Reed did not dwell on the nature of the yellow fever agent, he and his coworkers were the first to show that viruses could be spread by insect vectors such as mosquitoes.

1908:   **Karl Landsteiner** (1868–1943) and **Erwin Popper** proved that poliomyelitis was caused by a virus. Landsteiner and Popper were the first to prove that viruses could infect humans as well as animals.

1911:   **Francis Peyton Rous** (1879–1970) demonstrated that a virus (*Rous sarcoma virus*) can cause cancer in chickens (Nobel Prize, 1966) (see 1981). Rous was the first person to show that a virus could cause cancer.

1915:   **Frederick Twort** (1877–1950) discovered viruses infecting bacteria.

1917:   **Felix d'Herelle** (1873–1949) independently discovered viruses of bacteria and coined the term **bacteriophage**. The discovery of bacteriophages provided an invaluable opportunity to study virus replication at a time prior to the development of tissue culture when the only way to study viruses was by infecting whole organisms.

1935:   **Wendell Stanley** (1887–1955) crystallized TMV and showed that it remained infectious (Nobel Prize, 1946). Stanley's work was the first step towards describing the molecular structure of any virus and helped to further illuminate the nature of viruses.

1938:   **Max Theiler** (1899–1972) developed a live attenuated vaccine against yellow fever (Nobel Prize, 1951). Theiler's vaccine was so safe and effective that it is still in use today! This work saved millions of lives and set the model for the production of many subsequent vaccines.

1939:   **Emory Ellis** (1906–) and **Max Delbruck** (1906–1981) established the concept of the 'one step virus growth cycle' essential to the understanding of virus replication (Nobel Prize, 1969). This work laid the basis for the understanding of virus replication – that virus particles do not 'grow' but are instead assembled from preformed components.

1940:   **Helmuth Ruska** (1908–1973) used an electron microscope to take the first pictures of virus particles. Along with other physical studies of viruses, direct visualization of **virions** was an important advance in understanding virus structure.

1941:   **George Hirst** demonstrated that influenza virus agglutinates red blood cells. This was the first rapid, quantitative method of measuring eukaryotic viruses. Now viruses could be counted!

1945: **Salvador Luria** (1912–1991) and **Alfred Hershey** (1908–1997) demonstrated that **bacteriophages** mutate (Nobel Prize, 1969). This work proved that similar genetic mechanisms operate in viruses as in cellular organisms and laid the basis for the understanding of antigenic variation in viruses.

1949: **John Enders** (1897–1985), **Thomas Weller** (1915–) and **Frederick Robbins** (1916–) were able to grow poliovirus *in vitro* using human tissue culture (Nobel Prize, 1954). This development led to the isolation of many new viruses in tissue culture.

1950: **André Lwoff** (1902–1994), **Louis Siminovitch** and **Niels Kjeldgaard** discovered **lysogenic** bacteriophage in *Bacillus megaterium* irradiated with ultraviolet light and coined the term **prophage** (Nobel Prize, 1965). Although the concept of lysogeny had been around since the 1920s, this work clarified the existence of **temperate** and **virulent bacteriophages** and led to subsequent studies concerning the control of gene expression in prokaryotes, resulting ultimately in the operon hypothesis of Jacob and Monod.

1952: **Renato Dulbecco** (1914–) showed that animal viruses can form plaques in a similar way to **bacteriophages** (Nobel Prize, 1975). Dulbecco's work allowed rapid quantitation of animal viruses using assays which had only previously been possible with bacteriophages.

Alfred Hershey (1908–1997) and **Martha Chase** demonstrated that DNA was the genetic material of a **bacteriophage**. Although the initial evidence for DNA as the molecular basis of genetic inheritance was discovered using a bacteriophage, this principle of course applies to all cellular organisms (though not all viruses!).

1957: **Heinz Fraenkel-Conrat** (1910–1999) and **R.C. Williams** showed that when mixtures of purified tobacco mosaic virus (TMV) RNA and coat protein were incubated together, virus particles formed spontaneously. The discovery that virus particles could form spontaneously from purified subunits without any extraneous information indicated that the particle was in the free energy minimum state and was therefore the favoured structure of the components. This stability is an important feature of virus particles.

Alick Isaacs and **Jean Lindemann** discovered interferon. Although the initial hopes for interferons as broad spectrum antiviral agents equivalent to antibiotics have faded, interferons were the first cytokines to be studied in detail.

Carleton Gajdusek proposed that a 'slow virus' is responsible for the **prion** disease kuru (Nobel Prize, 1976) (see 1982). Gajdusek showed that the course of kuru is similar to that of scrapie, that kuru can be transmitted to chimpanzees and that the agent responsible is an atypical virus.

1961:   **Sydney Brenner**, **Francois Jacob** and **Matthew Meselson** demonstrate that bacteriophage T4 uses host cell ribosomes to direct virus protein synthesis. This discovery revealed the fundamental molecular mechanism of protein translation.

1963:   **Baruch Blumberg** discovered *Hepatitis B virus* (HBV) (Nobel Prize, 1976). Blumberg went on to develop the first vaccine against the HBV, considered by some to be the first vaccine against cancer because of the strong association of hepatitis B with liver cancer.

1967:   **Mark Ptashne** isolates and studies the λ repressor protein. Repressor proteins as regulatory molecules were first postulated by Jacob and Monod. Together with Walter Gilbert's work on the *E. coli* lac repressor protein, Ptashne's work illustrated how repressor proteins are a key element of gene regulation and control the reactions of genes to environmental signals.

   Theodor Diener discovered **viroids**, agents of plant disease which have no protein capsid. Viroids are infectious agent consisting of a low molecular weight RNA that contains no protein capsid responsible for many plant diseases.

1970:   **Howard Temin** (1934–1994) and **David Baltimore** independently discovered reverse transcriptase in retroviruses (Nobel Prize, 1975). The discovery of reverse transcription established a pathway for genetic information flow from RNA to DNA, refuting the so-called 'central dogma' of molecular biology.

1972:   **Paul Berg** created the first recombinant DNA molecules, circular SV40 DNA genomes containing λ phage genes and the galactose operon of *E. coli* (Nobel prize, 1980). This was the beginning of recombinant DNA technology.

1973:   **Peter Doherty** and **Rolf Zinkernagl** demonstrated the basis of antigenic recognition by the cellular immune system (Nobel Prize, 1996). The demonstration that lymphocytes recognize both virus antigens and major histocompatibility antigens in order to kill virus-infected cells established the specificity of the cellular immune system.

1975:   **Bernard Moss**, **Aaron Shatkin** and colleagues showed that messenger RNA contains a specific nucleotide cap at its 5′ end which affects correct processing during translation. These discoveries in reovirus and vaccinia were subsequently found to apply to cellular mRNAs – a fundamental principle.

1976:   **J. Michael Bishop** and **Harold Varmus** determined that the **oncogene** from *Rous sarcoma virus* can also be found in the cells of normal animals, including humans (Nobel Prize, 1989). Proto-oncogenes are essential for normal development but can become cancer genes when cellular regulators are damaged or modified, e.g. by virus **transduction**

1977:   **Richard Roberts**, and independently **Phillip Sharp**, showed that adenovirus genes are interspersed with non-coding segments that do not specify protein structure (**introns**) (Nobel Prize, 1993). The discovery of gene splicing in adenovirus was subsequently found to apply to cellular genes – a fundamental principle.

Frederick Sanger and colleagues determined the complete sequence of all 5375 nucleotides of the bacteriophage φX174 **genome** (Nobel Prize, 1980). This was the first complete genome sequence of any organism to be determined.

1979: Smallpox was officially declared to be eradicated by the World Health Organization (WHO). The last naturally occurring case of smallpox was seen in Somalia in 1977. This was the first microbial disease ever to be completely eliminated.

1981: **Yorio Hinuma** and colleagues isolated *Human T-cell leukaemia virus* (HTLV) from patients with adult T-cell leukaemia. Although several viruses are associated with human tumours, HTLV was the first unequivocal human cancer virus to be identified.

1982: **Stanley Prusiner** demonstrated that infectious proteins he called **prions** cause scrapie, a fatal neurodegenerative disease of sheep (Nobel Prize, 1997). This was the most significant advance in our understanding of what were previously called 'slow virus' diseases and are now known as transmissible spongiform encepthalopathies (TSEs).

1983: **Luc Montaigner** and **Robert Gallo** announced the discovery of *Human immunodeficiency virus* (HIV), the causative agent of AIDS. Only 2–3 years after the start of the AIDS epidemic the agent responsible was identified.

1985: US Department of Agriculture (USDA) granted the first ever licence to market a genetically modified organism (GMO) – a virus to vaccinate against swine herpes. The first commercial GMO.

1986: **Roger Beachy**, **Rob Fraley** and colleagues demonstrated that tobacco plants transformed with the gene for the coat protein of *Tobacco mosaic virus* are resistant to TMV infection. This work resulted in a better understanding of virus resistance in plants, a major goal of plant breeders for many centuries.

1989: *Hepatitis C virus* (HCV), the source of most cases of nonA, nonB hepatitis, was definitively identified. This was the first infectious agent to be identified by molecular cloning of the genome rather than by more traditional techniques (see 1994).

1990: First (approved) human gene therapy procedure was carried out on a child with severe combined immune deficiency (SCID), using a retrovirus vector. Although not successful, this was the first attempt to correct human genetic disease.

1993: Nucleotide sequence of the smallpox virus genome completed (185 578 bp). Initially, it was intended that destruction of remaining laboratory stocks of smallpox virus would be carried out when the complete genome sequence had been determined. However, this decision has now been post-poned (1999).

1994:   **Yuan Chang**, **Patrick Moore** and their collaborators identified *Human herpesvirus 8* (HHV-8), the causative agent of Kaposi's sarcoma. Using a poly-merase chain reaction (PCR)-based technique, representational difference analysis, this novel pathogen was identified.

1999:   Number of confirmed cases of people living with HIV/AIDS worldwide reaches 33 million. The AIDS pandemic continues to grow. Confirmed cases are an underestimate of the true total worldwide.

Nucleotide sequence of the largest known virus genome completed: *Paramecium bursaria* Chlorella virus 1. This 330 742 bp sequence represents the technical advances in sequencing which have occurred since the first genome sequence was completed in 1977.

ANSWERS TO SELF-ASSESSMENT QUESTIONS

CHAPTER 1

(1.1) Are the following statements true or false?

TRUE   (a) Viruses are submicroscopic, obligate intracellular parasites. This simple definition excludes all other types of micro-organism.

FALSE   (b) Virus particles (virions) do NOT 'grow' or undergo division.

TRUE   (c) Viruses lack the genetic information which encodes apparatus necessary for the generation of metabolic energy.

TRUE   (d) Viruses lack the genetic information which encodes apparatus necessary for protein synthesis (ribosomes).

FALSE   (e) Prions are infectious agents believed to consist of a single PROTEIN component.

(1.2) Are the following statements true or false?

FALSE   (a) Virus particles cannot generally be seen using light microscopes.

TRUE   (b) Edward Jenner first vaccinated a patient against smallpox on 14 May 1796.

TRUE   (c) Louis Pasteur invented the term 'virus' in the 1890s.

TRUE   (d) Dimitri Iwanowski showed that viruses could pass through filters fine enough to retain the smallest known bacteria.

FALSE   (e) Viruses which infect bacteria are called BACTERIO-PHAGES.

(1.3) These are Koch's postulates:

TRUE   (a) The agent must be present in every case of the disease.

TRUE   (b) The agent must be isolated from the host and grown *in vitro*.

TRUE   (c)   The disease must be reproduced when a pure culture of the agent is inoculated into a healthy susceptible host.

TRUE   (d)   The same agent must be recovered once again from the experimentally infected host.

(1.4) The following are immunological methods of studying viruses (true or false?):

TRUE   (a)   Complement fixation.

FALSE   (b)   Northern blots use hybridization to analyse RNA.

FALSE   (c)   Southern blots use hybridization to analyse DNA.

TRUE   (d)   Western blot.

FALSE   (e)   PCR (polymerase chain reaction) is a method of amplifying small quantities of nucleic acid.

(1.5) Are the following statements true or false?

FALSE   (a)   Electron microscopes allow direct examination of viruses at magnifications of up to 100 000 times.

TRUE   (b)   X-ray diffraction by crystalline forms of purified virus can be used to determine their atomic structure.

FALSE   (c)   The atomic structures of comparatively few viruses have been determined due to technical difficulties.

FALSE   (d)   Viruses DO NOT originate by spontaneous generation.

FALSE   (e)   The limitations of NMR mean that only relatively small molecules can be examined – considerably smaller than even the smallest virus particles.

CHAPTER 2

(2.1) Are the following statements true or false?

FALSE   (a)   Nucleic acids are SENSITIVE to physical damage such as shearing by mechanical forces and to chemical modification.

TRUE   (b)   The protein subunits in a virus capsid are multiply redundant, i.e. present in many copies per particle.

TRUE   (c)   The forces which drive the assembly of virus particles include hydrophobic and electrostatic interactions.

FALSE   (d)   The protein subunits in virus capsids are rarely held together by covalent bonds.

FALSE   (e)   In addition to protecting the genome from physical, chemical, or enzymatic damage, the outer shells of a virus particle initiate the process of infection by binding to receptors on host cells.

(2.2) Are the following statements true or false?

TRUE   (a)   A helix can be constructed by stacking repeated components with a constant relationship to one another.

TRUE   (b)   A helix can be defined by two parameters: amplitude and pitch.

FALSE   (c)   A helix can be defined mathematically by the equation:
$$P = \mu \times p$$

FALSE   (d)   The 'amplitude' of a helix is its diameter.

FALSE   (e)   Bacteriophage M13 particles are about 900 nm long, but their precise length varies depending on their nucleic acid content.

(2.3) Are the following statements true or false?

FALSE   (a)   The particles of many plant viruses have helical symmetry, but some have icosahedral symmetry.

TRUE   (b)   There are no known non-enveloped helical viruses of animals.

TRUE   (c)   Rhabdovirus particles have a helical nucleocapsid.

TRUE   (d)   Bacteriophage M13 is a member of the *Inovirus* genus.

FALSE   (e)   Bacteriophage M13 requires the F pilus on the surface of *E. coli* for infection.

(2.4) Are the following statements true or false?

FALSE   (a)   An icosahedron is a solid shape consisting of 20 triangular faces arranged around the surface of a sphere.

FALSE   (b)   An icosahedron has an axis of TWOFOLD rotational symmetry through the centre of each edge.

FALSE   (c)   An icosahedron has an axis of THREEFOLD rotational symmetry through the centre of each face.

FALSE   (d)   An icosahedron has an axis of FIVEFOLD rotational symmetry through the centre of each corner.

FALSE   (e)   Some simple icosahedral virus capsids contain only 60 subunits (e.g. ϕX174), most contain more than this (e.g. $T = 3$ viruses have 180 subunits).

(2.5) All the following virus groups have icosahedral symmetry (true or false?):

FALSE   (a)   Orthomyxoviruses are pleiomorphic (variable), enveloped viruses.

FALSE   (b)   Paramyxoviruses are pleiomorphic (variable), enveloped viruses.

TRUE   (c)   Picornaviruses have icosahedral symmetry.

FALSE   (d)   Rhabdoviruses are helical, enveloped viruses.

FALSE   (e)   Tobamoviruses are helical, non-enveloped viruses.

(2.6) Are the following statements true or false?

FALSE (a) The lipid composition of a virus envelope is SIMILAR to that of the host cell.

TRUE (b) Virus envelopes are acquired during extrusion (budding) of the particle through the host cell membrane.

FALSE (c) Budding can occur from the host cell surface, cytoplasmic or even nuclear membranes.

FALSE (d) Some enveloped viruses have underlying icosahedral symmetry.

FALSE (e) Most envelope proteins are encoded by the virus, although some virus envelopes contain a proportion of host cell proteins.

(2.7) All the following virus groups possess lipid envelopes (true or false?):

TRUE (a) Orthomyxoviruses

TRUE (b) Paramyxoviruses

FALSE (c) Picornaviruses

TRUE (d) Rhabdoviruses

FALSE (e) Tobamoviruses.

(2.8) Are the following statements true or false?

TRUE (a) Matrix proteins are internal virion proteins that link the internal nucleocapsid assembly to the envelope.

TRUE (b) Matrix proteins are often very abundant in the virus particle.

TRUE (c) External glycoproteins are usually the major antigens of enveloped viruses.

TRUE (d) External glycoproteins are usually the virus attachment proteins of enveloped viruses.

TRUE (e) The influenza virus M_2 peptide is a transmembrane protein.

(2.9) Are the following statements true or false?

FALSE (a) Poxvirus particles have elements of helical symmetry, but overall are too complex to define in simple terms.

TRUE (b) Poxvirus particles contain more than 100 different proteins.

FALSE (c) The tailed phages of *E. coli* are released from the host cell by LYSIS.

TRUE (d) The tailed phages of *E. coli* have separate assembly pathways for the head and tail sections of the particle.

TRUE (e) Reovirus capsids are composed of a double protein shell.

(2.10) Genome packaging (true or false?):

FALSE (a) is specific for virus nucleic acids, but viruses make mistakes!

TRUE (b) requires interaction with a specific virus–encoded capsid or nucleocapsid protein.

TRUE	(c)	requires specific nucleotide sequences in the virus genome, although the secondary structure of the genome is also important in some cases.
TRUE	(d)	requires positively charged groups to overcome negative electrostatic charges on the virus genome.
TRUE	(e)	in TMV is initiated by the OAS region of the genome.

CHAPTER 3

(3.1) Are the following statements true or false?

TRUE	(a)	Virus genomes vary in size from 3500 nucleotides to approximately 380 kilobase pairs.
FALSE	(b)	The genetic code of a virus must be SIMILAR to that of the host organism so that it can be decoded by the host cell biochemical machinery.
TRUE	(c)	Virus genomes consisting of (+)sense RNA are infectious when the purified vRNA is applied to cells in the absence of any virus proteins (except for retroviruses).
TRUE	(d)	'Reverse genetics' makes possible the manipulation of (−)sense RNA virus genomes.
TRUE	(e)	Infection of cells caused by nucleic acid alone is referred to as transfection.

(3.2) Are the following statements true or false?

FALSE	(a)	'Superinfection' is infection of a single cell by more than one virus particle.
FALSE	(b)	The probability of recombination between two genetic markers is PROPORTIONAL to the distance between them.
TRUE	(c)	In viruses with segmented genomes, 'reassortment groups' are usually equivalent to the individual genome segments.
TRUE	(d)	Populations of virus genomes consisting of mixtures of molecular variants are known as quasi-species.
TRUE	(e)	Site-specific molecular biological methods are commonly used to mutagenize virus genomes.

(3.3) Are the following statements true or false?

FALSE	(a)	Mutation rates in herpesvirus genomes may be as LOW as 10^8 to 10^{11} per nucleotide incorporated, similar to those seen in cellular genomes.
FALSE	(b)	Mutation rates in retrovirus genomes may be as HIGH as 10^3 to 10^4 per nucleotide incorporated, due to the low fidelity of reverse transcriptase.

TRUE   (c)   Every new HIV provirus formed contains, on average, at least one new mutation.

FALSE   (d)   Temperature-sensitive (t.s.) mutants tend to be unstable and frequently revert to the original phenotype since they are usually single base substitutions and frequently disadvantage viruses compared with the wild-type sequence.

TRUE   (e)   t.s. mutations usually result from mis-sense mutations in proteins.

(3.4) Are the following statements true or false?

TRUE   (a)   Deletion mutants are very useful for assigning structure-function relationships to virus genomes, since they are easily mapped by physical analysis.

TRUE   (b)   Deletion mutants can only revert to wild-type by recombination, which only occurs at low frequencies.

TRUE   (c)   Complementation may be asymmetric or symmetrical.

FALSE   (d)   Phenotypic mixing is where individual progeny viruses from a mixed infection contain PROTEINS derived from both parental viruses but are genetically unaltered.

FALSE   (e)   Only retrovirus have completely diploid genomes, i.e. two alleles of each gene.

(3.5) Are the following statements true or false?

FALSE   (a)   Herpesvirus genomes vary in size from 105 to 235 kbp.

TRUE   (b)   Herpesvirus genomes consist of linear, double-stranded DNA.

TRUE   (c)   In *Herpes simplex virus* (HSV), each gene is expressed from its own promoter.

TRUE   (d)   The HSV genome is approximately 152 kbp.

TRUE   (e)   The HSV genome contains about 80 genes, densely packed and with overlapping reading frames.

(3.6) Are the following statements true or false?

TRUE   (a)   Parvovirus genomes consist of linear, non-segmented, single-stranded DNA.

TRUE   (b)   The ends of parvovirus genomes are palindromic sequences of about 115 nt required for replication.

TRUE   (c)   Polyomaviruses are about 5 kbp in size and contain six genes.

TRUE   (d)   In the virus particle, polyomavirus DNA assumes a super-coiled form and is associated with cellular histones.

TRUE   (e)   The polyomavirus genome contains overlapping reading frames on both strands of the DNA.

(3.7) (+)sense RNA virus genomes (true or false?):

FALSE   (a)   can be up to 30 kbp in length (Coronaviruses).

TRUE   (b)   are usually modified at the 5′ end, by a methylated cap or a covalently attached protein.

FALSE   (c)   are sometimes polyadenylated at the 3′ end, not always.

FALSE   (d)   are sometimes expressed as a polyprotein, not always.

FALSE   (e)   do NOT require splicing for expression, since they are replicated in the cytoplasm.

(3.8) (−)sense RNA virus genomes (true or false?):

TRUE   (a)   are sometimes segmented, but not in all cases.

FALSE   (b)   may have an ambisense coding strategy, e.g. bunyaviruses, arenaviruses.

TRUE   (c)   are never capped at the 5′ end.

TRUE   (d)   are never polyadenylated at the 3′ end.

FALSE   (e)   are NEVER circular.

(3.9) Retroviruses (true or false?):

FALSE   (a)   Reverse transcriptase is also encoded by hepadnaviruses and caulimoviruses.

TRUE   (b)   are the only RNA viruses whose genome is produced by cellular transcriptional machinery.

TRUE   (c)   are the only (+)sense RNA viruses whose genome does not serve directly as mRNA immediately after infection.

TRUE   (d)   have high mutation rates, due to the low fidelity of reverse transcriptase.

TRUE   (e)   have a high rate of recombination, due to reverse transcription.

(3.10) Are the following statements true or false?

TRUE   (a)   Segmentation of virus genomes reduces the probability of strand breakage due to shearing.

FALSE   (b)   Hepadnaviruses have SMALL genomes of about 3.5 kbp.

TRUE   (c)   The *Cauliflower mosaic virus* (CaMV) genome consists of a gapped, circular double-stranded DNA molecule.

TRUE   (d)   The *Cauliflower mosaic virus* (CaMV) genome is generated by reverse transcription.

FALSE   (e)   Viruses MAY have had a common ancestor, but the existence of virus superfamilies does not prove this – alternative explanations such as convergent evolution are possible.

CHAPTER 4

(4.1) Virus replication involves the following distinct phases (true or false?):

TRUE (a) Initiation of infection.

TRUE (b) Replication of the virus genome.

TRUE (c) Expression of the virus genome.

FALSE (d) Cleavage of the virus genome.

TRUE (e) Release of mature virions from the infected cell.

(4.2) Are the following statements true or false?

FALSE (a) The 'single-burst' experiment was performed by Ellis and Delbruck in 1939, not 1989!

TRUE (b) The 'single-burst' experiment demonstrates that new virus particles from the intracellular assembly of preformed components are released in a batch-like process.

TRUE (c) The 'single-burst' experiment demonstrates the essential phases of virus replication.

FALSE (d) The 'single-burst' experiment demonstrates the essential phases of virus replication.

TRUE (e) The 'Hershey-Chase' experiment demonstrates that nucleic acid is the genetic material of viruses, but this conclusion can be extended to all other organisms.

(4.3) Are the following statements true or false?

FALSE (a) Virus receptor molecules may be proteins or the sugar residues present on glycoproteins or glycolipids.

FALSE (b) Many viruses have more than one receptor molecule, e.g. different receptors on different cell types.

FALSE (c) No known plant virus uses a cellular receptor due to the surface structure of plant cells.

FALSE (d) Sialic acid is the influenza virus receptor. The human rhinovirus receptor is either ICAM-1 or the LDL receptor.

TRUE (e) The expression of receptors on the surface of cells is the major factor which determines the tropism of viruses.

(4.4) The following are mechanisms by which virus particles penetrate cells (true or false?):

TRUE (a) Translocation.

FALSE (b) Transfection is the infection of cells mediated by the introduction of nucleic acid rather than by virus particles.

FALSE (c) Exocytosis is one mechanism by which viruses are released from cells.

TRUE   (d)   Endocytosis.
TRUE   (e)   Fusion.

(4.5) Are the following statements true or false?

TRUE   (a)   Viral penetration of cells is an energy–dependent process.
TRUE   (b)   Influenza haemagglutinin is a virus fusion protein.
FALSE   (c)   Uncoating only occurs after penetration of the host cell.
FALSE   (d)   The product of uncoating is frequently (not always) a complex of nucleic acids and proteins.
FALSE   (e)   Nucleoproteins closely associated with virus genomes in the core of the particle are responsible for nuclear localization of virus genomes.

(4.6) Are the following statements true or false?

FALSE   (a)   There are SEVEN classes of virus genome structure.
FALSE   (b)   Class I viruses have double-stranded DNA genomes which may be linear or circular.
TRUE   (c)   Class II viruses have (−)sense single-stranded DNA genomes.
FALSE   (d)   Class VI viruses (retroviruses) have (+)sense single-stranded RNA genomes (with a DNA intermediate in the replication cycle).
FALSE   (e)   Class VII viruses have (+)sense single-stranded DNA genomes (with an RNA intermediate in the replication cycle).

(4.7) Are the following statements true or false?

TRUE   (a)   Adenoviruses encode their own DNA polymerase but are dependent on cellular factors for genome replication.
FALSE   (b)   Poxviruses encode their own DNA polymerase and are INDEPENDENT of cellular factors for genome replication (although some cellular factors are required for unknown steps in the maturation process).
FALSE   (c)   Reovirus genomes are transcribed by a viral enzyme present in the particle.
FALSE   (d)   Some RNA virus genomes replicate in the nucleus of the host cell, e.g. influenza virus.
TRUE   (e)   Retrovirus genomes in the form of a DNA provirus are transcribed by cellular RNA polymerase.

(4.8) The following viruses replicate their genomes in the cytoplasm of infected cells (true or false?):

TRUE   (a)   Picornaviruses, e.g. *Poliovirus*.
TRUE   (b)   Poxviruses, e.g. *Vaccinia virus*.
TRUE   (c)   Rhabdoviruses, e.g. *Rabies virus*.

TRUE   (d)   Paramyxoviruses, e.g. *Respiratory syncytial virus*.
FALSE   (e)   Hepadnaviruses, e.g. *Hepatitis B virus*.

(4.9) The following viruses replicate their genomes in the nucleus of infected cells (true or false?):

TRUE   (a)   Herpesviruses, e.g. *Epstein–Barr virus*.
TRUE   (b)   Parvoviruses, e.g. B19.
TRUE   (c)   Orthomyxoviruses, e.g. influenza virus.
FALSE   (d)   Rotaviruses, e.g. group A rotaviruses.
FALSE   (e)   Coronaviruses, e.g. OC43.

(4.10) Are the following statements true or false?

TRUE   (a)   Maturation usually involves structural changes in the virus particle.
TRUE   (b)   Maturation frequently involves protease cleavage of virus proteins.
TRUE   (c)   Enveloped viruses acquire their lipid membranes by budding through cellular membranes.
TRUE   (d)   Virus envelope proteins are acquired during the process of budding.
TRUE   (e)   Virus envelope proteins are involved in release from as well as attachment to host cells.

CHAPTER 5

(5.1) Are the following statements true or false?

FALSE   (a)   The course of virus replication is determined by tight control of gene expression.
TRUE   (b)   Transcription promoters are *cis*-acting sequences located adjacent to the genes whose transcription they control.
TRUE   (c)   Transcription factors are *trans*-acting proteins which bind to specific sequences present anywhere in the cell.
TRUE   (d)   Transcription of bacterial operons typically produces polycistronic mRNAs.
FALSE   (e)   Gene expression in bacteria is regulated at the level of transcription and at subsequent (post-transcriptional) stages of gene expression.

(5.2) Viruses have counteracted their genetic limitations by evolving of a range of solutions, including (true or false?):

TRUE   (a)   Powerful positive *cis*- and *trans*-acting signals which promote gene expression.

TRUE   (b)   Powerful *cis*-acting negative signals which repress gene expression.

TRUE   (c)   Highly compressed genomes with overlapping reading frames common.

TRUE   (d)   Control signals which are frequently nested within other genes.

TRUE   (e)   Several strategies designed to create multiple polypeptides from a single mRNA.

(5.3) Are the following statements true or false?

TRUE   (a)   Bacteriophage λ can alternate between the lysogenic and lytic growth cycles.

FALSE   (b)   The λ N protein acts as a POSITIVE transcription regulator (antiterminator).

TRUE   (c)   In the absence of the N protein, RNA polymerase stops at the nut site.

FALSE   (d)   The *cI* repressor protein binds to BOTH O_R AND O_L.

TRUE   (e)   Lysogeny is maintained by autoregulation of *cI* transcription.

(5.4) Are the following statements true or false?

TRUE   (a)   Transcription of eukaryotic cellular genes results in monocistronic mRNAs, each transcribed from its own promoter.

TRUE   (b)   Post-transcriptional control of gene expression in eukaryotes is achieved by splicing of hnRNA and differential export of mRNA from the nucleus to the cytoplasm.

FALSE   (c)   Eukaryotic mRNAs are translated with variable efficiency mainly due to the efficiency with which sequences surrounding the AUG initiation codon are recognized by ribosomes.

TRUE   (d)   The stability of eukaryotic mRNAs depends on the speed at which they are degraded.

TRUE   (e)   Translation enhancers perform a function analogous to that of transcription enhancers.

(5.5) Are the following statements true or false?

TRUE   (a)   Polyomaviruses are heavily dependent on cellular machinery for gene expression.

FALSE   (b)   Herpesviruses make three classes of mRNA: immediate-early (IE) mRNAs (*trans*-acting regulators of virus transcription); Early mRNAs (further non-structural regulatory proteins and some minor structural proteins); Late mRNAs (major structural proteins).

TRUE   (c)   Geminivirus genomes are replicated and expressed in the nucleus of infected cells because they are heavily reliant on host cell functions.

TRUE   (d) Reovirus transcription occurs inside virus core particles.

TRUE   (e) Segmented virus genomes are usually transcribed to produce monocistronic mRNAs.

(5.6) Viruses with (+)sense RNA genomes (true or false?):

FALSE   (a) are largely INDEPENDENT of cellular mechanisms for control of gene expression.

FALSE   (b) SOME are translated to produce a long polyprotein, OTHERS are transcribed to produce subgenomic RNAs.

FALSE   (c) SOME are translated to produce a long polyprotein, OTHERS are transcribed to produce subgenomic RNAs.

FALSE   (d) SOME are non-segmented, others segmented.

FALSE   (e) can produce varying ratios of the polypeptides they encode by mechanisms such as alternative cleavages of polyproteins and variable translation efficiency of subgenomic RNAs.

(5.7) Are the following statements true or false?

TRUE   (a) Viruses with non-segmented (−)sense genomes produce monocistronic mRNAs.

TRUE   (b) Viruses with (−)sense genomes all contain a virus-specific transcriptase/replicase within the virus nucleocapsid.

FALSE   (c) Viruses with non-segmented (−)sense genomes can produce variable ratios of the polypeptides they encode, e.g. paramyxoviruses (Figure 5.10).

TRUE   (d) Retroviruses are the only RNA viruses whose genomes (in the form of the DNA provirus) are transcribed by cellular RNA polymerase.

TRUE   (e) *Hepadnavirus* and *Caulimovirus* genomes contain a number of overlapping reading frames.

(5.8) Are the following statements true or false?

TRUE   (a) SV40 large T-antigen binds to the origin of replication in the virus genome.

TRUE   (b) SV40 large T-antigen represses transcription of the virus early genes.

FALSE   (c) SV40 large T-antigen does not promote export of virus mRNAs from the nucleus to the cytoplasm.

FALSE   (d) The HTLV tax protein binds to cellular transcription factors and to the provirus CRE sequences, but not to virus mRNAs.

FALSE   (e) The HIV tat protein binds to the TAR sequence in HIV mRNAs.

(5.9) Are the following statements true or false?

TRUE   (a)   With the exception of retroviruses, no RNA virus genome undergoes splicing.

TRUE   (b)   The HTLV rex protein promotes the export of virus structural protein mRNAs from the nucleus.

FALSE   (c)   The abbreviation 'IRES' stands for 'internal ribosomal entry site'.

FALSE   (d)   SOME (+)sense RNA viruses contain an IRES element, others do not.

FALSE   (e)   Very few eukaryotic cellular mRNAs contain an IRES element.

(5.10) Are the following statements true or false?

TRUE   (a)   Ribosomal frameshifting allows viruses to produce several different proteins from a polycistronic mRNA.

TRUE   (b)   Ribosomal frameshifting allow viruses to produce varying amounts of different proteins from a polycistronic mRNA.

TRUE   (c)   RNA pseudoknots are produced by *trans*-acting proteins such as the HIV tat protein.

TRUE   (d)   RNA pseudoknots increase the frequency of ribosomal frameshifting.

TRUE   (e)   Suppression of termination codons allows some viruses to produce multiple proteins from a polycistronic mRNA.

CHAPTER 6

(6.1) Plant viruses (true or false?):

FALSE   (a)   are responsible for an estimated US$60 000 000 000 (!) worth of damage each year.

TRUE   (b)   can be transmitted by infected seeds.

TRUE   (c)   may be transmitted to new hosts as wind-blown dust or as rain-splashed mud.

FALSE   (d)   sometimes replicate in insect vectors (propagative transmission), e.g. plant rhabdoviruses.

FALSE   (e)   may or may not cause systemic infections involving the whole plant.

(6.2) Are the following statements true or false?

FALSE   (a)   Movement proteins allow plant viruses to be transmitted from infected cells to neighbouring cells.

TRUE   (b)   Damage to virus-infected plants occurs due to necrosis of cells, hypoplasia and hyperplasia.

TRUE   (c)   The hypersensitive response in plants is functionally analogous to the production of interferons in animals.

TRUE   (d)   The hypersensitive response in plants tends to limit the occurrence of systemic infection.

TRUE   (e)   Virus-resistant plants have been created by genetic manipulation resulting in the endogenous expression of virus genes.

(6.3) Are the following statements true or false?

TRUE   (a)   The major impact of the humoral immune response on virus infections is the eventual clearance of virus from the body.

FALSE   (b)   Virus particles ARE directly neutralized by antibodies and phagocytosed by white blood cells.

TRUE   (c)   Overall, cell-mediated immunity is more important than humoral immunity in controlling virus infections.

TRUE   (d)   Natural killer (NK) cells are the first cell-mediated defence mechanism active against virus infection.

FALSE   (e)   Cytotoxic T lymphocytes (CTLs) ARE MHC-restricted, i.e. recognize a specific antigen only in the context of MHC class II antigen plus the T-cell receptor/CD3 complex on the surface of the CTL.

(6.4) Are the following statements true or false?

FALSE   (a)   Interferon production was first observed from chick chorioallantoic membranes in 1957.

FALSE   (b)   Biochemical purification of interferons from natural sources was difficult because interferons are highly potent and therefore non-abundant molecules.

TRUE   (c)   There are three distinct types of interferon: α, β and γ.

FALSE   (d)   Only IFNβ is synthesized only by fibroblasts; IFNα and IFNγ are synthesized predominantly by lymphocytes.

FALSE   (e)   Double-stranded RNA is a potent inducer of interferon synthesis; all other nucleic acids do not induce IFN synthesis.

(6.5) Are the following statements true or false?

TRUE   (a)   All interferons have similar antiviral capacities, but act differently as cellular regulators.

TRUE   (b)   2′,5′-oligo A activates RNAse L, which digests all RNAs.

TRUE   (c)   PKR phosphorylates eIF2α, which is required for the initiation of translation.

TRUE   (d)   Interferons are used to treat chronic viral hepatitis.

TRUE   (e)   Several viruses have evolved mechanisms which enable them to resist the effects of interferons.

(6.6) Are the following statements true or false?

TRUE   (a) Mucosal membranes are favourable routes of access for viruses to the tissues of the body.

TRUE   (b) 'Coughs and sneezes spread diseases.'

TRUE   (c) The natural environment is a considerable barrier to virus infections.

FALSE   (d) Primary LOCALIZED infection by viruses is frequently followed by SYSTEMIC secondary infection.

FALSE   (e) Spread of virus to the nervous system usually PRECEDED by primary viraemia.

(6.7) Viruses have evolved many tricks to fool the immune system (true or false?):

TRUE   (a) Antigenic variation.

FALSE   (b) DOWNREGULATION of MHC class I gene expression.

FALSE   (c) DOWNREGULATION of accessory molecules involved in immune recognition.

TRUE   (d) Infection of immunocompromised sites within the body.

FALSE   (e) Few viruses infect the cells of the skin and this does not enable them to escape the immune system.

(6.8) Are the following statements true or false?

TRUE   (a) Abortive infection of cells can have significant pathological consequences, e.g. transformation.

TRUE   (b) In acute infections, much viral replication occurs before the onset of any symptoms.

TRUE   (c) In persistent infections, the virus adjusts its replication and pathogenicity to avoid killing the host.

TRUE   (d) Persistent infections may result from the production of defective-interfering (D.I.) particles.

TRUE   (e) Latent infections are typified by strictly limited gene expression without ongoing virus replication.

(6.9) Are the following statements true or false?

FALSE   (a) Subunit vaccines are generally the LEAST effective and MOST expensive virus vaccines.

FALSE   (b) The hepatitis B virus vaccine currently in use is produced by genetic engineering.

TRUE   (c) Inactivated virus vaccines are sometimes not as effective as 'live' virus vaccines because they fail to stimulate mucosal and cell-mediated immunity.

TRUE   (d) The majority of successful virus vaccines are based on attenuated viruses.

TRUE   (e)   Retroviruses have been successfully used as vectors for gene therapy.

(6.10) Are the following statements true or false?

FALSE   (a)   Prevention of virus infection by drug treatment is rarely effective compared with vaccination.

TRUE   (b)   Any of the stages of viral replication can be a potential target for antiviral chemotherapy.

TRUE   (c)   The majority of antiviral drugs in use are nucleoside/nucleotide analogues.

FALSE   (d)   Ribavirin is active against a wide spectrum of viruses.

TRUE   (e)   The frequency with which viruses become resistant to antiviral drugs depends on the drug and the virus concerned and varies considerably.

CHAPTER 7

(7.1) Are the following statements true or false?

TRUE   (a)   Most disease states are multi-factorial.

TRUE   (b)   Inflammation, fever, headaches and skin rashes are frequently not caused by virus replication, but the immune response to virus infection.

TRUE   (c)   The vast majority of virus infections do not result in disease.

TRUE   (d)   Eukaryotic cells must constantly synthesize a variety of macromolecules which require continual replacement.

FALSE   (e)   Virus nucleic acids do not act as toxins.

(7.2) The cytopathic effects of virus infection include (true or false?):

TRUE   (a)   Altered shape.

TRUE   (b)   Detachment from the substrate.

TRUE   (c)   Lysis.

TRUE   (d)   Membrane fusion and altered permeability.

TRUE   (e)   Apoptosis.

(7.3) Are the following statements true or false?

FALSE   (a)   Shutoff is the sudden and dramatic cessation of HOST CELL macromolecular synthesis.

FALSE   (b)   Shutoff in poliovirus-infected cells occurs owing to protease degradation of the p220 component of eIF-4F, a complex of proteins required for cap-dependent translation of messenger RNAs by ribosomes.

TRUE   (c)   Lysis of adenovirus–infected cells is caused by virus–encoded molecules with a toxin–like action.

FALSE   (d)   Virus–induced membrane fusion may cause cell death but not transformation.

FALSE   (e)   The HIV env protein is responsible for syncytium formation.

(7.4) Are the following statements true or false?

FALSE   (a)   Some human herpesviruses are highly cytopathic, e.g. HSV, but others are not, e.g. EBV.

TRUE   (b)   Retroviruses cause a variety pathogenic conditions including paralysis, arthritis, anaemia in addition to cell transformation.

FALSE   (c)   Lentiviruses are NOT associated with cell transformation.

TRUE   (d)   HIV and other lentiviruses escape immune recognition by infecting monocytes.

FALSE   (e)   Some laboratory-adapted isolates of HIV are highly cyto-pathic in $CD4^+$ cells but may primary isolates of the virus are not.

(7.5) The following mechanisms may be involved in the pathogenesis of AIDS (true or false?):

TRUE   (a)   Antigenic variation.

TRUE   (b)   T-cell anergy.

TRUE   (c)   Apoptosis.

TRUE   (d)   Superantigens from opportunistic infections MAY be involved, although this has not been proved.

FALSE   (e)   Insertional activation of oncogenes causes cell transformation, not AIDS.

(7.6) Are the following statements true or false?

FALSE   (a)   Subacute sclerosing panencephalitis (SSPE) occurs following about 1 in 300 000 cases of measles.

TRUE   (b)   Dengue haemorrhagic fever is largely due to immune–mediated damage of virus-infected cells.

FALSE   (c)   Reye's syndrome MAY be caused or worsened by administration of aspirin during the initial illness.

FALSE   (d)   The cause of Kawasaki disease is not known.

TRUE   (e)   Guillain–Barré syndrome is a rare demyelinating disease of unknown aetiology.

(7.7) Transformed cells may display (true or false?):

TRUE   (a)   loss of anchorage dependence.

TRUE   (b)   loss of contact inhibition.

TRUE   (c)   colony formation in semi-solid media.

TRUE   (d)   decreased requirements for growth factors.

FALSE   (e) Transformed cells display normal or decreased expression of p53, or express altered p53 proteins.

(7.8) Are the following statements true or false?

FALSE   (a) Transformation is a change in the morphological, biochemical, or growth parameters of a cell. Carcinogenesis or oncogenesis multi-step process in which cellular transformation may be only the first, although essential, step along the way.

FALSE   (b) Most acutely transforming retroviruses are replication defective, Rous sarcoma virus, the first to be discovered (1911), is replication competent.

TRUE   (c) p53 causes the cell cycle to arrest at the G_1 phase.

FALSE   (d) Rb causes the cell cycle to arrest at the G_1 phase.

FALSE   (e) SV40 T antigen binds to p53 AND Rb. Adenovirus E1A and the HPV E7 protein bind Rb.

(7.9) The normal functions of oncogenes may be (true or false?):

TRUE   (a) Cytoplasmic protein kinases.

TRUE   (b) Extracellular growth factors.

TRUE   (c) G proteins involved in signal transduction.

TRUE   (d) Transcription factors.

TRUE   (e) Tyrosine kinases.

(7.10) Are the following statements true or false?

TRUE   (a) At least six viruses which are associated with the formation of human tumours (HHV-4/EBV, HBV, HCV, HHV-8, HPVs, HTLV).

FALSE   (b) EBV has a dual cell tropism for human epithelial cells (PRODUCTIVE infection) and B-lymphocytes (NON-PRODUCTIVE infection).

FALSE   (c) EBV infection is associated with at least four human tumours: Burkitt's lymphoma, nasopharyngeal carcinoma, B-cell lymphomas and some clonal forms of Hodgkin's disease, but not HCG.

TRUE   (d) Chronic HBV carriers are at 100–200 times the risk of non-carriers of developing hepatocellular carcinoma.

TRUE   (e) Chronic active hepatitis caused by *Hepatitis C virus* (HCV) infection is associated with hepatocellular carcinoma.

CHAPTER 8

(8.1) Are the following statements true or false?
TRUE   (a) Satellites encode their own coat proteins.
TRUE   (b) Viroids use the coat protein of their helper virus.
FALSE (c) There is little or no nucleotide sequence similarity between satellites and their helper virus genomes.
TRUE   (d) Viroids are 200–400 nucleotides long.
TRUE   (e) All viroids have a conserved region involved in their replication.

(8.2) Are the following statements true or false?
FALSE (a) The mechanisms by which viroids cause disease is not known, but it is not by interfering with cellular DNA replication.
FALSE (b) *Hepatitis delta virus* (HDV) δAg-S is necessary for HDV replication.
FALSE (c) HDV δAg-L is necessary for the assembly and release of HDV-containing particles.
TRUE   (d) HDV has some of the properties of a satellite virus and some of a viroid.
FALSE (e) HDV infection cannot occur without HBV co-infection.

(8.3) The following diseases are caused by prions (true or false?):
FALSE (a) Alzheimer's syndrome is a NON-TRANSMISSIBLE amyloid disease.
FALSE (b) Coconut cadang–cadang disease is cause by a VIROID.
TRUE   (c) Chronic wasting disease (CWD).
TRUE   (d) Creutzfeldt–Jakob disease (CJD).
TRUE   (e) Fatal familial insomnia (FFI).

(8.4) Are the following statements true or false?
FALSE (a) Scrapie was first described more than two hundred years ago.
TRUE   (b) Scrapie is endemic in the UK and USA.
FALSE (c) Transmissible mink encephalopathy (TME) has been reported in the USA, Canada, Finland, Germany and Russia.
TRUE   (d) More than 179 000 cases of BSE have been reported in the UK and at least 70 people have died of vCJD.
FALSE (e) BSE is NOT caused by scrapie-infected feed since the BSE and scrapie agents are biochemically and biologically distinct.

(8.5) Are the following statements true or false?

TRUE (a) There are three sources of human TSEs: sporadic, iatrogenic/acquired and familial/inherited.

TRUE (b) Sporadic Creutzfeldt-Jakob disease (CJD) accounts for about 90% of human TSE.

FALSE (c) Kuru is an acquired form of TSE, resulting from ritual cannibalism.

TRUE (d) The incidence of CJD is similar worldwide.

TRUE (e) Only about 1% of sporadic CJD cases are transmissible to mice.

(8.6) Prion infectivity is inactivated by the following treatments (true or false?):

FALSE (a) Heating to 135°C for 30 min hardly affects infectivity.

FALSE (b) After heating to 600°C for 15 min some infectivity is still retained.

FALSE (c) DNAse treatment.

FALSE (d) RNAse treatment.

TRUE (e) Phenol, which denatures proteins.

(8.7) PrP^C (true or false?):

TRUE (a) is a 254 amino acid protein.

TRUE (b) is encoded by a cellular gene.

TRUE (c) is converted by PrP^{Sc} to a protease-resistant form.

FALSE (d) PrP^C consists of 43% α-helix and no β-sheet. PrP^{Sc} consists of 30% α-helix and 43% β-sheet.

TRUE (e) is resistant to short-wave ultraviolet radiation and to ionizing radiation.

(8.8) Are the following statements true or false?:

TRUE (a) Transgenic animals which do not possess an endogenous prion gene are immune to the effects of PrP^{Sc}.

FALSE (b) Most transgenic animals which do not possess an endogenous prion gene ('knockouts') do not develop any obvious symptoms.

TRUE (c) Human PrP differs from mouse PrP at 28 of 254 amino acids.

FALSE (d) The BSE agent is distinct from that of scrapie and has a unique 'fingerprint' in inbred strains of mice.

TRUE (e) The 'species barrier' prevents the efficient transfer of infectious prions from one species to another.

(8.9) Are the following statements true or false?

TRUE   (a) The URE3 protein of yeast has the properties of a prion.

TRUE   (b) The URE3 phenotype of yeast can be 'cured' by treatment with guanidium.

TRUE   (c) Prion-like proteins have also been found in fungi.

FALSE   (d) There is no evidence that prions cause disease in plants.

FALSE   (e) The prion hypothesis is the most likely interpretation for TSEs, but other interpretations are still formally possible.

INDEX

·THE PRINCIPLES OF MOLECULAR VIROLOGY CD
STANDARD EDITION

Wherever the ✎ icon appears in the text, an accompanying learning resource can be found on the compact disk (CD) included with this book. To use the CD on a PC, put the disk into the CD-ROM drive, double-click on the My Computer icon, double-click on the CD-ROM icon and double-click on the Start.htm file. To use the CD on a Macintosh, put the disk into the CD-ROM drive, double-click on the CD-ROM icon on the desktop and double-click on the Start.htm file. If you need further help, click on the file 'README.txt'.

The CD contains virtual interactive tutorials and experiments, self-assessment questions and numerical exercises, links to many useful on-line resources, along with the Appendix section of the book, including a Glossary, Abbreviations and Pronunciation, Classification of Sub-Cellular Infectious Agents and a History of Virology. However, to gain the maximum benefit from the disk, you will need internet access. The resources in the 'Virology Online' section have been selected to encourage you to move beyond the text of the book and find information about any topic you may wish to investigate. Not sure what any word or name in the text means? Type it into the search forms listed in 'Virology Online' and you will be surprised how much information is available.

However, readers should be aware that the quality and accuracy of information they may find on the internet varies greatly. All of the resources suggested on the CD are of the highest quality, although neither the author nor Academic Press can guarantee that they will remain freely available indefinitely. Information accessed through search engines is another matter − it is up to users to judge the quality of resources found in this way:

- Who wrote the information? A knowledgeable academic in a respected university or a teenager in their bedroom?
- When did they write it? This year or six years ago − is there even a date on the page?
- What is their motivation for making the information available? Commercial or non-commercial?

By considering these quality issues, readers can expand the capacity of this book indefinitely.

All of the information on the *Principles of Molecular Virology* CD is copyright and may not be reproduced in any form.

For technical support, contact the Harcourt Technical Support Center at the numbers indicated below. Service is available in English only between the hours of 7am and 6pm US Central Time (15:00 to 02:00 GMT), Mondays through Fridays.

Toll free in the US and Canada (877)809-6433
Direct dial (817)820-3710
Toll free tax in the US only (800)354-1774
Direct fax (817)820-5100
Email: tscap@hbtechsupport.com